Diagnosis and Endoscopic Management of Digestive Diseases

Rita Conigliaro • Marzio Frazzoni
Editors

Diagnosis and Endoscopic Management of Digestive Diseases

New Tools and Strategies

Springer

Editors
Rita Conigliaro
S. Agostino Estense Hospital
Modena
Italy

Marzio Frazzoni
S. Agostino Estense Hospital
Modena
Italy

ISBN 978-3-319-42356-2 ISBN 978-3-319-42358-6 (eBook)
DOI 10.1007/978-3-319-42358-6

Library of Congress Control Number: 2017930183

Printed on acid-free paper

This Springer imprint is published by Springer Nature
The registered company is Springer International Publishing AG
The registered company address is: Gewerbestrasse 11, 6330 Cham, Switzerland

To our sons

Foreword

Modern times are characterized by unprecedented complexity and speed of changes. Gastroenterologists are daily faced with unusual cases, comorbidities, critical conditions, advanced age, and complex therapies. Know-how in various disciplines such as pathophysiology, biochemistry, genetics, pharmacology, and traditional and laparoscopic surgery is currently required for caring patients with GI tract disorders. Moreover, gastroenterologists are daily challenged with new devices and novel exciting but demanding tools and techniques.

The book edited by Rita Conigliaro and Marzio Frazzoni was written by internationally recognized experts in the various fields of GI endoscopy and digestive tract pathophysiology and consists in an updated review of the most relevant topics concerning diagnostic and therapeutic endoscopy as well as manometric and reflux-monitoring techniques. Evidence of the clinical relevance of endoscopic, manometric, and reflux-monitoring tools and techniques currently includes not only observational studies but also randomized controlled trials and meta-analyses. The reader will find evidence of the most updated developments of diagnostic and therapeutic endoscopy throughout the book, such as confocal laser endomicroscopy, endoscopic submucosal dissection, endoscopic suturing and myotomy, and cholangioscopy, as well as updated reports of the most exciting advances in digestive tract pathophysiological investigations including high-resolution manometry and impedance-pH monitoring. Moreover, an in-depth look to coming-soon progresses can be found in all chapters, so the reader will have the chance to think about and be watchful on the near future in gastroenterology.

Rita Conigliaro and Marzio Frazzoni are to be commended for their efforts to give us an updated review of GI endoscopy and digestive tract pathophysiology. Their enthusiasm, scientific honesty, and thoroughness represent a model for young gastroenterologists.

Giuliano Bedogni, MD
Former Director
Digestive Endoscopy Unit
Santa Maria Nuova Hospital
Reggio Emilia
Italy

Contents

Confocal Laser Endomicroscopy in GI Tract

1

Helga Bertani, Laurent Palazzo, Vincenzo Giorgio Mirante, and Flavia Pigò

1.1 Introduction

Technologic advances in endoscopic imaging have improved the visualization of mucosal layer, allowing to distinguish neoplastic vs nonneoplastic tissue; however, the imaging is far from a perfect tool. Although histology is a highly accurate technique, it has few limitations: false-negative results in case of ulcers or inflammation, delayed final diagnosis and treatment, and increased costs in pathology in analysis with consequently repeated procedures. Moreover in some GI districts, the accuracy of cytopathology results is low like pancreatic cyst and bile duct due to the difficulties in acquiring tissue. Nevertheless histology is a postmortem analysis without informations about in vivo processes (blood flow, mucosal junction exchanges).

Confocal laser endomicroscopy (CLE), a recent advance of endoluminal imaging, allows an in vivo visualization of mucosal layer with a detailed visualization of tissue and subcellular structures with magnification up to 500–1000-folds. CLE has the potential to predict the final diagnosis (neoplastic vs nonneoplastic) and consequently to guide the next therapeutic procedure without the delay of a pathology response. Indeed, mucosa can be studied at a micron resolution providing an "optical biopsy". Forthcoming developments include the in vivo study of angiogenesis and inflammation in healthy and neoplastic tissues.

H. Bertani, MD (✉) • V.G. Mirante • F. Pigò
Digestive Endoscopy Unit, Baggiovara Hospital, Modena, Italy
e-mail: helga.bertani@gmail.com

L. Palazzo
Department of Gastroenterology and Endoscopy, Trocadero Clinic, Paris, France

R. Conigliaro, M. Frazzoni (eds.), *Diagnosis and Endoscopic Management of Digestive Diseases*, DOI 10.1007/978-3-319-42358-6_1

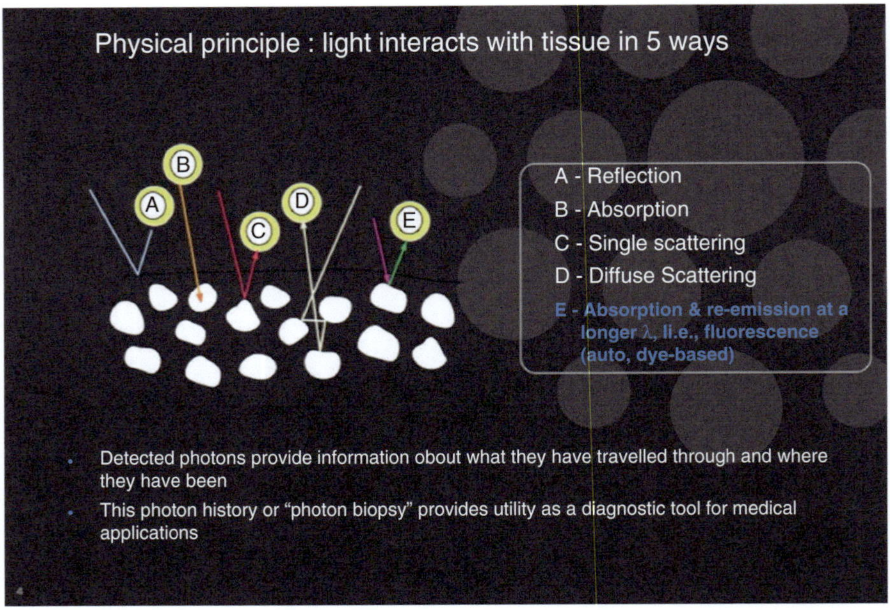

Fig. 1.1 (1) Reflection, (2) absorption, (3) single scattering, (4) diffuse scattering, (5) absorption and reemission at a different wavelength of fluorescence (Courtesy of Pr. Satish Singh, MD Department of Medicine & Biomedical Engineering, Boston University)

1.2 Physics

The physics of the CLE is based on tissue light interactions. Light interacts with tissue in five different ways (Fig. 1.1): (1) reflection, (2) absorption, (3) single scattering, (4) diffuse scattering, and (5) absorption and reemission at a different wavelength of fluorescence.

This last phenomenon can be an autofluorescence or a dye-based fluorescence. The light source is a blue laser beam with variable wavelength (488–660 nm) focused into the plane of interest, and the returned light is filtered by means of a small pinhole that rejects out-of-focus light. The illumination and detection systems are in the same focal plane and are termed "confocal." After passing the pinhole, the fluorescent light is detected by a photodetector device that stabilizes images from a system software transforming the light signal into an electrical one that is recorded by a computer. All detected signals from the illuminated spot are captured and measured. The gray-scale image created is an optical section representing one focal plane within the examined specimen. Because confocal images depend on fluorescence, a fluorescent dye (contrast agent) is required to make the objects visible. The contrast agents can be applied systemically (fluorescein) or topically (acriflavine and cresyl violet). Most studies in humans have been performed with intravenous administration of fluorescein sodium. As fluorescein distribution is outside the cell in intercellular space, it contrasts cellular and subcellular details, connective tissue, and vessel architecture at high resolution but does not stain the nuclei. The safety of the fluorescein as contrast agent has been demonstrated in ophthalmology; it has been used for years for ophthalmological imaging of blood vessels. Wallace et al. [1] reported a cross-sectional survey study about the safety of fluorescein in CLE procedures. 2272 patients were enrolled and no serious adverse events were reported. Minor adverse events occurred in 1.4 % (transient hypotension, nausea, injection site erythema, mild epigastric pain), but none of them required additional intervention than observation. Acriflavine, another contrast agent, is applied topically and predominantly stains nuclei, but they are not allowed for human use, by FDA and EMEA.

1.3 Systems

In 2003, at the beginning of CLE research, two systems were available: one system inserted in the tip of the scope (eCLE, Pentax Corporation, Tokyo, Japan) and the other, a probe-based system, a separate device from the endoscope, able to be introduced in the working channel of any standard endoscope (pCLE, Cellvizio, Mauna Kea Tech, Paris, France). Currently, only the last one is commercially available and approved to perform CLE (Fig. 1.2).

1.4 Gastrointestinal Applications

In the following pages, we will describe all the current applications of CLE in gastrointestinal tract and literature results.

1.4.1 Barrett's Esophagus (BE)

Barrett's esophagus, defined as an abnormal change in squamous epithelium of the esophagus into an intestinal columnar epithelium (Fig. 1.3), is considered a premalignant condition and the most important risk factor for the development of esophageal adenocarcinoma.

The incidence of esophageal adenocarcinoma has been rapidly rising, increasing from threefold to sixfold since 1990 [2]. International guidelines suggest endoscopic surveillance with random four-quadrant biopsies every 1–2 cm through the extension of intestinal metaplasia for the detection of dysplasia (high grade/low grade) or early intraepithelial cancer (Seattle protocol) [3]. However, surveillance endoscopy has several limitations as dysplastic changes occurring in Barrett's esophagus are not easily identifiable by standard endoscopy. Moreover there is much controversy: first about the real efficacy of such an intense four-quadrant biopsy sampling protocol and second biopsies obtained using this technique are prone to sampling error, and interobserver agreement is low even between advanced operators and even among expert pathologists [4]. Nevertheless, the need for histology confirmation of neoplasia eliminates the ability to direct therapy during the

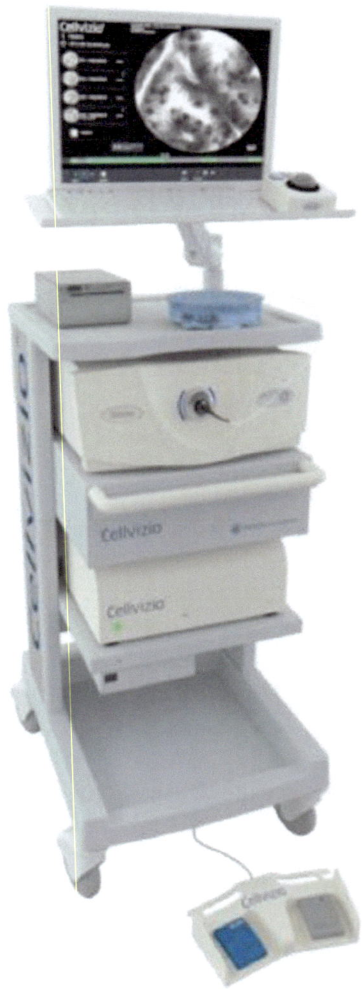

Fig. 1.2 pCLE, Cellvizio, Mauna Kea Tech, Paris, France

index endoscopy. Thus repeated procedures are needed, the first for the diagnosis and then for the therapy. A multiple biopsy protocol could also interfere with the next therapeutic steps.

EMR or ESD could be more difficult without adequate "lifting sign" due to scar tissue after repeated biopsies.

pCLE since its debut has demonstrated a really good accuracy in distinguishing visible neoplastic changes in epithelial cancers that occur at a cellular level. Randomized clinical studies have shown that eCLE or pCLE with white light endoscopy (WLE) can reduce up to 65 % of the number of biopsies needed to reach the same diagnostic yield of WLE alone [5, 6].

The interobserver agreement has been reported to be 86 % with a kappa estimate of 0.72 (CI 95 % 0.58–0.86) [7]. The observers in this study also rated individual

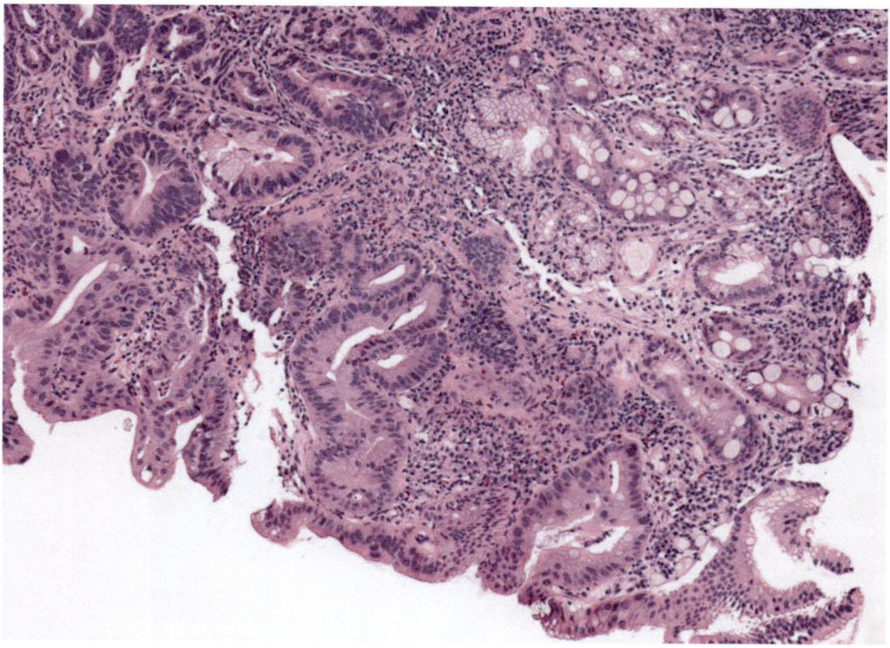

Fig. 1.3 Barrett's esophagus: intestinal metaplasia

features suggestive of neoplasia, such as irregular epithelial thickness, epithelial inhomogeneity, dark epithelial structures (lack of fluorescein uptake), crypt/villi fusion, and irregular vessels. These individual features had good specificity but lower sensitivity, and none of them appeared to compete with the overall diagnostic assessment.

In 2011 a classification has been proposed by a group of experts, the Miami classification, for real-time diagnosis of Barrett's neoplasia with pCLE, and later it has been widely accepted and validated in randomized controlled trials. BE pCLE criteria are uniform villiform architecture and columnar epithelial cells with dark goblet cells. In high-grade dysplasia (HGD), villiform structures have irregularly shaped crypts and dilated capillary vessels. In early adenocarcinoma (EAC), a complete loss of crypt and villiform architecture is observed with irregular and dilated capillaries [8] Fig. 1.4a, b.

A meta-analysis based on eight studies involving 709 patients and 4008 specimens showed a pooled sensitivity and specificity of CLE (in a per-patient analysis) for the detection of neoplasia of 89 % and 75 %, respectively [9].

Another recent application of confocal endomicroscopy is a role in guiding therapeutic endoscopic procedure (1) to localize and predict pathology, (2) to target biopsies and resections in surveillance and treatment, (3) to guide which therapy to use, and (4) to assess treatment adequacy and gauge need for further treatment [10].

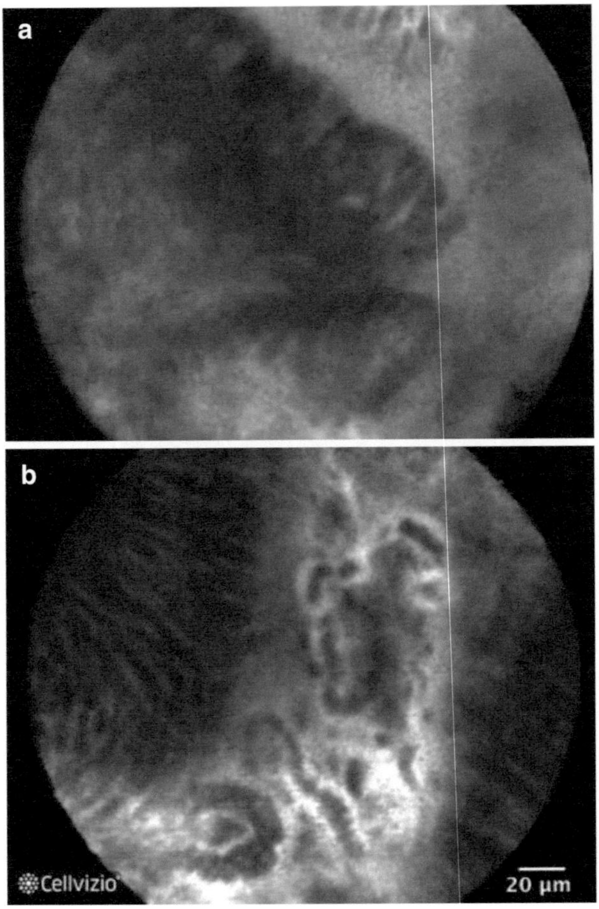

Fig. 1.4 (**a**) pCLE image of low-grade dysplasia with loss of crypt and villiform architecture. (**b**) pCLE image of low-grade dysplasia with irregular and dilated capillaries

1.4.2 Gastritis and Early Gastric Cancer

Gastric cancer remains the world's second leading cause of cancer-related deaths, with a mortality rate of 16.3 per 100,000 in men and 7.9 per 100,000 in women [11], and in eastern countries, the risk of gastric cancer is dramatically high. One of the strategies, to improve prognosis, essentially depends on the earlier detection of preneoplastic changes in mucosal layer because intraepithelial neoplasia and early gastric cancer have a dramatically better prognosis than the advanced one. Currently, the diagnosis of these lesions is based on pathologic assessment. Virtual chromoendoscopy and trimodal imaging endoscopy have demonstrated a significant value for the detection of early gastric neoplasia, whereas the detection of intraepithelial gastric neoplasia (GIN) has been less mentioned and investigated [12].

pCLE demonstrated a high accuracy for detecting gastric carcinomas compared with conventional histological biopsy, providing an excellent definition of the gastric pit pattern with high diagnostic accuracy on the detection of gastric atrophy and gastric intestinal metaplasia as well as *Helicobacter pylori* infection [13–15]. According to the study by Li, the sensitivity and specificity of gastric pit patterns and vessel architecture classification with pCLE for predicting atrophic gastritis were 88.51 % and 99.19 %, respectively. The sensitivity and specificity for predicting intestinal metaplasia were 92.34 % and 99.34 %, respectively. The overall sensitivity and specificity for predicting neoplasia were 89.89 % and 99.44 %, respectively. The use of CLE could possibly reduce the number of unnecessary biopsies and mistaken diagnoses before ESD [16–18]. The interobserver agreement was "substantial" (kappa = 0.70) for the differentiation of neoplasia versus non-neoplasia [19].

Another possible future application in the stomach is the "molecular CLE" that consists in the employment of fluorescein-labeled peptides that can be used for evaluating the expression of receptors in carcinomas in order to individualize the treatment regimens, but also for improving the diagnostic accuracy of endoscopic procedures by identifying otherwise invisible mucosal lesions. These novel applications need further evaluations about efficacy and safety because most of the studies have been conducted in animal facilities or in vitro, while only a limited number of trials have actually been carried out in vivo [20].

1.4.3 Celiac Disease

Many papers have been published about the role of CLE in the study of jejunal mucosa in celiac disease. Alterations of villa in terms of length, numbers, and distribution are easily recognized [21, 22].

1.4.4 Inflammatory Bowel Disease

The use of CLE in colon disease ranges from classifications of colorectal polyps to the study of inflammatory bowel disease (IBD). In particular patients affected by ulcerative colitis (UC) are at increased risk of developing colorectal cancer, so guidelines recommend surveillance including targeted biopsies of suspected lesions and multiple random biopsies. However, the sensitivity of this protocol for the detection of neoplasia is still low. Chromoendoscopy, virtual chromoendoscopy (NBI), and pCLE have been proposed to improve the detection of dysplastic lesions. Kiesslich et al. using the eCLE system reported a sensitivity of 97.4 %, specificity of 99.4 %, and accuracy of 99.2 % to predict the presence of neoplastic changes [23, 24]. Van den Broek et al. [25] reported similar data but lower sensitivity (65 %), specificity (82 %), and accuracy (81 %) due probably to a different system, learning curve in providing images and technical skills. Hurlstone et al. [26] assessed the clinical feasibility and predictive power of

CLE for in vivo differentiation between ALM and DALM in UC. The study evidenced high accuracy of the technique and consequently the possibility to differentiate patient eligible for endoscopic treatment from patients fit for surgery. Recently, De Palma et al. [27] reported the use of CLE applied in real-time inflammation activity assessment. The inflammation activity assessment includes polyps' architecture, cellular infiltration, and vessel architecture. These studies showed that images taken with CLE provide informations that were equivalent to conventional histology, differentiating between active and nonactive UC during ongoing colonoscopy. Recently the use of CLE has been applied also to functional studies in IBD, to evaluate epithelial gaps resulting from intestinal cell shedding rate higher than in healthy patients undergoing colonoscopy. Liu et al. [28] reported that patients with IBD had a significantly higher epithelial gap densities in the terminal ileum compared with controls without IBD. A novel and future application of CLE is the prediction of therapeutic response to TNF-α inhibitors. The utility and safeness of new contrast agent (fluorescent antibodies specific for TNF-alpha receptors) need to be confirmed in other studies [29–31].

1.4.5 Polyps

Colorectal cancer has been recognized as the second most common cause of cancer-related death in the United States [32]. Standard endoscopic inspection cannot by itself distinguish between neoplastic and nonneoplastic lesions; thus, all detected lesions need to be removed and then evaluated by a pathologist, and this approach still remains the gold standard. The first report of the potential role of CLE in predicting pathology of the colon polyps was by Kiesslich et al. [23]. They reported an accuracy in the prediction of intraepithelial neoplasia of 92 % (sensitivity of 97 % and specificity of 99 %). Hurlstone et al. [26] subsequently confirmed Kiesslich data, in particular confirmed the role of CLE in the visualization of high-quality cellular, subsurface vascular, and stromal imaging enabling prediction of intraepithelial neoplasia with accuracy of 99 %. Polglase et al. [33] also confirmed similar results. Recently Xie published that in polyps with diameter > 10 mm, the sensitivity of CLE was 97.1 % and specificity 100 % [34]. A study by Gomez et al. [7] reported also a moderate-to-good interobserver agreement between international collaborative colleagues for distinguishing neoplasia from nonneoplastic tissue. Buchner et al. reported a learning curve of the technique with accuracy of 82 % after 60 procedures [35]. In a meta-analysis that involved 15 studies and 719 patients, the pooled sensitivity of all studies was 0.94 [95 % confidence intervals (CI), 0.88–0.97], and pooled specificity was 0.95 (95 % CI, 0.89–0.97). Real-time CLE yielded higher sensitivity (0.96 vs 0.85, $P<0.001$) and specificity (0.97 vs 0.82, $P<0.001$) than blinded CLE. For real-time CLE, endoscopy-based systems had better sensitivity (0.96 vs 0.89, $P<0.001$) and specificity (0.99 vs 0.82, $P<0.0001$) than probe-based systems [36].

1.4.6 Pancreas

Pancreatic cystic lesions are relatively common findings in the general population due to the widespread use of cross-sectional imaging. They are a heterogeneous group of lesions as some show a benign behavior and others have a premalignant or malignant potential. A different management should be applied for each type: benign cysts are usually referred for follow-up (based on imaging), while premalignant or malignant lesions should be surgically resected. Endoscopic ultrasound (EUS) is used to evaluate pancreatic lesions and to identify its features as it offers a good visualization of the lesion and its relation with pancreatic main duct. When combined with fine-needle aspiration and cystic fluid analysis, the diagnosis potential is increased, although its accuracy for differentiating benign and malign tumors remains modest [37].

EUS-guided needle-based confocal laser endomicroscopy (nCLE) is a confocal procedure based on a confocal miniprobe (AQ-flex Cellvizio Technology, Mauna Kea Tech, France) thin enough to be passed through a 19-G FNA needle. The miniprobe (0.632 mm diameter) preloaded and screwed by a locking device in the EUS needle is guided endosonographically in the target lesion, and then the miniprobe is pushed under the EUS guidance in gentle contact with the cyst wall. It potentially provides in vivo images of the pancreas at a cellular level, offering the possibility to precisely define a lesion.

The first multicenter study was the INSPECT study [38] with the primary aim to develop descriptive image interpretation criteria and a classification of nCLE findings in pancreatic cysts through a review of prospectively obtained nCLE videos from proven malignant and benign cases. Secondary aims included assessing procedure-related adverse events, technical feasibility of nCLE, and developing a first atlas of nCLE images in pancreatic cysts. A total of 66 patients underwent nCLE imaging, and images were available for 65 patients, eight of whom were subsequently excluded due to insufficient information for consensus reference diagnosis. The presence of epithelial villous structures based on nCLE was associated with pancreatic cystic neoplasm [intraductal papillary mucinous neoplasm (IPMN)] ($P = 0.004$) and provided a sensitivity of 59 %, specificity of 100 %, positive predictive value (PPV) of 100 %, and negative predictive value (NPV) of 50 %. The overall complication rate was 9 % and included pancreatitis (one mild case, one moderate case), transient abdominal pain ($n = 1$), and intracystic bleeding not requiring any further measures ($n = 3$). These preliminary data suggested that nCLE has a high specificity in the detection of IPMN, but may be limited by a low sensitivity.

The second published multicenter study (CONTACT study) [39] aimed to define the criteria of serous cystadenoma (SCA) and to differentiate mucinous from serous pancreatic lesion using nCLE. A total of 31 patients with a solitary pancreatic cystic lesion of unknown diagnosis were prospectively included at three centers. The final diagnosis was based on either a stringent gold standard (surgical specimen and/or positive cytopathology) or a committee consensus. Six not-blinded investigators reviewed nCLE sequences from patients with the most stringent final diagnosis and

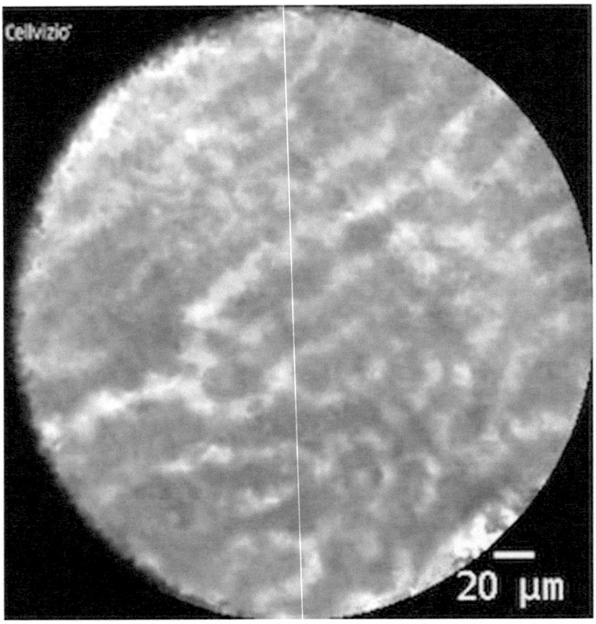

Fig. 1.5 A superficial vascular network pattern visualized on nCLE which corresponds to a dense and subepithelial capillary vascularization visible only in SCA

identified a single feature that was only present in SCA. The findings were correlated with the pathology of archived specimens. After a training session, four blinded independent observers reviewed, with a separate independent video set, and the yield and interobserver agreement for the criterion were assessed. A superficial vascular network pattern visualized on nCLE was identified as the criterion. It corresponded on pathological specimen to a dense and subepithelial capillary vascularization only seen in SCA (Fig. 1.5).

The accuracy, sensitivity, specificity, positive predictive value, and negative predictive value of this sign for the diagnosis of SCA were 87 %, 69 %, 100 %, 100 %, and 82 %, respectively. Interobserver agreement was substantial ($k=0.77$). This new nCLE criterion seems highly specific for the diagnosis of SCA.

Recently a single-center trial by Nakai et al. combined nCLE with an EUS-guided cystoscopy (DETECT study). The goal of this study was to assess the feasibility, safety, and diagnostic yield of the combination of cystoscopy and nCLE in the clinical diagnosis of pancreatic cystic lesion. Thirty patients were included. The procedure was technically successful with the exception of one probe exchange failure. In two patients (7 %), post-procedure pancreatitis developed. Specific features associated with the clinical diagnosis of mucinous cysts were identified: mucin on cystoscopy and papillary projections and dark rings on nCLE. The sensitivity of cystoscopy was 90 % (9/10) and that of nCLE was 80 % (8/10), and the combination was 100 % (10/10) in 18 high-certainty patients. The combination of dual through-the-needle imaging (cystoscopy and nCLE) of pancreatic cysts appears to have strong concordance with the clinical diagnosis of pancreatic cyst [40].

1.4.7 Biliary Tract

Despite the technological developments in the field of imaging as well as available options for endoscopic evaluation through endoscopic retrograde cholangiopancreatography (ERCP), the diagnostic yield in biliary and pancreatic duct strictures and preoperative diagnosis of undetermined biliary strictures are still suboptimal.

The probe usually used for confocal imaging of the pancreatobiliary system is the CholangioFlex miniprobe (Mauna Kea Technologies, Paris, France) that requires a working channel of at least 1.2 mm and has a working length of 4 m. The lateral resolution of the probe is 3.5 μm with a field of view of 325 μm.

The first study aimed to classify confocal patterns related to biliary strictures in the so-called Miami classification study. This study was an attempt to identify as well as standardize the interpretation of finding on pCLE of the biliary system in cases on indeterminate biliary strictures. The combination of thick white bands with dark clumps or epithelial structures provided a 94 % diagnostic sensitivity and 46 % diagnostic specificity. On the other hand, the combination of white bands with thick white bands or fluorescein leakage or dark clamps provided a 61 % diagnostic sensitivity and a 100 % diagnostic specificity [8].

When using a cholangioscope, pCLE had a sensitivity of 96 % (95 % CI, 84–100 %) and a specificity of 76 % (95 % CI, 53–91 %), while when using a catheter, the sensitivity was 100 % (95 % CI, 83–100 %) and the specificity was 62 % (95 % CI, 45–78 %), but there was no statistical difference in the accuracy between these delivery techniques, but the operator confidence about the diagnosis was much higher when using cholangioscopy when compared to a catheter-based approach for pCLE of biliary strictures (43.2 % vs 9.8 %, respectively) [41]. In a randomized trial for the comparison between catheter-guided (fluoroscopy only) pCLE and cholangioscopy-guided pCLE, the accuracy of cholangioscopy-guided pCLE was 82 % compared to 78 % for catheter-guided pCLE. Of note, the sample size of the study was small [42]. The addition of pCLE with ERCP in the evaluation of indeterminate pancreatobiliary strictures can increase the detection of [43] with a sensitivity of (98 % vs 45 %) and NPV (97 % vs 69 %), although it decreased the specificity (67 % vs 100 %) and the PPV (71 % vs 100 %) when compared to index pathology [44].

Although conventionally the use of pCLE for the evaluation of biliary strictures is through a side-viewing duodenoscope, a case series showed pCLE through direct peroral cholangioscopy in 22 out of 24 patients with biliary strictures [45]. In this case series, they classified patients based on the pre-pCLE evaluation for the probability of a malignant etiology for biliary stricture into a range from very unlikely to certainly based on the clinical evaluation as well as imaging, pCLE was found to be complementary to peroral cholangioscopy and ERCP in cases where a malignant etiology was suspected and did not affect the management decision, but it might be sufficient for the confirmation of a malignant etiology when tissue acquisition is not required. pCLE in hilar strictures has also been proven to be of use in a series of 19 patients with the correct identification of all cases with neoplasia, but one false-positive case was reported [46].

Two years later a refinement of the Miami classification named the Paris classification was published [47]. The aim of the Paris classification was to decrease the number of false-positive results when evaluating indeterminate strictures of the biliary system as in inflammatory strictures. Caillol et al. [48] identified four characteristics on biliary pCLE that were associated with benign inflammatory strictures: vascular congestion, dark granular patterns with scales, increased inter-glandular space, and thickened reticular structure. In this study the authors sought to explain the false-positive cases in 60 cases that were enrolled in a registry and found that pCLE diagnosis was either influenced by the ERCP impression or the presence of less than three malignant Miami classification criteria. In a validation study for the Paris classification, it was found to increase the specificity to 73 % compared to 67 % when using the Miami criteria [8]; a similar finding was obtained in a second study [49].

Giovannini et al. [50] evaluated the effect of biliary stenting in 54 patients with indeterminate biliary stenosis and found that biliary stenting decreased the accuracy of pCLE when using the Miami criteria, similar findings were replicated where a decrease in the sensitivity from 88 to 75 %, and specificity from 83 to 71 % was found in those who had cholangitis or a stent inserted prior to pCLE imaging [51]. Although this requires validation in other series, it might be prudent to perform pCLE prior to biliary stenting in cases with biliary strictures of unknown etiology. Also, of note, in the study by Caillol et al. [47], they noted that stricture dilation could induce fluorescein leakage, thus giving the impression of a malignant stricture, while it was subsequently found to be benign.

A recent consensus report by 16 physicians validated seven statements with regard to the use of pCLE in biliary strictures: (1) CLE can be used to evaluate biliary strictures, and the probe can be delivered via a catheter or a cholangioscope; (2) CLE is more accurate than ERCP with brush cytology and/or forceps biopsy in determining malignant or benign strictures, using established criteria; (3) The accuracy of CLE in indeterminate biliary strictures may be decreased by prior presence of plastic stent; (4) The NPV of CLE is very high; (5) The use of CLE can assist clinical decision-making such as excluding malignancy; (6) CLE should be cited as a valuable tool for an increased diagnostic yield in official guidelines; (7) The "black bands" that can be seen in pCLE images have been shown to be collagen fibrils that predictably increase in pathologic tissue [52]. A preliminary analysis of the multicenter FOCUS trial demonstrated that the clinical impression of physicians and pCLE during the workup of biliary strictures outperform tissue sampling where the combination of brush cytology and biopsy would have missed five malignant strictures out of 36 patients [53].

Adding histology/cytology to pCLE resulted in a marginal increase in sensitivity (from 89 to 93 %) but did not change specificity (79 %) compared to the addition of pCLE alone [54].

1.4.8 Primary Sclerosing Cholangitis (PSC)

In a series of 15 patients, 19 strictures, both extra and intrahepatic, were evaluated by ERCP and pCLE. Due to the inflammatory nature of PSC, the authors used a scoring system based on the Miami classification. When there were two of five malignant criteria, the lesion was classified as "suspicious." When there was one criterion, the lesion was classified as "reactive," and the finding of a reticular pattern was deemed as "benign." The findings on pCLE were compared to ERCP, cholangioscopy, histology/cytology, liver explants, fluorescence in situ hybridization (FISH), or 12 months of follow-up. Visualization was successful in 95 % of the procedures; pCLE was found to have a sensitivity of 100 % (95 % CI, 40–100 %), a specificity of 50 % (95 % CI, 9–90 %), a PPV of 67 % (95 % CI, 24.5–94 %), and a NPV of 100 % (95 % CI, 20–100 %). The authors suggested the high-negative predictive value of pCLE could guide in the interval of surveillance in patients with dominant biliary strictures [55, 56].

1.4.9 Solid Organs

With the availability of new probes, CLE allows virtual biopsies of solid organs and other intraperitoneal structures during EUS, laparoscopy, or natural-orifice transluminal endoscopic surgery (NOTES) procedures providing thus a pathological diagnosis based on the morphological features of the solid tissue.

The first report [57] about the use of a probe designed to be used like a handheld laparoscope (FIVE1, Optiscan, Notting Hill, Australia) was used in a liver of a healthy mice and in pathological tissue in human liver disease of a rodent model. Thus, chronic hepatitis, steatosis, and fibrosis were studied using different fluorescent-staining protocols, and images in rodents were collected after topical application or bolus injection of fluorescent agents. No toxic effects on the animals had been observed. Most images were deemed good to excellent quality, and the correlation with ex vivo histopathology was substantial. In the same study group, a handheld probe was used in 25 patients [58] to examine their liver diseases during mini laparoscopy under conscious sedation. Subsurface serial images allowed the visualization of hepatocytes, bile ducts, sinusoids, and collagen fibers in vivo. Typical appearances of liver diseases were identified. Confocal diagnosis of moderate-to-severe steatosis and pericellular fibrosis correlated well with histopathologic analysis of subsequent biopsies (83.3 % and 84.6 %, respectively).

Recently the AQ-flex probe was used through a 19-G needle in solid organs. Mennone and colleagues [59] evaluated, in in vivo feasibility study, the ability of nCLE to distinguish between normal and cirrhotic liver tissue in a non-survival rat model. In this study three healthy and four cirrhotic rats were examined under general anesthesia using three prototypes of confocal miniprobes with different working distances. During laparotomy features were acquired on the surface of the liver capsule and through a 19-gauge needle inserted into the liver parenchyma.

Real-time sequences were recorded after intravenous injection of fluorescein. Biopsy specimens were taken for standard histopathology. All the three miniprobes identified different features like cords of hepatocytes radiating toward central venules in normal livers and distorted hepatic architecture in cirrhotic livers.

Another feasibility study of nCLE in a porcine model by Becker [60] was applied in various abdominal organs such as the pancreas, lymph node, spleen, and liver. At three academic centers, ten pigs were examined in a non-survival experiment with the animals under general anesthesia. Either EUS-guided organ puncture or NOTES procedure was technically feasible allowing real-time in vivo images at histologic resolutions when compared to standard histopathology.

Subsequent human clinical trials were focused on the evaluation of the pancreas and of its pathological features. The first multicenter pilot study [38] evaluated the feasibility of nCLE in sixteen pancreatic cysts and two pancreatic masses. No complications occurred after the puncture of pancreatic solid mass. The final diagnosis of the solid lesions was established after surgical resection in one case (pancreatic endocrine tumor) and by cytology in the other case (adenocarcinoma). Of the two solid masses, image quality was respectively deemed good (NET) and moderate (adenocarcinoma). Karstensen et al. [61] published a feasibility study in 25 patients with pancreatic masses studied with nCLE preloaded into the needle at the same location of EUS-FNA. No adverse advents were registered, but the diagnostic value was considered limited. In a second paper [62], the same group evaluated prospectively 20 patients with pancreatic masses selected for EUS-FNA. Also for these patients, the FNA was performed at the same location studied with nCLE. Features like dark aggregates and pseudoglandular structures were observed in all pancreatic adenocarcinomas.

An interesting field of application of pCLE consists in the use of fluorescein-labeled antibodies that have shown the feasibility of in vivo immunohistological staining. Moreover, the fluorescein-labeled antibodies direct to a specific target could evaluate the expression of cellular receptors. The detection of these receptors in solid neoplasia might potentially be correlated to the efficacy of treatment regimens (tailored therapy).

Nakai and colleagues [63] evaluated whether this method was feasible using needle-based confocal laser endomicroscopy (nCLE) for extraluminal investigation of the pancreas in conjunction with topical administration of antihuman EGFR-fluorescein-conjugated monoclonal antibodies and antihuman surviving-fluorescein-conjugated monoclonal antibodies. In pancreatic cancer the expression of EGFR and of anti-apoptosis protein surviving is significantly upregulated. Although the number of pigs was limited, the technique was feasible. However, the resolution of the pictures obtained was low. Other problems were the immunogenic nature of antibodies, long half-life in serum, and slow penetration into tissues due to their high molecular weight. Furthermore, antibodies are expensive to produce in high amounts.

Another experimental study [64] showed a precise identification of perigastric lymph nodal metastasis using CLE systems to detect fluorescein-labeled hepatic cells in original noncancer animal model. Various tumor cell lines coupled with dye substances can be injected in the submucosa of the GI tract to migrate to regional lymph nodes and allow for testing node navigation technologies or advanced optical imaging systems. They choose hepatic cells as they are easy to be collected in a large amount and for their ability to be differentiated from the lymphoid tissue by IHC. This model enables the potential of cancer-specific fluorescent antibodies of recognizing cancer cells in real time. This model is reproducible and simulated metastatic spread of gastric cancer.

CLE technology was used also to make several important observations on functional and molecular features of apoptosis. Goetz and colleagues [65] reported hepatocyte apoptosis studied with confocal endomicroscopy: different features were seen in living rodents following distinct morphological, functional, and molecular features of apoptosis in intact liver in vivo and at high resolution. In another study [66], the injection of fluorescent apoptosis marker was used to study the effect of high-linear energy transfer radiation on the HCC tumor model orthotopically transplanted.

Conclusion

In conclusion CLE may be a useful virtual biopsy of GI organs. Real-time confocal laser endomicroscopy has the potential to improve sampling error and potentially reduce the number of procedure needed for a diagnosis in more difficult organs to access such as the bile duct and pancreas. In situations in which there is no on-site cytopathologist available, endomicroscopy could facilitate cytology acquisition. Therefore, safety issues still need further evaluations. However, a limited number of trials have actually been carried especially in solid organs. However, this finding has to be confirmed in larger studies. Further studies are needed to assess the diagnostic accuracy and if nCLE in focal masses is clinically relevant in selected cases.

References

1. Wallace MB, Meining A, Canto MI, Fockens P, Miehlke S, Roesch T, Lightdale CJ, Pohl H, Carr-Locke D, Löhr M, Coron E, Filoche B, Giovannini M, Moreau J, Schmidt C, Kiesslich R. The safety of intravenous fluorescein for confocal laser endomicroscopy in the gastrointestinal tract. Aliment Pharmacol Ther. 2010;31(5):548–52. doi:10.1111/j.1365-2036.2009.04207.x. Epub 2009 Nov 30. PMID: 20002025.
2. Cameron AJ. Epidemiology of columnar-lined esophagus and adenocarcinoma. Gastroenterol Clin North Am. 1997;26:487–94.
3. Evans JA, Early DS, Fukami N, Ben-Menachem T, Chandrasekhara V, Chathadi KV, Decker GA, Fanelli RD, Fisher DA, Foley KQ, Hwang JH, Jain R, Jue TL, Khan KM, Lightdale J, Malpas PM, Maple JT, Pasha SF, Saltzman JR, Sharaf RN, Shergill A, Dominitz JA, Cash BD. The role of endoscopy in Barrett's esophagus and other premalignant conditions of the esophagus. ASGE Standards of Practice Committee, Standards of Practice Committee of the American Society for Gastrointestinal Endoscopy. Gastrointest Endosc. 2012;76(6):1087–94. doi:10.1016/j.gie.2012.08.004. No abstract available. PMID: 23164510.
4. Skacel M, Petras RE, Gramlich TL, Sigel JE, Richter JE, Goldblum JR. The diagnosis of low-grade dysplasia in Barrett's esophagus and its implications for disease progression. Am J Gastroenterol. 2000;95(12):3383–7.

5. Sharma P, Meining AR, Coron E, et al. Real-time increased detection of neoplastic tissue in Barrett's esophagus with probe-based confocal laser endomicroscopy: final results of an international multicenter, prospective, randomized, controlled trial. Gastrointest Endosc. 2011;74:465–72.
6. Canto MI, Anandasabapathy S, Brugge W, et al. In vivo endomicroscopy improves detection of Barrett's esophagus–related neoplasia: a multicenter international randomized controlled trial (with video). Gastrointest Endosc. 2014;79:211–21.
7. Gómez V, Buchner AM, Dekker E, van den Broek FJ, Meining A, Shahid MW, Ghabril MS, Fockens P, Heckman MG, Wallace MB. Interobserver agreement and accuracy among international experts with probe-based confocal laser endomicroscopy in predicting colorectal neoplasia. Endoscopy. 2010;42(4):286–91. doi:10.1055/s-0029-1243951. Epub 2010 Mar 30. PMID: 20354938.
8. Wallace M, Lauwers GY, Chen Y, Dekker E, Fockens P, Sharma P, Meining A. Miami classification for probe-based confocal laser endomicroscopy. Endoscopy. 2011;43(10):882–91. doi:10.1055/s-0030-1256632. Epub 2011 Aug 4. Review.PMID:21818734.
9. Wu J, Pan YM, Wang TT, Hu B, et al. Confocal laser endomicroscopy for detection of neoplasia in Barrett's esophagus: a meta-analysis. Dis Esophagus. 2014;27:248–54.
10. Konda VJ, Chennat JS, Hart J, Waxman I. Confocal laser endomicroscopy: potential in the management of Barrett's esophagus. Dis Esophagus. 2010;23(5):E21–31. doi:10.1111/j442–2050.2010.01088.x. Epub 2010 Jul 8. PMID: 20626448.
11. Brenner H, Rothenbacher D, Arndt V. Epidemiology of stomach cancer. Methods Mol Biol. 2009;472:467–77. doi:10.1007/978-1-60327-492-0_23.
12. Gweon TG, Park JM, Lim CH, Kim JS, Cho YK, Kim SW, Choi MG. Trimodal imaging endoscopy reduces the risk of synchronous gastric neoplasia. Eur J Gastroenterol Hepatol. 2015;27(3):215–20. doi:10.1097/MEG.0000000000000278. PMID: 25569570.
13. Imaeda A. Confocal laser endomicroscopy for the detection of atrophic gastritis: a new application for confocal endomicroscopy? J Clin Gastroenterol. 2015;49(5):355–7. doi:10.1097/MCG.0000000000000309. No abstract available. PMID: 25811115.
14. Lim LG, Yeoh KG, Srivastava S, Chan YH, Teh M, Ho KY. Comparison of probe-based confocal endomicroscopy with virtual chromoendoscopy and white-light endoscopy for diagnosis of gastric intestinal metaplasia. Surg Endosc. 2013;27(12):4649–55. doi:10.1007/00464-013-3098-x. Epub 2013 Jul 27. PMID: 23892761.
15. Li Z, Zuo XL, Yu T, Gu XM, Zhou CJ, Li CQ, Ji R, Li YQ. Confocal laser endomicroscopy for in vivo detection of gastric intestinal metaplasia: a randomized controlled trial. Endoscopy. 2014;46(4):282–90. doi:10.1055/s-0033-1359215. Epub 2014 Jan 28. PMID: 24473908.
16. Li WB, Zuo XL, Li CQ, Zuo F, Gu XM, Yu T, Chu CL, Zhang TG, Li YQ. Diagnostic value of confocal laser endomicroscopy for gastric superficial cancerous lesions. Gut. 2011;60(3):299–306. doi:10.1136/gut.2010.223586. Epub 2010 Dec 30. PMID: 21193460.
17. Jeon SR, Cho WY, Jin SY, Cheon YK, Choi SR, Cho JY. Optical biopsies by confocal endomicroscopy prevent additive endoscopic biopsies before endoscopic submucosal dissection in gastric epithelial neoplasias: a prospective, comparative study. Gastrointest Endosc. 2011;74(4):772–80. doi:10.1016/j.gie.2011.05.005. Epub 2011 Jul 29.
18. Bok GH, Jeon SR, Cho JY, Cho JH, Lee WC, Jin SY, Choi IH, Kim HG, Lee TH, Park EJ. The accuracy of probe-based confocal endomicroscopy versus conventional endoscopic biopsies for the diagnosis of superficial gastric neoplasia (with videos). Gastrointest Endosc. 2013;77(6):899–908. doi:10.1016/j.gie.2013.01.018. Epub 2013 Mar 6. PMID: 23473002.
19. Li Z, Zuo XL, Li CQ, Liu ZY, Ji R, Liu J, Guo J, Li YQ. New classification of gastric pit patterns and vessel architecture using probe-based confocal laser endomicroscopy. J Clin Gastroenterol. 2016;50(1):23–32. doi:10.1097/MCG.0000000000000298. PMID: 25751373.
20. Goetz M, Hoetker MS, Diken M, et al. In vivo molecular imaging with cetuximab, an anti-EGFR antibody, for prediction of response in xenograft models of human colorectal cancer. Endoscopy. 2013;45(6):469–77.doi:10.1055/s-0032-1326361. Epub 2013 Apr 11 PMID 23580409.

21. Trovato C, Sonzogni A, Ravizza D, et al. Celiac disease: in vivo diagnosis by confocal endomicroscopy. Gastrointest Endosc. 2007;65:1096–9.
22. Leong RW, Nguyen NQ, Meredith CG, et al. In vivo confocal endomicroscopy in the diagnosis and evaluation of celiac disease. Gastroenterology. 2008;135:1870–5.
23. Kiesslich R, Gossner L, Goetz M, Dahlmann A, Vieth M, Stolte M, Hoffman A, Jung M, Nafe B, Galle PR, Neurath MF. In vivo histology of Barrett's esophagus and associated neoplasia by confocal laser endomicroscopy. Clin Gastroenterol Hepatol. 2006;4(8):979–87. Epub 2006 Jul 13.PMID: 16843068.
24. Moussata D, Goetz M, Gloeckner A, Kerner M, Campbell P, Hoffman A, Biesterfeld S, Flourie B, Saurin JC, Galle PR, Neurath MF, Watson AJ, Kiesslich R. Confocal laser endomicroscopy is a new imaging modality for recognition of intramucosal bacteria in inflammatory bowel disease in vivo. Gut. 2011;60:26–33.
25. Van den Broek FJ, van Es JA, van Eeden S, Stokkers PC, Ponsioen CY, Reitsma JB, Fockens P, Deker E. Pilot study of probe-based confocal laser endomicroscopy during colonoscopic surveillance of patients with longstanding ulcerative colitis. Endoscopy. 2011;43(2):116–22. Epub 2010 Dec 16.
26. Hurlstone DP, Thomson M, Brown S, Tiffin N, Cross SS, Hunter MD. Confocal endomicroscopy in ulcerative colitis: differentiating dysplasia-associated lesional mass and adenoma-like mass. Clin Gastroenterol Hepatol. 2007;5(10):1235–41. Epub 2007 Aug 8.
27. De Palma GD. Confocal laser endomicroscopy in the "in vivo" histological diagnosis of the gastrointestinal tract. World J Gastroenterol. 2009;15(46):5770–5. PMID: 19998496.
28. Liu JJ, Wong K, Thiesen AL, Mah SJ, Dieleman LA, Claggett B, Saltzman JR, Fedorak RN. Increased epithelial gaps in the small intestines of patients with inflammatory bowel disease: density matters. Gastrointest Endosc. 2011;73(6):1174–80. doi:10.1016/j.gie.2011.01.018. Epub 2011 Mar 11. PMID: 21396639.
29. Atreya R, Neumann H, Neufert C, Waldner MJ, Billmeier U, Zopf Y, Willma M, App C, Münster T, Kessler H, Maas S, Gebhardt B, Heimke-Brinck R, Reuter E, Dörje F, Rau TT, Uter W, Wang TD, Kiesslich R, Vieth M, Hannappel E, Neurath MF. In vivo imaging using fluorescent antibodies to tumor necrosis factor predicts therapeutic response in Crohn's disease. Nat Med. 2014;20(3):313–8. doi:10.1038/nm.3462. Epub 2014 Feb 23. PMID: 24562382.
30. Noth R, Stüber E, Häsler R, Nikolaus S, Kühbacher T, Hampe J, Bewig B, Schreiber S, Arlt A. Anti-TNF-α antibodies improve intestinal barrier function in Crohn's disease. J Crohns Colitis. 2012;6(4):464–9. doi:10.1016/j.crohns.2011.10.004. Epub 2011 Nov 11. PMID: 22398062.
31. af Björkesten CG, Nieminen U, Sipponen T, Turunen U, Arkkila P, Färkkilä M. Mucosal healing at 3 months predicts long-term endoscopic remission in anti-TNF-treated luminal Crohn's disease. Scand J Gastroenterol. 2013;48(5):543–51. doi:10.3109/00365521.2013.772230. Epub 2013 Mar 12. PMID: 23477356.
32. Hawk ET, Levin B. Colorectal cancer prevention. J Clin Oncol. 2005;23(2):378–91. Review. PMID: 15637400.
33. Polglase AL, McLaren WJ, Skinner SA, Kiesslich R, Neurath MF, Delaney PM. A fluorescence confocal endomicroscope for in vivo microscopy of the upper- and the lower-GI tract. Gastrointest Endosc. 2005;62(5):686–95. PMID: 16246680.
34. Xie XJ, Li CQ, Zuo XL, Yu T, Gu XM, Li Z, Ji R, Wang Q, Li YQ. Differentiation of colonic polyps by confocal laser endomicroscopy. Endoscopy. 2011;43(2):87–93. doi:10.1055/s-0030-1255919. Epub 2010 Oct 29. PMID: 21038291.
35. Buchner AM, Gomez V, Heckman MG, Shahid MW, Achem S, Gill KR, Jamil LH, Kahaleh M, Lo SK, Picco M, Riegert-Johnson D, Raimondo M, Sciemeca D, Wolfsen H, Woodward T, Wallace MB. The learning curve of in vivo probe-based confocal laser endomicroscopy for prediction of colorectal neoplasia. Gastrointest Endosc. 2011;73(3):556–60. doi:10.1016/j.gie.2011.01.002. Erratum in: Gastrointest Endosc. 2011 Jun;73(6):1333. Laith, Jamil [corrected to Jamil, Laith H]. PMID: 21353852.
36. Su P, Liu Y, Lin S, Xiao K, Chen P, An S, He J, Bai Y. Efficacy of confocal laser endomicroscopy for discriminating colorectal neoplasms from non-neoplasms: a systematic review and meta-analysis. Colorectal Dis. 2013;15(1):e1–12. doi:10.1111/codi.12033. Review. PMID: 23006609.

37. Brugge WR, Lewandrowski K, Lee-Lewandrowski E, Centeno BA, Szydlo T, Regan S, del Castillo CF, Warshaw AL. Diagnosis of pancreatic cystic neoplasms: a report of the cooperative pancreatic cyst study. Gastroenterology. 2004;126(5):1330–6. PMID: 15131794.
38. Konda VJ, Meining A, Jamil LH, Giovannini M, Hwang JH, Wallace MB, Chang KJ, Siddiqui UD, Hart J, Lo SK, Saunders MD, Aslanian HR, Wroblewski K, Waxman I. A pilot study of in vivo identification of pancreatic cystic neoplasms with needle-based confocal laser endomicroscopy under endosonographic guidance. Endoscopy. 2013;45(12):1006–13. doi:10.1055/s-0033-1344714. Epub 2013 Oct 25. PMID: 24163192.
39. Napoléon B, Lemaistre AI, Pujol B, Caillol F, Lucidarme D, Bourdariat R, Morellon-Mialhe B, Fumex F, Lefort C, Lepilliez V, Palazzo L, Monges G, Filoche B, Giovannini M. A novel approach to the diagnosis of pancreatic serous cystadenoma: needle-based confocal laser endomicroscopy. Endoscopy. 2015;47(1):26–32. doi:10.1055/s-0034-1390693. Epub 2014 Oct 17. PMID: 25325684.
40. Nakai Y, Iwashita T, Park do H, Samarasena JB, Lee JG, Chang KJ. Diagnosis of pancreatic cysts: EUS-guided, through-the-needle confocal laser-induced endomicroscopy and cystoscopy trial: DETECT study. Gastrointest Endosc. 2015;81(5):1204–14. doi:10.1016/j.gie.2014.10.025. Epub 2015 Jan 26. PMID: 25634486.
41. Slivka A, Chen YK, Pleskow DK, Stevens PD, Shah RJ, Chuttani 60 R, Meining A. Real-time microscopic evaluation of indeterminate strictures: comparison of cholangioscopy vs catheter delivery for probe-based confocal laser endomicroscopy (pCLE) – a multicenter experience using cellvizio. Gastrointest Endosc. 2011;1:61 AB146–7. doi:10.1016/j.gie.2011.03.108.
42. Pratico C, Leblanc S, Vienne A, Duchmann JC, Mangialavori L, Chaussade S, Prat F. Diagnostic performance of catheter-based compared with cholangioscopy-based endomicroscopy of indeterminate biliary strictures. Gastrointest Endosc. 2013;1:AB323.
43. Giovannini M, Bories E, Monges G, Pesenti C, Caillol F, Delpero JR. Results of a phase I-II study on intraductal confocal microscopy (IDCM) in patients with common bile duct (CBD) stenosis. Surg Endosc. 2011;25(7):2247–53. doi:10.1007/s00464-010-1542-8. Epub 2011 Mar 18. PMID: 21424206.
44. Meining A, Chen YK, Pleskow D, Stevens P, Shah RJ, Chuttani R, Michalek J, Slivka A. Direct visualization of indeterminate pancreaticobiliary strictures with probe-based confocal laser endomicroscopy: a multicenter experience. Gastrointest Endosc. 2011;74(5):961–8. doi:10.1016/j.gie.2011.05.009. Epub 2011 Jul 29. PMID: 21802675.
45. Mehraban N, Simien M, Linder JD, Tarnasky PR. Clinical utility of biliary confocal laser endomicroscopy. Gastrointest Endosc. 2012;1:AB377. doi:10.1016/j.gie.2012.03.994.
46. Cesaro P, Tringali A, Caillol F, Monges GM, Familiari P, Perri V, Spada C, Giovannini M, Costamagna G. In-vivo miniprobe-based Confocal fluorescence Endomicroscopy (Cellvizio) for hilar biliary strictures: an experience of two centres. Dig Liver Dis. 2011;43:S145. doi:10.1016/S1590-8658(11)60221-1.
47. Caillol F, Filoche B, Gaidhane M, Kahaleh M. Refined probe-based confocal laser endomicroscopy classification for biliary strictures: the Paris classification. Dig Dis Sci. 2013;58(6):1784–9. doi:10.1007/s10620-012-2533-5. Epub 2013 Jan 12. PMID: 23314855.
48. Kahaleh M, Giovannini M, Jamidar P, Gan SI, Cesaro P, Caillol F, Filoche B, Karia K, Smith I, Gaidhane M, Slivka A. Probe-based confocal laser endomicroscopy for indeterminate biliary strictures: refinement of the image interpretation classification. Gastroenterol Res Pract. 2015;2015:675210. doi:10.1155/2015/675210. Epub 2015 Mar 12. PMID: 25866506.
49. Sarah L, Berson A, Dhooge M, Esch A, Tabouret T, Chaussade S, Prat F. Accuracy of confocal laser endomicroscopy for the diagnosis of indeterminate biliary strictures: comparison of the Miami and Paris classifications. Gastroenterology. 2014;1:S-9. doi:10.1016/S0016-5085(14)60032-9.
50. Giovannini M, Caillol F, Monges GM, Bories E, Pesenti C, Turrini O, Delpero JR. Probe Based Confocal Laser Endomicroscopy (pCLE) in the bile duct for indeterminate stenosis: be careful with the biliary stenting!!! Gastrointest Endosc. 2012;1:AB392–3. doi:10.1016/j.gie.2012.03.1040.

51. Caillol F, Bories E, Poizat F, Pesenti C, Esterni B, Monges G, Giovannini M. Endomicroscopy in bile duct: inflammation interferes with pCLE applied in the bile duct: a prospective study of 54patients. United European Gastroenterol J. 2013;1(2):120–7. doi:10.1177/2050640613483462. PMID: 24917949.
52. Wang KK, Carr-Locke DL, Singh SK, Neumann H, Bertani H, Galmiche JP, Arsenescu RI, Caillol F, Chang KJ, Chaussade S, Coron E, Costamagna G, Dlugosz A, Ian Gan S, Giovannini M, Gress FG, Haluszka O, Ho KY, Kahaleh M, Konda VJ, Prat F, Shah RJ, Sharma P, Slivka A, Wolfsen HC, Zfass A. Use of probe-based confocal laser endomicroscopy (pCLE) in gastrointestinal applications. A consensus report based on clinical evidence. United European Gastroenterol J. 2015;3(3):230–54. doi:10.1177/2050640614566066. Review. Erratum in: United European Gastroenterol J. 2015 Aug;3(4):404. PMID: 26137298.
53. Slivka A, Gan I, Jamidar P, Costamagna G, Cesaro P, Giovannini M, Caillol F, Kahaleh M. Validation of the diagnostic accuracy of probe-based confocal laser endomicroscopy for the characterization of indeterminate biliary strictures: results of a prospective multicenter international study. Gastrointest Endosc. 2015;81(2):282–90. doi:10.1016/j.gie.2014.10.009. PMID: 25616752.
54. Slivka A, Gan SI, Giovannini M, Jamidar PA, Costamagna G, Cesaro P, Kahaleh M. Accuracy of optical biopsy using probe based confocal laser endomicroscopy (PCLE) in patients with indeterminate biliary strictures: interim results with modified criteria of a large multicentric study. Gastrointest Endosc. 2014;1:AB264. doi:10.1016/j.gie.2014.02.443.
55. Heif M, Yen RD, Fukami N, Brauer BC, Wani S, Shah RJ. Probe-based confocal laser endomicroscopy for dominant stenoses in patients with primary sclerosing cholangitis. Gastrointest Endosc. 2012;1:AB397. doi:10.1016/j.gie.2012.03.1054.
56. Chang S, Kang B, Liu X, Dai Y, Chen D. The combined in uence of surface modification, size distribution, and interaction time on the cytotoxicity of CdTe quantum dots in PANC-1 cells. Acta Biochim Biophys Sin (Shanghai). 2012;44:241–8. PMID: 22236580. doi:10.1093/abbs/gmr126.
57. Goetz M, Deris I, Vieth M, Murr E, Hoffman A, Delaney P, Galle PR, Neurath MF, Kiesslich R. Near-infrared confocal imaging during mini-laparoscopy: a novel rigid endomicroscope with increased imaging plane depth. J Hepatol. 2010;53(1):84–90. doi:10.1016/j.jhep.2010.01.039. Epub 2010 Apr 8. PMID: 20452700.
58. Goetz M, Kiesslich R, Dienes HP, Drebber U, Murr E, Hoffman A, Kanzler S, Galle PR, Delaney P, Neurath MF. In vivo confocal laser endomicroscopy of the human liver: a novel method for assessing liver microarchitecture in real time. Endoscopy. 2008;40(7):554–62. doi:10.1055/s-2008-1077296. PMID: 18609449.
59. Mennone A, Nathanson MH. Needle-based confocal laser endomicroscopy to assess liver histology in vivo. Gastrointest Endosc. 2011;73(2):338–44. doi:10.1016/j.gie.2010.10.002. Epub 2010 Dec 8. PMID: 21145055.
60. Becker V, Wallace MB, Fockens P, von Delius S, Woodward TA, Raimondo M, Voermans RP, Meining A. Needle-based confocal endomicroscopy for in vivo histology of intra-abdominal organs: first results in a porcine model (with videos). Gastrointest Endosc. 2010;71(7):1260–6. doi:10.1016/j.gie.2010.01.010. Epub 2010 Apr 24. PMID: 20421104.
61. Karstensen J, Cartana T, Pia K, Saftoiu A, Vilmann P. Endoscopic ultrasound-guided needle confocal laser endomicroscopy in pancreatic masses. Endosc Ultrasound. 2014;3 Suppl 1:S2–3. PMID: 26425525.
62. Karstensen JG, Cârţână T, Klausen PH, Hassan H, Popescu CF, Săftoiu A, Vilmann P. Endoscopic ultrasound-guided needle-based confocal laser endomicroscopy: a pilot study for use in focal pancreatic masses. Pancreas. 2015;44(5):833–5. doi:10.1097/MPA.0000000000000345. No abstract available. PMID: 26061561.
63. Nakai Y, Shinoura S, Ahluwalia A, Tarnawski AS, Chang KJ. In vivo visualization of epidermal growth factor receptor and surviving expression in porcine pancreas using endoscopic ultrasound guided fine needle imaging with confocal laser-induced endomicroscopy. J Physiol Pharmacol. 2012;63(6):577–80. PMID: 23388473.

64. Diana M, Robinet E, Liu YY, Legnèr A, Kong SH, Schiraldi L, Marchegiani F, Halvax P, Swanstrom L, Dallemagne B, Marescaux J. Confocal imaging and tissue-specific fluorescent probes for real-time in vivo immunohistochemistry. Proof of the concept in a gastric lymph node metastasis model. Ann Surg Oncol. 2016;23(Suppl 5):567–573. PMID: 26511264.
65. Goetz M, Ansems JV, Galle PR, Schuchmann M, Kiesslich R. In vivo real-time imaging of the liver with confocal endomicroscopy permits visualization of the temporospatial patterns of hepatocyte apoptosis. Am J Physiol Gastrointest Liver Physiol. 2011;301(5):G764–72. doi:10.1152/ajpgi.00175.2011. Epub 2011 Jul 21. PMID: 21778462.
66. Altmeyer A, Ignat M, Denis JM, Messaddeq N, Gueulette J, Mutter D, Bischoff P. Cell death after high-LET irradiation in orthotopic human hepatocellular carcinoma in vivo. In Vivo. 2011;25(1):1–9. PMID: 21282728.

2 OTSC System in All Possible Applications

Rita Conigliaro, Santi Mangiafico, Giuseppe Iabichino,
Monica Arena, and Carmelo Luigiano

2.1 Introduction

The OTSC® system (Ovesco Endoscopy AG, Tübingen, Germany) consists of a nitinol alloy, which allows a high grade of elasticity and was designed to overcome the limitations of traditional through-the-scope (TTS) clips allowing a significantly larger mechanical circumferential compression of large tissue areas, surrounding the vessel without direct trauma.

When released from the applicator, the shape-memory effect and the high grade of elasticity of the nitinol alloy cause closure of the clip. The shape-memory alloy effects a permanent closing force of the OTSCs between 8 and 9 newtons. Because of the superelastic effect of nitinol, the force is permanently applied. Phantom tests and animal survival studies have shown that this closing force is necessary to reach sufficient compression of tissue.

OTSC has shown its encouraging results in management of various clinical situations also critical as the closure of gastrointestinal fistulas, iatrogenic perforations during endoscopy, anastomotic leaks and post bariatric surgery, bleeding lesions, complications and closure of gastrostomies during natural orifice transluminal endoscopic surgery.

Therefore in this chapter we present all the possible applications of the OTSC devices including.

R. Conigliaro, MD (✉) • S. Mangiafico
Digestive Endoscopy Unit, Baggiovara Hospital, Modena, Italy
e-mail: rita.conigliaro@teletu.it

G. Iabichino • M. Arena • C. Luigiano
Digestive Endoscopy Unit, San Paolo Hospital, Milano, Italy

R. Conigliaro, M. Frazzoni (eds.), *Diagnosis and Endoscopic Management of Digestive Diseases*, DOI 10.1007/978-3-319-42358-6_2

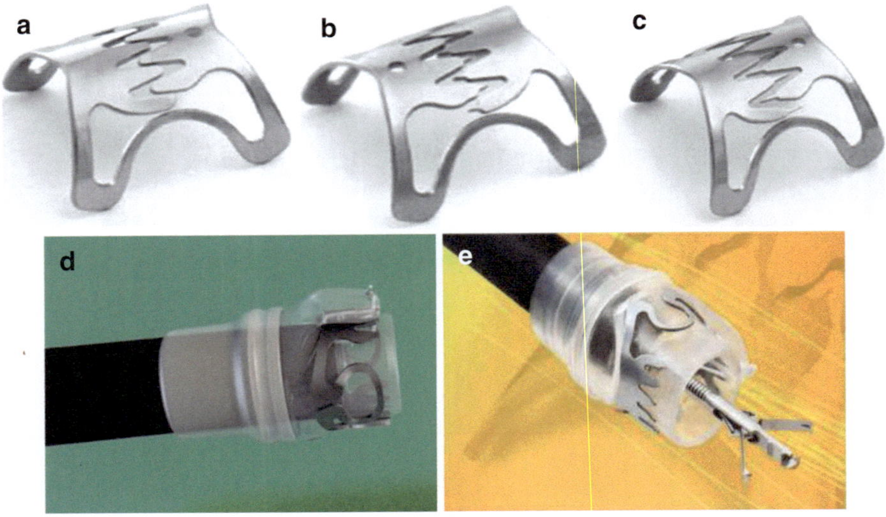

Fig. 2.1 OTSC system. (**a**) Atraumatic: short teeth for vessels. OTSC. (**b**) Traumatic regular type: pointed teeth for fistula' s wall. OTSC. (**c**) Traumatic gastric-type clip (gc): longer pointed teeth for gastric wall. OTSC. (**d**) Atraumatic clip installed on the tip of an endoscope. OTSC (**e**) the tip of the endoscope loaded with clip and a "twin Gasper" sometimes used to get the tissue

2.2 Technical Concepts

The over-the-scope clip system must be mounted onto the tip of the scope by the applicator with a loading coil, which assists in the opening of the clip. The applicator consists of a cylindrical cap, a wire, and a protection cap. When the clip is opened, it fits to the shape of the cylindrical cap. The cap is mounted onto the tip of the endoscope.

Two different configurations are available: the "atraumatic" version with blunt teeth and the "traumatic" version with two types of sharp teeth ("regular" and "gastric" types) (Fig. 2.1).

The application for bleeding is shown in Fig. 2.2.

The application for the treatment of fistulas is similar, but two types of forceps as shown in Fig. 2.3 can also be used.

2.3 OTSC in GI Bleeding

Gastrointestinal bleeding is a frequent event in clinical practice. Upper gastrointestinal bleeding (UGIB) and lower gastrointestinal bleeding (LGIB) are usually distinguished according to the proximal or distal origin of bleeding with respect to the ligament of Treitz.

Acute UGIB is a common condition worldwide with an estimated annual incidence of 40–150 cases per 100,000 population [3, 4], 4–6 times more frequent than

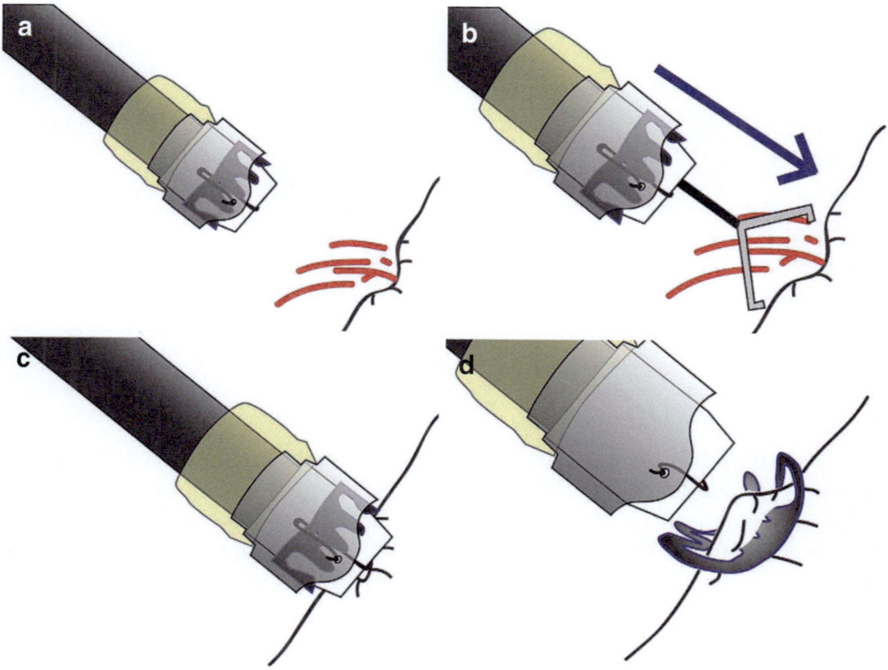

Fig. 2.2 Application procedure. The endoscope is inserted with the mounted and loaded clipping device (**a**). The tip of the endoscope is adapted to the lesion, with the optional use of application aids like a forceps/grasper, and additional tissue is suctioned into the applicator cap (**b**). The tissue is in close proximity to the applicator, and the clip is fired by stretching the wire with the hand wheel (**c**). The clip captures the tissue that is suctioned into the applicator cap, and then it removes the scope from the lesion and proceeds with the correct positioning inspection (**d**). The arms of the clip protruded approximately 4.5 mm into the lumen of the GI tract

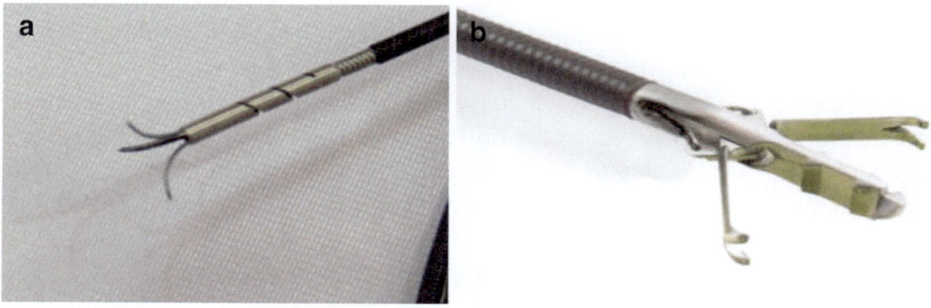

Fig. 2.3 Forceps/graspers: Anchor type (**a**) twin type (**b**)

Table 2.1 Most common causes of UIGB

	%
Peptic ulcer	28–59
Erosive	1–47
Variceal bleeding	4–20
Esophagitis	3–12
Mallory–Weis	4–7
Neoplasm	2–4
Others (Dieulafoy's lesions, angiodysplasias, gastric antral vascular ectasia, portal hypertensive gastropathy)	2–7
None	16–20

LGIB; it frequently leads to hospital admission and has significant associated morbidity and mortality, especially in the elderly. The most common causes of acute UGIB are nonvariceal UGIB (NVUGIB) [3, 4]. This includes peptic ulcers, 28–59 % (duodenal ulcer 17–37 % and gastric ulcer 11–24 %); mucosal erosive disease of the esophagus/stomach/duodenum, 1–47 %; Mallory–Weiss syndrome, 4–7 %; upper GI tract malignancy, 2–4 %; other diagnoses, 2–7 %; or no cause identified, 7–25 % [3, 4]. Moreover, in 16–20 % of acute UGIB cases, the cause of bleeding is multifactorial (Table 2.1).

LGIB is less common than UIGB, and the incidence is approximately 36 per 100,000 population [5] with a mortality of up to 3.9 % within 1 year [6, 7], although this may rise as high as 13 % by 5 years [8]. The mean age at presentation is in the range 63–77 years [9]. Up to 85 % of patients have self-limiting episodes [10], but re-bleeding can occur in up to 19 % of cases within a year [8].

The commonest cause of lower GI bleeding requiring hospital admission is diverticulosis, accounting for approximately 20–40 % of the cases [8], as well as more than 50 % of re-bleeding admission [12]. Right-sided diverticulitis is particularly likely to cause bleeding [13]. Ischemic colitis is the second most common cause, representing 12–16 % of cases [13, 14]. Common causes also include hemorrhoids and carcinomas of the colon and rectum [12]. Less common causes are bleeding following polypectomy, inflammatory bowel disease, and infective colitis. A few cases are due to radiation proctitis. Angiodysplasias are less common, but the source of these can be in the small bowel, and bleeding is often severe in such cases [11].

Endoscopic therapy for active UGIB can dramatically reduce the risk of re-bleeding or ongoing bleeding, the need for surgery, the number of units of packed erythrocytes required for transfusion, and the length of hospital stay [15, 16].

The goal of therapeutic endoscopy in patients with UGIB is to stop bleeding and prevent re-bleeding.

Endoscopic techniques include injection therapy, ablative therapy, and mechanical therapy. Commonly and less commonly used and experimental therapies for NUGIB are reported in Table 2.2.

Table 2.2 Endoscopic therapies for NUIGB

Common therapies for nonvariceal UGIB	Uncommon therapies for nonvariceal UGIB
Injection therapy *Dilute epinephrine* *Sclerosants* *Ablative therapy* *Contact methods* *Thermocoagulation—heater probe* *Electrocoagulation—BICAP, Gold Probe™* *Noncontact methods* *Argon plasma coagulation* *Mechanical therapy* *Hemoclips* *Band ligation*	*Injection therapy* *Normal saline* *Thrombin* *Fibrin sealant* *Cyanoacrylate glue* *Ablative therapy* *Cryotherapy* *Photocoagulation—Nd:YAG laser* *Mechanical therapy* *Detachable snare—Endo-loop™ (Olympus Corporation, Lake Success, NY)* *Suturing device* *Dual-therapy devices* *Probe combining electrocautery with needle injection* *Device combining electrocautery with mechanical therapy* *Topical therapy* *Hemospray* *Endoclot*

Although several types of endoscopic treatment for bleeding peptic ulcers have been described, including injection therapy, thermal coagulation, hemostatic clips, fibrin sealant (or glue), argon plasma coagulation, and combination therapy (typically injection of epinephrine combined with another treatment modality), relatively a few prospective comparative trials have been performed. Currently, most patients are treated with either thermal coagulation therapy or hemostatic clips, with or without the addition of injection therapy.

Meta-analyses have shown that combination endoscopic therapy (dilute epinephrine injection combined with a second hemostasis modality including injectable, thermal contact probe, or clips) is superior to injection therapy alone, but not to clips or contact thermal therapy alone [17, 18]. There may be practical reasons to pre-inject dilute epinephrine before other therapies for high-risk endoscopic stigmata. Injection of epinephrine may slow or stop bleeding allowing improved visualization for application of subsequent therapy. Adverse events associated with combination endoscopic hemostasis are infrequent and include induction of bleeding (1.7 %) and perforation (0.6 %) [18].

Recent international consensus guidelines recommend combination therapy (dilute epinephrine injection combined with contact thermal therapy, clips, or injection of a sclerosant) as appropriate treatment in patients with peptic ulcer bleeding with high-risk endoscopic stigmata [19–21].

Despite major advances in its management over the past decade, including intravenous high-dose proton pump inhibitors, NVUGIB is still associated with considerable morbidity, mortality, and health economic burden [22]. Of particular note is re-bleeding, a major predictor of morbidity and mortality that has not been significantly improved according to data registered in the last 15 years [4, 23]. Although huge advances have been made in terms of therapeutic endoscopic devices, complete hemostasis of complicated lesions (i.e., large vessels or fibrotic ulcers) still represents a challenging task.

Mechanical or thermal therapy fails to stop bleeding in 5–12 % of cases [18, 24]. The limits of current endoscopic therapies are linked to different variables such as type, size, and location of the lesion and exposed large vessels. High-risk lesions may be technically difficult to manage, resulting in failure of endoscopic treatment.

From a technical point of view, the limits of hemoclips application are well known. The limited diameter of the working channel of the endoscope results in a relatively small size of through-the-scope clips allowing compression of limited amounts of tissue, especially in the presence of scarred and hardened tissue or inflammatory mucosa. Accordingly, the hemostatic effect may not be sufficient for large-size vessels, and there is often the need to apply more than one clip to achieve an effective hemostasis [25, 26]. Furthermore correct application in the antrum and duodenal bulb is technically challenging [27].

Preliminary data suggested a possible role of OTSC in GI bleeding. Kirschniak et al. [28] treated 12 patients with upper GI bleedings; most of them were caused by peptic ulcer disease. Primary hemostasis was achieved in all cases. In two cases, a secondary bleeding occurred. In one case, it was observed 12 h after OTSC treatment of a Mallory–Weiss lesion, and in the other case, it occurred 7 days after treatment of bleeding duodenal ulcer. This study demonstrated the efficacy of OTSC in upper GI bleeding; however, authors did not specify the characteristics of the lesions treated in terms of Forrest classification, location, and size, debarring the assessment of its possible advantage versus standard endoscopic therapy.

A recent study demonstrated efficacy and safety of the OTSC for the treatment of patients with severe acute upper and lower GI bleeding unresponsive to conventional treatment, resulting in a salvage endoscopic treatment during NVUGIB emergencies [29]. In that study, 23 cases with GI bleeding unresponsive to conventional endoscopic treatment modalities were treated with OTSC. Primary hemostasis with OTSC was achieved in 22/23 patients. In one patient with a posterior wall duodenal ulcer, emergency-selective radiological embolization was required to stop bleeding after failure of the OTSC procedure. Re-bleeding was observed in two cases; both cases were successfully re-treated endoscopically. Authors concluded that OTSC is an effective and safe endoscopic tool for treatment of patients with severe acute NVUGIB unresponsive to conventional treatment modalities, although the proportion of high-risk patients was not stated.

These data were confirmed in two recent studies. One study reported 12 patients with severe gastrointestinal bleeding due a duodenal ulcer ($n=6$), gastric ulcer ($n=2$), Dieulafoy's lesion ($n=2$), anastomotic ulceration ($n=1$), and Mallory–Weiss tear ($n=1$). All patients had failed hemostatic therapy using traditional endoscopic methods. Hemostasis was achieved in all patients. REBLEEDING occurred in two patients 1 day after OTSC placement. Subsequently, the patient with a Mallory–Weiss tear was successfully treated with an injection of saline/epinephrine and the placement of conventional clips. The patient with gastrojejunal anastomotic ulcers was readmitted with melena 7 days after placement of the OTSC. Repeat EGD showed active bleeding from a large, circumferential ischemic anastomotic ulcer. No endoscopic intervention was undertaken, and the patient proceeded to radiological embolization and then to surgery for reconstruction of the anastomosis. There were no complications associated with the application of OTSCs [30].

The second recent study reported a series of a total of nine patients. Six of them had undergone previous endoscopic hemostasis therapy. The median size of the ulcers was 2.5 cm. All the ulcers and tumors demonstrated the presence of a visible vessel on endoscopy. The technical success rate of OTSC was 100 %, and endoscopic hemostasis was achieved in all patients. Two patients experienced re-bleeding, which required further intervention, and hence, the clinical effectiveness was 78 % [31]. In these two studies, the authors concluded that OTSC should be considered in patients with refractory bleeding after failure of conventional methods of endoscopic hemostasis, before surgery or angiographic embolization. Analyzing the results of these two studies, we could suppose that previous endoscopic treatment, i.e., clip, could hamper OTSC application resulting in re-bleeding.

Another case series reported the utility of OTCS to provide endoscopic hemostasis for bleeding posterior duodenal ulcers [32]. In this study, four patients with massive gastrointestinal bleeding due to ulcers located in the posterior bulb and actively oozing were treated with OTSC after failure of initial therapy with injection of epinephrine/saline solution and clip placement. Hemostasis was successfully achieved in all four cases. The authors concluded the OTSC is effective for obliterating ulcers with bleeding vessel located in a difficult position (i.e., the posterior duodenum); although heater probe is an effective alternative method to treat such lesions, this treatment modality is available in the USA and some Asian countries only but not in most European countries. However, using a heater probe can result in a higher risk of perforation [33]. The authors also claimed that the placement of OTSC was easy [32].

A more recent study reported a series of patients in whom OTSC represented the first-line endoscopic treatment in patients with high-risk nonvariceal upper gastrointestinal bleeding [34]. During the study period, 40 consecutive patients with severe acute NVUGIB were treated with OTSC as first-line endoscopic treatment. Indications for OTSC treatment included gastric ulcer with large vessel (Forrest IIa) ($n=8$, 20 %), duodenal ulcer (Forrest Ib) ($n=7$, 18 %), duodenal ulcer with large vessel (Forrest IIa) ($n=6$, 15 %), Dieulafoy's lesion ($n=6$, 15 %), and other secondary indications ($n=13$, 32 %). Sixteen (40 %) patients had gastric or duodenal ulcer [20 mm (20–29 mm: $n=10$, 25 %]; [30 mm: $n=6$, 15 %)]. Technical success and primary hemostasis were achieved in all patients (100 %). None of the patients had re-bleeding or required surgical or radiological embolization treatment. No other complications were observed during the 30-day follow-up period. The authors concluded that OTSC placement represents a first-line endoscopic treatment being effective, safe, and technically easy to perform.

In summary, OTSC system utilizes a very contractile, superelastic nickel titanium alloy, which provides tissue apposition that is far superior to that of traditional clipping. Based on published data, the OTSC system appears promising for the treatment of bleeding lesions with large-diameter visible vessels, challenging high-risk bleeding lesions such as Dieulafoy's lesion or those located in awkward positions, such as the greater curvature of the stomach or the posterior duodenal wall or which may not always be amenable to treatment with standard endoscopic devices.

It is believed that hemostasis is achieved by a combination of two mechanisms: (I) sealing the blood vessel and (II) closing an ulcer. However, the main mechanism appears to be "tissue compression," which occurs by compressing the surrounding tissue around the vessel. However even if it is possible to close an ulcer by applying the OTSC directly on a bleeding vessel, it is believed that the abovementioned "tissue compression" mechanism better explains the hemostatic mechanisms.

Moreover, most gastroscopes have working channels on the left side making it difficult to apply endoscopic hemostasis to lesions located on the right or in the posterior duodenum. In addition, standard clips often fall off from these lesions and also induce more bleeding by lacerating the vessel.

The duration of the clipping procedure itself depends on the ability to get in touch with the lesion and sufficient adaptation of the applicator cap to the lesion. The correct and secure application of the OTSC depends on the correct fitting of the application cap to the lesion. With the help of application aids like forceps or graspers, the lesion can be fixed, and then the scope can be pushed onto the lesion. Because there is no visualization possible at the moment of application, the endoscopist must be sure to be in the correct position.

Despite the early promising results regarding the OTSC device, we need more prospective clinical trials to demonstrate its superiority relative to traditional clips and closure devices.

Nevertheless, it is clear that the OTSC system is already part of the therapeutic armamentarium of the advanced endoscopist, and we expect this device to be used more frequently in clinical practice.

2.4 The New Device DC ClipCutter

A potential complication of the OTSC system is that once it is deployed it cannot be removed. Some publication has recently demonstrated three rescue methods to remove the clip in case of misapplication [35–37].

The "official device" of Ovesco Endoscopy AG is the DC ClipCutter: the clip is locally brought to the melting point through the application of a brief pulse of current.

The remOVE DC System consists of three units: (Fig. 2.4)

A. remOVE Impulse DC (DC generator)
B. remOVE DC Cutter (bipolar endoscopic instrument)
C. remOVE Securcap (cap for the safe extraction of the clip fragments)

Until now, in addition to some report stated on the porcine model [38], only one paper has been published with the application in humans [39]. A total of 11 patients underwent endoscopic removal of an OTSC. The clip was cut at two opposing sites

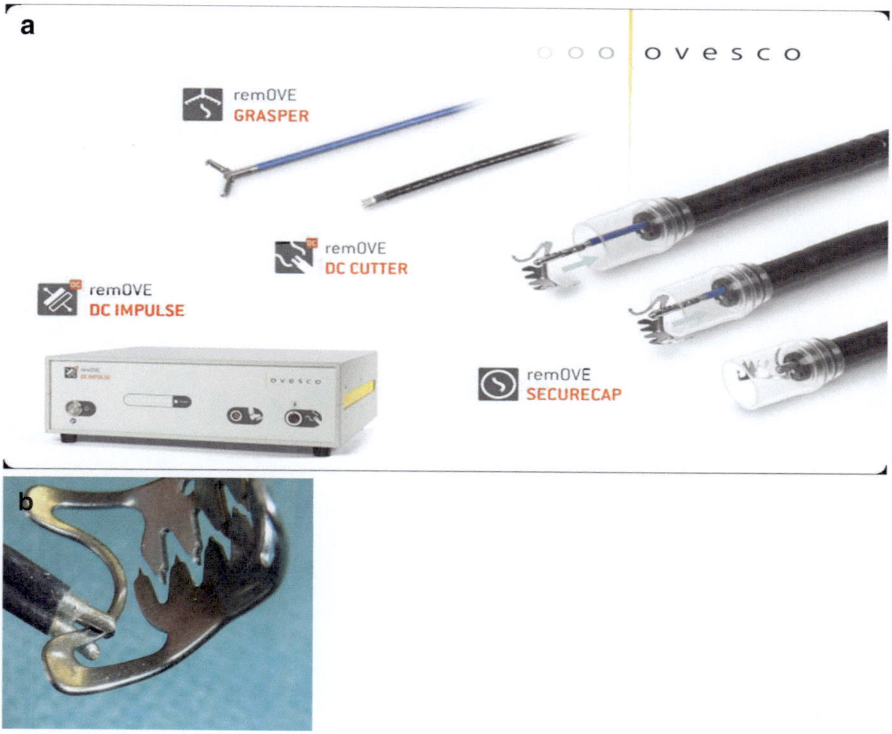

Fig. 2.4 The remOVE DC system (**a**) The cutter kipping the clip during the cutting (**b**)

by a prototype of DC ClipCutter getting the success rate, to complete the cutting and removal in 91 % of cases.

No major complications were observed.

2.5 Performance of Over-The-Scope Clip System in the Endoscopic Closure of Iatrogenic Gastrointestinal Perforations and Postsurgical Leaks

Over the years, the absolute number of diagnostic and especially therapeutic endoscopies has grown tremendously.

Endoscopic technological developments led to the performance of more advanced therapeutic procedures with higher risk of complications [40].

Surgeons also began to perform more complex gastrointestinal interventions. Consequently, endoscopists are increasingly facing gastrointestinal (GI) defects, such as anastomotic leaks, fistulas, and perforations. Anastomotic leak is defined as disruption at a surgical anastomosis resulting in a fluid collection, fistula is defined as abnormal communication between a natural or pathological cavity with the external or two natural cavities between them, and perforation is defined as an unintentional, acute iatrogenic, full-thickness defect in the GI tract [41, 42].

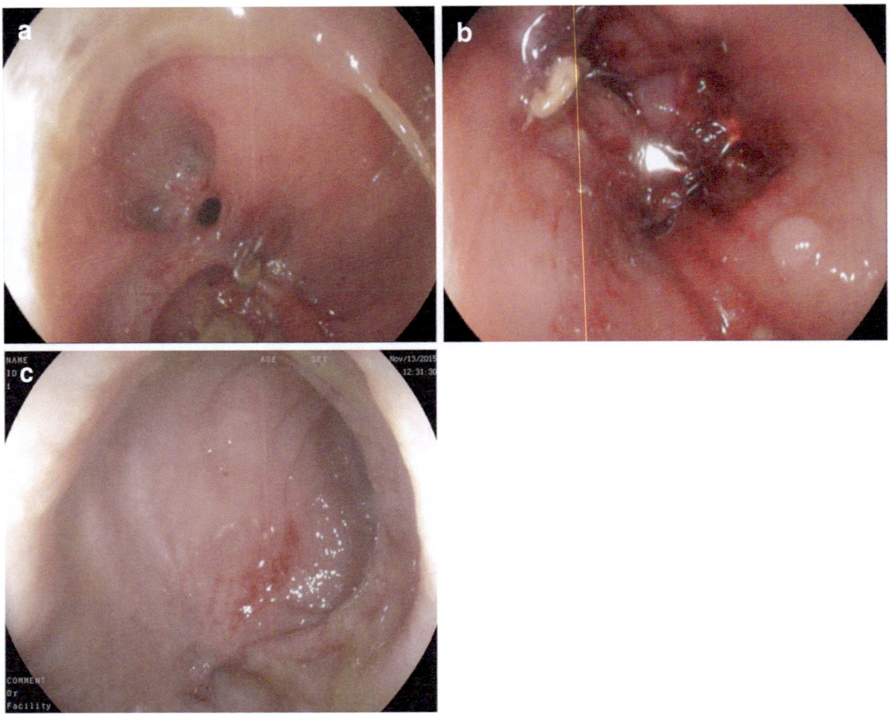

Fig. 2.5 (**a**) Perianastomotic fistula. (**b**) The OTS clip positioned to closing the fistula. (**c**) After 2 months, the fistula completely healed

Surgical treatment has been the mainstay of therapy for GI defects. However, surgical repair, especially for perforations, is associated with higher morbidity (25–36 %) and mortality (7–10 %) risks, which are accompanied by the risks of general anesthesia, prolonged recovery, and increased costs [43–46].

Therefore, endoscopic management of these complications is gaining more popularity and became a good option in selected cases.

Several endoscopic techniques have been described for closure of GI defects by using several devices, such as clips, endoloops and rubber bands, and fibrin glue, and methods, such as plugging by a prolene mesh and application of cyanoacrylate and placement of covered self-expandable metal stents (CSEMSs) or self-expandable plastic stents [47–51]. However, the success rate of these procedures varies between 55 and 69 %, and additional surgical management is often required [52]

More recently the placement of a new endoscopic Over-The-Scope Clip (OTSC®) system (Ovesco Endoscopy GmbH, Tübingen, Germany) has been described as illustrated above. The GI defect is suctioned into the cap, and the clip is then deployed, approximating the edges (Fig. 2.5). The OTSC device also contains two types of grasping forceps that can be inserted through the operative channel of the scope and used to pull both tissue edges into the cap before the clip released (Fig. 2.3). The use of OTSC has some advantages and limitations. The first technical limitation of OTSC system is large diameter, until 12 mm, that in patient with GI defect and endoluminal stenosis does not allow passage of the scope with mounted devices. Another limitation, compared to the through-the-scope (TTS) clips, is that in cases of necessity to place two or more devices, it is mandatory to remove every time the scope and proceed to assembly a new system. The advantages of OTSC over TTS devices are the larger defects that can be closed by one clip (limited by cap diameter and flexibility of the tissue being pulled into the cap) and the greater compression and higher closure force. The OTSC system also has a higher rate of full-thickness closure, therefore an improved safety profile with regard to closure-related infectious complications.

Clinical experience shows that clips usually fall off after several weeks or months, depending on the amount of tissue grasped. Since OTSC clips are fully biocompatible, they may stay in place indefinitely and does not subsequently preclude magnetic resonance imaging [53].

Complications with the use of OTSC device are rare; isolated cases of esophageal perforation, acute cholangitis, inadvertent tongue piercing, and intestinal obstruction (from accidental inclusion of opposing walls into the OTSC) have been reported [54–57].

2.6 Perforation

Perforation is the most feared adverse event of GI endoscopy, and its incidence varies depending on multiple patient-related and procedure-related factors [58, 59].

With more advanced interventional endoscopic procedures, endoscopists may be faced more often with perforations; indeed most cases of iatrogenic perforations occur during therapeutic procedures. The reported perforation rates are 0.3–0.5 % in endoscopic mucosal resection (EMR) and 4–10 % in endoscopic submucosal dissection (ESD) [60].

The standard treatment for acute endoscopic perforations is surgical repair. However, immediate endoscopic closure is less invasive, does not require anesthesia, and minimizes leakage of GI contents.

The OTSC system can capture and close larger defects up to 30 mm. From the technical point of view, the setting of acute endoscopic perforation is optimal for OTSC use: the lesion is fresh and without fibrotic alterations or inflammation. Until now, no randomized controlled clinical study has been performed to compare the OTSC system with other approaches. Several case series have demonstrated successful use of the OTSC in closure of acute perforations with clinical success rates ranging from 65 to 100 % in healing the GI defect (Table 2.3) [28, 54, 56, 61–71]. The largest numbers of patients with gastrointestinal perforations treated with OTSC have been reported in two multicenter studies. Voermans et al. reported successful closure without need for surgery in 32 of 36 patients (89 %) with acute iatrogenic perforations of the gastrointestinal tract <3 cm in size within 24 h of onset of perforation [56]. Recently, Haito-Chavez et al. published a multicenter international retrospective study of 188 patients who underwent attempted OTSC

Table 2.3 Studies reporting over-the-scope clip closure of gastrointestinal perforation

Author	Year	Study design	Number	Overall success (%)	Size of defect
Kirschniak et al. [22]	2007	Retrospective	4	4/4 (100 %)	4–8 mm
Repici et al. [23]	2009	Retrospective	2	2/2 (100 %)	N.S.
Seebach et al. [4]	2010	Retrospective	4	3/4 (75 %)	N.S.
Kirschniak et al. [24]	2011	Retrospective	11	11/11 (100 %)	N.S.
Sandmann et al. [25]	2011	Retrospective	3	3/3 (100 %)	N.S.
Baron et al. [15]	2012	Retrospective	5	4/5 (80 %)	N.S.
Gubler et al. [26]	2012	Prospective	14	13/14 (93 %)	6–30 mm
Hagel et al. [27]	2012	Retrospective	17	11/17 (65 %)	2–40 mm
Voermans et al. [17]	2012	Prospective	36	32/36 (89 %)	N.S.
Nishiyama et al. [28]	2013	Retrospective	11	10/11 (90 %)	5–40 mm
Schlag et al. [29]	2013	Prospective	6	6/6 (100 %)	7–30 mm
Changela K et al. [30]	2014	Retrospective	3	3/3 (100 %)	20 mm
Haito- Chavez et al. [31]	2014	Retrospective	40	36/40 (90 %)	7 mm (median)
Farnick et al. [32]	2015	Prospective	18	15/18 (83 %)	1–30 mm

placement for GI defects, and in the 40 cases with perforation analyzed, technical success was achieved in 39 cases (97.5 %), immediate clinical success was achieved in 37 (94.9 %), and 36 patients (90 %) had a long-term clinical success [70].

The position paper for diagnosis and management of iatrogenic perforation occurring during diagnostic or therapeutic digestive endoscopic procedures of the European Society of Gastrointestinal Endoscopy (ESGE) recommends the use of OTSC system as first-line therapy for large esophageal (<20 mm) gastric (<30 mm), duodenal, and colonic perforations [72].

2.7 Postsurgical Leaks

Anastomotic and staple line leaks occur in 0.4–5.2 % of patients having Roux-en-Y gastric bypass, 1.6–13.6 % of patients undergoing gastric resection for malignant neoplasms, and 3–33 % of patients having a colon resection for colorectal cancer [73–79]

Postsurgical complications such as fistula and leaks are conventionally submitted to surgical repair. However, surgical re-intervention has a significant morbidity and mortality, prolongs hospital stay, and increases costs [80]

The main goal of endoscopic therapy is the interruption of the flow of luminal contents across a gastrointestinal defect. Covered removable SEMS and OTSC are recent innovations that provide minimally invasive closure. Most of the stents usually used for the management of leakages in benign indications are fully covered in order to optimize removability. It results in a high migration rate with risk of recurrence [51].

Table 2.4 Studies reporting Over-The-Scope Clip closure of postsurgical leak

Author	Year	Study design	Number	Overall success (%)	Size of defect
Parodi et al. [42]	2010	Prospective	6	4/6 (67 %)	10–20 mm
Pohl et al. [43]	2010	Retrospective	2	1/2 (50 %)	N.S.
Seebach et al. [4]	2010	Retrospective	3	2/3 (67 %)	N.S.
Albert et al. [44]	2011	Retrospective	6	5/6 (83.3.6 %)	N.S.
Sandmann et al. [25]	2011	Retrospective	3	2/3 (67 %)	N.S.
Manta et al. [45]	2011	Retrospective	12	11/12 (92 %)	6–25 mm
Surace et al. [46]	2011	Prospective	18	7/18 (39 %)	N.S.
Arezzo et al. [47]	2012	Prospective	10	6/10 (60 %)	6–12 mm
Baron et al. [15]	2012	Retrospective	3	1/3 (33 %)	N.S.
Disibeyaz et al. [48]	2012	Retrospective	5	3/5 (57 %)	6–20 mm
Galizia et al. [49]	2012	Retrospective	3	3/3 (100 %)	N.R.
Menningen et al. [50]	2013	Retrospective	6	5/6 (83 %)	<20 mm
Haito-Chavez et al. [31]	2014	Retrospective	30	22/30 (73.3 %)	8 mm (median)
Winder et al. [51]	2015	Retrospective	6	6/6 (100 %)	8 mm (median)
Farnick et al. [32]	2015	Prospective	16	9/16 (56 %)	1–30 mm

The successful closure of leaks with OTSC has varied widely between 33 and 100 % in published series (Table 2.4) [54, 63, 64, 70, 71, 81–91]. Difficulties arise in the treatment of chronic leaks. The failure of this technique is more frequent when the leak edges are fibrotic and in patients who had undergone several surgical approaches. Indeed, Albert et al. found that success was high and durable when the time from diagnosis to application of the clip was within 1 week, resulting in a success rate of 100 % in postoperative lesions [44]. With increasing time from detection of the lesion to endoscopic treatment, the tissue was more difficult to grasp, and the success rate decreased to less than 60 % [44]. Haito-Chavez et al. analyzed 30 cases with long-term follow-up of OTSC placement for leaks, and technical success was achieved in 27 patients, immediate clinical success was achieved in 26 patients (96.3 %), and the overall long-term clinical success was achieved in 22 patients (73.3 %) [31]. In the three cases without technical success, the fibrotic or necrotic borders were cited as the most common cause of failure [70]

2.8 Gastrointestinal Fistulas

Gastrointestinal fistulas occur after surgical intervention, secondary to inflammatory or infectious disorders, after radiation therapy, or following removal of percutaneous tubes [91].

Despite the advent of the OTSC system, closure of GI fistulas using endoscopic methods remains difficult, and the successful closure of fistulas varies between 25 and 100 % in published series (Table 2.5) [54, 63, 64, 70, 71, 81–90]. A systematic review by Weiland et al. evaluated several studies using the OTSC system for

Table 2.5 Studies reporting Over-The-Scope Clip closure of gastrointestinal fistulas

Author	Year	Study design	Number	Overall success	Size of defect
Parodi et al. [42]	2010	Prospective	3	3/3 (100 %)	10–15 mm
Albert et al. [44]	2011	Retrospective	4	1/4 (25 %)	N.S.
Kirschniak et al. [24]	2011	Retrospective	8	3/8 (37.5 %)	N.S.
Sandmann et al. [25]	2011	Retrospective	4	4/4 (100 %)	N.S.
Arezzo et al. [47]	2012	Prospective	4	4/4 (100 %)	5–12 mm
Baron et al. [15]	2012	Retrospective	14	10/17 (59 %)	N.S.
Disibeyaz et al. [48]	2012	Retrospective	3	1/3 (33 %)	10–15 mm
Nishiyama et al. [28]	2013	Retrospective	4	3/4 (75 %)	10–28 mm
Menningen et al. [50]	2013	Retrospective	8	6/8 (75 %)	N.S.
Haito-Chavez et al. [31]	2014	Retrospective	30	33/91 (42.9 %)	5 mm (median)
Winder et al. [51]	2015	Retrospective	17	17/22 (77.3 %)	5 mm (median)
Law et al. [52]	2015	Retrospective	27	25/47 (53 %)	N.S.

endoscopic closure of GI fistulas and reported a high rate of technical success (84.6 %) but a durable clinical success of 69 % [92].

Haito-Chavez et al. reported the results of the OTSC system for the treatment of GI fistula in 91 patients with a median follow-up of 121 days, and technical success was achieved in 85 patients (93.4 %), immediate clinical success was achieved in 77 patients (90.6 %), and the overall long-term clinical success was achieved in only 39 patients (42.9 %) [90].

Law et al. in a retrospective review of 47 patients, who underwent OTSC placement for closure of GI fistulas, reported an initial technical success of 89 % (42/47 cases) but an overall long-term clinical success achieved in only 25 cases (53 %) [91].

The induration and fibrosis associated with chronic fistulas may result in failure of adequate tissue apposition. Adjunctive measures have been evaluated in addition to OTSC placement to promote fistula closure. Attempts to denude or disrupt the epithelialized tract by mechanical (e.g., standard cytology brush) or thermal (e.g., argon plasma coagulation) processes have been described and might hinder optimal OTSC opposition and successful fistula closure [54, 70, 93] The OTSC system may be effective in combination with adjunctive therapies, such as covered SEMS placement and application of cyanoacrylate or other tissue adhesives, to resolve the underlying disorder [54, 90, 93].

2.9 Over-The-Scope Clip Full-Thickness Resection Device (OTSC FTRD)

The novel "full-thickness resection device" (FTRD, Ovesco Endoscopy, Tübingen, Germany) is the first combined system for full-thickness resection of colon lesions with the closure and resection of the tissue integrated in a single procedure.

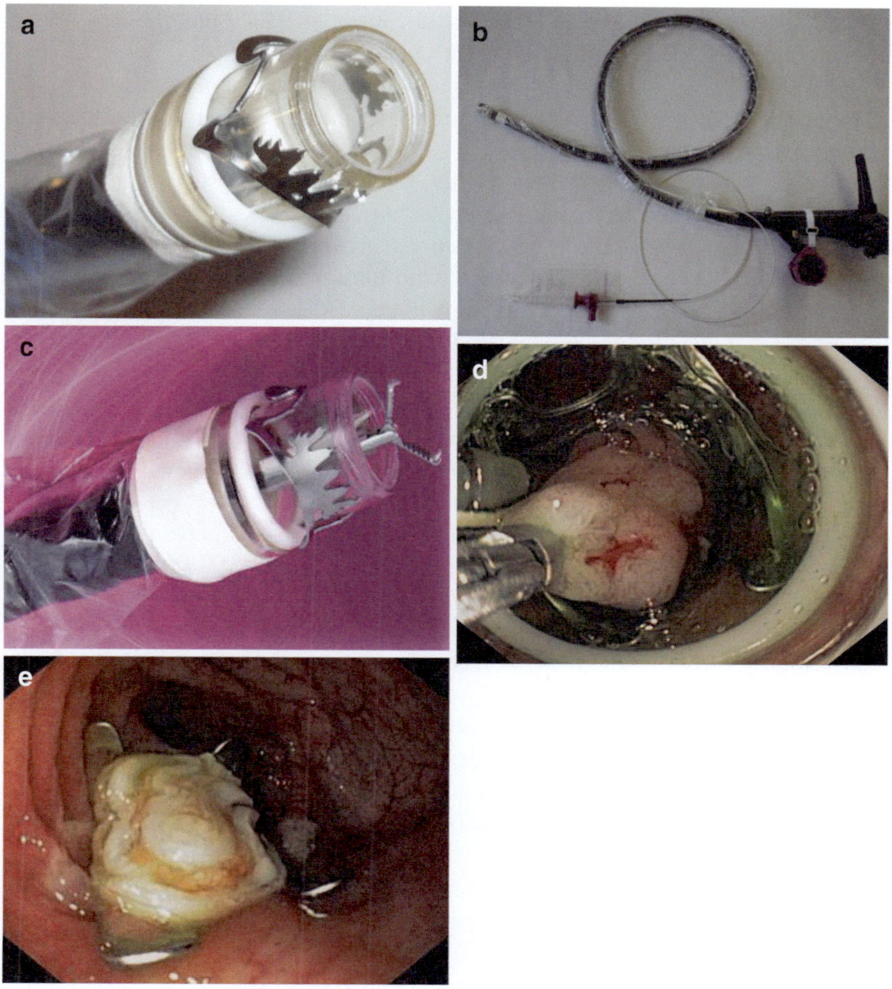

Fig. 2.6 OTSC FTRD system. (**a**) Cap with preloaded clip, (**b**) FTRD system assembled, mounted and ready for use. (**c**) Forceps to grasp the tissue introduced into the working channel. (**d**) Lesion pulled into the cap with forceps. (**e**) The Over-The-Scope Clip deployed; and the tissue above the clip resected

The OTSC FTRD was designed for one-step colon endoscopic FTR (EFTR) after OTSC application. Similar to the OTSC system, it can be mounted over a standard colonoscope and consists of a long transparent applicator cap carrying a modified 14 mm OTSC. The FTRD system is shown in Fig. 2.6. Compared to the conventional OTSC system, the cap is much longer (23 mm vs. 6 mm) and can therefore incorporate more tissue.

A 13 mm monofilament high-frequency (HF) snare is a preloaded on the tip of the cap. The handle of the snare runs on the outer surface of the scope underneath a plastic sheath. For resection, grasping forceps (or a tissue anchor) are advanced through the working channel of the scope; the lesion is pulled into the cap thereby creating a full-thickness duplication of the colonic wall.

Immediately after clip deployment, the tissue above the clip is resected with the snare above the clip. The device was firstly introduced in 2011 and evaluated in several porcine studies [94–97].

To date, there are five published studies, the first reporting successful EFTR of three recurrent non-lifting colonic adenomas [98]. A video case has been published demonstrating successful EFTR of an adenoma arising from a diverticulum [99].

A case series concerning 25 patients who underwent EFTR in the colon and rectum has recently been reported: immediate or delayed perforation or major bleeding was not reported. Technical success was 83.3 % and R0 resection rate 75 % [100].

In all series published, the majority of indications were non-lifting adenomas, or the recurrences and the sites were everywhere in the colorectum. Other indications are the resection of small subepithelial tumors in different locations with a mean tumor size of 15 mm.

A published data suggest that the FTRD system is feasible, effective, and safe. The major limitation of the system is the maximum size of the lesion to be resected. It is true that this limit strongly depends on the mobility of the colonic wall; indeed a resection specimen of up to 5.4 cm has been reported in experimental porcine study colon [94], while the median diameter in the mentioned clinical study was 24 mm (range 12–40 mm) [100].

This technique represents a minimally invasive endoluminal approach, which could become the ideal treatment for lesions with low risk of tumor seeding like advanced adenomas, "small" mesenchymal tumors, even a subset of early carcinomas, or neuroendocrine tumor [101, 102].

The advantages are:

- To allow to evaluate and get properly the R0 resection in T1 lesions with infiltration of the submucosa
- Give the option to safely and completely remove small submucosal lesions
- Having the possibility to get full-thickness intestinal biopsies

However some disadvantages are:

- Lower maneuverability of the colonoscope with the mounted device, so sometimes it is difficult to achieve proximal lesions
- Limits of size related to the diameter of the device
- Applicability only in the colon, because pharyngeal intubation would be dangerous and the gastric wall thickness does not allow a complete resection "full thickness"

The limit of the size of the device involves:

(a) The difficulty to resect larger lesions or hard scar tissue.
(b) The difficulty to evaluate well the wound edges with the risk of an R1 resection

In this context, until now, the percentage of R0 resections are around 75 % vs. 88 % of endoscopic submucosal dissection (ESD) [103]

At this point, it should be stated that all innovative techniques need to be investigated systematically. The majority of available studies are preclinical with a very limited amount of animal models or retrospective noncontrolled small clinical series; surely this depends partly because the device is recent. However, it is known that in Germany there are some prospective multicenter and single-center ongoing studies [104].

Conclusions

In summary, the recent developments and studies have brought the OTSC system into clinical routine for selected indications. While the role of OTSC system is widely accepted and there are many published literature for application in fistulas and bleeding, the EFTR system has yet to be widely applied in order to take stock of cost benefit.

This progress has again pushed the frontiers of endoluminal resections toward transmural interventions. However, prospective clinical trials are necessary to define applications and technical improvements regarding resection/closure devices and platforms.

References

1. Mori H, Kobara H, Fujihara S, Nishiyama N, Kobayashi M, Masaki T, Izuishi K, Suzuki Y. Rectal perforations and fistulae secondary to a glycerin enema: closure by over-the scope-clip. World J Gastroenterol. 2012;18:3177–80.
2. Iacopini F, Di Lorenzo N, Altorio F, Schurr MO, Scozzarro A. Over-the-scope clip closure of two chronic fistulas after gastric band penetration. World J Gastroenterol. 2010;16:1665–9.
3. van Leerdam ME. Epidemiology of acute upper gastrointestinal bleeding. Best Pract Res Clin Gastroenterol. 2008;22:209–24.
4. Hearnshaw SA, Logan RF, Lowe D, et al. Acute upper gastrointestinal bleeding in the UK: patient characteristics, diagnoses and outcomes in the 2007 UK audit. Gut. 2011;60:1327–35.
5. Laine L, Yang H, Chang SC, Datto C. Trends for incidence of hospitalization and death due to GI complications in the United States from 2001 to 2009. Am J Gastroenterol. 2012;107(8):1190–5.
6. Strate LL, Ayanian JZ, Kotler G, Syngal S. Risk factors for mortality in lower intestinal bleeding. Clin Gastroenterol Hepatol. 2008;6(9):1004–10.
7. Nagata N, Niikura R, Aoki T, Shimbo T, Itoh T, Goda Y, Suda R, Yano H, Akiyama J, Yanase M, Mizokami M, Uemura N. Increase in colonic diverticulosis and diverticular hemorrhage in an aging society: lessons from a 9-year colonoscopic study of 28, 192 patients in Japan. Int J Colorectal Dis. 2014;29(3):379–85.
8. Aoki T, Nagata N, Niikura R, Shimbo T, Tanaka S, Sekine K, Kishida Y, Watanabe K, Sakurai T, Yokoi C, Akiyama J, Yanase M, Mizokami M, Uemura N. Recurrence and mortality among patients hospitalized for acute lower gastrointestinal bleeding. Clin Gastroenterol Hepatol. 2015;13(3):488–94.
9. Longstreth GF. Epidemiology and outcome of patients hospitalized with acute lower gastrointestinal hemorrhage: a population-based study. Am J Gastroenterol. 1997;92(3):419–24.
10. Farrell JJ, Friedman LS. Gastrointestinal bleeding in the elderly. Gastroenterol Clin North Am. 2001;30(2):377–407.
11. Farrell JJ, Friedman LS. Review article: the management of lower gastrointestinal bleeding. Aliment Pharmacol Ther. 2005;21(11):1281–98.

12. Gayer C, Chino A, Lucas C, Tokioka S, Yamasaki T, Edelman DA, Sugawa C. Acute lower gastrointestinal bleeding in 1,112 patients admitted to an urban emergency medical center. Surgery. 2009;146(4):600–6.
13. Ghassemi KA, Jensen DM. Lower GI bleeding: epidemiology and management. Curr Gastroenterol Rep. 2013;15(7):333–5.
14. Hreinsson JP, Gumundsson S, Kalaitzakis E, Bjornsson ES. Lower gastrointestinal bleeding: incidence, etiology, and outcomes in a population-based setting. Eur J Gastroenterol Hepatol. 2013;25(1):37–43.
15. Cappell MS, Friedel D. Initial management of acute upper gastrointestinal bleeding: from initial evaluation up to gastrointestinal endoscopy. Med Clin North Am. 2008;92:491–509.
16. Kovacs TO. Management of upper gastrointestinal bleeding. Curr Gastroenterol Rep. 2008;10:535–42.
17. Barkun AN, Martel M, Toubouti Y, et al. Endoscopic hemostasis in peptic ulcer bleeding for patients with high-risk lesions: a series of metaanalyses. Gastrointest Endosc. 2009;69:786–99.
18. Marmo R, Rotondano G, Piscopo R, et al. Dual therapy versus monotherapy in the endoscopic treatment of high-risk bleeding ulcers: a meta-analysis of controlled trials. Am J Gastroenterol. 2007;102:279–89.
19. Barkun AN, Bardou M, Kuipers EJ, et al. International consensus recommendations on the management of patients with nonvariceal upper gastrointestinal bleeding. Ann Intern Med. 2010;152:101–13.
20. Laine L, Jensen DM. Management of patients with ulcer bleeding. Am J Gastroenterol. 2012;107:345–60.
21. Sung JJ, Chan FK, Chen M, et al. Asia-Pacific Working Group consensus on non-variceal upper gastrointestinal bleeding. Gut. 2011;60:1170–7.
22. Jairath V, Barkun AN. Improving outcomes from acute upper gastrointestinal bleeding. Gut. 2012;61(9):1246–9.
23. Rockall TA, Logan RF, Devlin HB, et al. Incidence of and mortality from acute upper gastrointestinal haemorrhage in the United Kingdom. Steering Committee and members of the National Audit of Acute Upper Gastrointestinal Haemorrhage. BMJ. 1995;311:222–6.
24. Chung IK, Ham JS, Kim HS, et al. Comparison of the hemostatic efficacy of the endoscopic hemoclip method with hypertonic saline epinephrine injection and a combination of the two for the management of bleeding peptic ulcers. Gastrointest Endosc. 1999;49:13–8.
25. Barkun A, Bardou M, Marshall JK, et al. Consensus recommendations for managing patients with nonvariceal upper gastrointestinal bleeding. Ann Intern Med. 2003;139:843–57.
26. Greenspoon J, Barkun A, Bardou M, et al. Management of patients with nonvariceal upper gastrointestinal bleeding. Clin Gastroenterol Hepatol. 2012;10:234–9.
27. Peng YC, Chen SY, Tung CF, et al. Factors associated with failure of initial endoscopic hemoclip hemostasis for upper gastrointestinal bleeding. J Clin Gastroenterol. 2006;40:25–8.
28. Kirschniak A, Subotova N, Zieker D, et al. The Over-The-Scope Clip (OTSC) for the treatment of gastrointestinal bleeding, perforations, and fistulas. Surg Endosc. 2011;25:2901–5. PubMed PMID: 21424197.
29. Manta R, Galloro G, Mangiavillano B, et al. Over-the-scope clip (OTSC) represents an effective endoscopic treatment for acute GI bleeding after failure of conventional techniques. Surg Endosc. 2013;27:3162–4.
30. Skinner M, Gutierrez JP, Neumann H, Wilcox CM, Burski C, Mönkemüller K. Over-the-scope clip placement is effective rescue therapy for severe acute upper gastrointestinal bleeding. Endosc Int Open. 2014;2(1):E37–40.
31. Chan SM, Chiu PW, Teoh AY, et al. Use of the over-the scope clip for treatment of refractory upper gastrointestinal bleeding: a case series. Endoscopy. 2014;46(5):428–31.
32. Mönkemüller K, Toshniwal J, Zabielski M, Vormbrock K, Neumann H. Utility of the "bear claw", or over-the-scope clip (OTSC) system, to provide endoscopic hemostatis for bleeding posterior duodenal ulcers. Endoscopy. 2012;44(Suppl 2 UCTN):E412–3.
33. Sung JY, Chung SC, Lo KK, et al. Heater-probe treatment of bleeding peptic ulcers. Surg Endosc. 1988;2:234–6.

34. Manno M, Mangiafico S, Caruso A, Barbera C, Bertani H, Mirante VG, Pigò F, Amardeep K, Conigliaro R. First-line endoscopic treatment with OTSC in patients with high-risk non-variceal upper gastrointestinal bleeding: preliminary experience in 40 cases. Surg Endosc. 2016;30:2026–9.
35. Neumann H, Diebel H, Mönkemüller K, et al. Description of a new, endoscopic technique to remove the over-the-scope-clip in an ex vivo porcine model (with video). Gastrointest Endosc. 2012;76:1009–13.
36. Mönkemüller K, Toshniwal J, Zabielski M. Endoscopic removal of an over-the-scope-clip ('bear claw'). Gastrointest Endosc. 2012;76:1077–8.
37. Schostek S, Ho CN, Melbert M, Krautwald M, Caputo A, Parisi G, Wehrmann M, Gottwald T, Schurr MO. DC current pulses for OTSC clip fragmentation: technology and experimental study. Surg Endosc. 2015;29(8):2418–22.
38. Arezzo A, Bullano A, Fisher H, Morino M. The way to remove an over-the-scope-clip (with video). Gastrointest Endosc. 2013;77:974–5.
39. Schmidt A, Riechen B, Damm M, Cahyadi O, Bauder M, Caca K. Endoscopic removal of over-the-scope clips using a novel cutting device : a retrospective case series. Endoscopy. 2014;46:762–6.
40. Peery AF, Dellon ES, Lund J, et al. Burden of gastrointestinal disease in the United States: 2012 update. Gastroenterology. 2012;143(5):1179–87. PubMed PMID: 22885331.
41. Caulfield H, Hyman NH. Anastomotic leak after low anterior resection: a spectrum of clinical entities. JAMA Surg. 2013;148(2):177–82.
42. Metcalf C. Enterocutaneous fistulae. J Wound Care. 1999;8(3):141–2. Review.
43. Lüning TH, Keemers-Gels ME, Barendregt WB, et al. Colonoscopic perforations: a review of 30,366 patients. Surg Endosc. 2007;21(6):994–7.
44. Svanes C. Trends in perforated peptic ulcer: incidence, etiology, treatment, and prognosis. World J Surg. 2000;24(3):277–83. Review.
45. Iqbal CW, Cullinane DC, Schiller HJ, et al. Surgical management and outcomes of 165 colonoscopic perforations from a single institution. Arch Surg. 2008;143(7):701–6.
46. van der Sluis FJ, Loffeld RJ, Engel AF. Outcome of surgery for colonoscopic perforation. Colorectal Dis. 2012;14(4):e187–90.
47. Rodella L, Laterza E, De Manszoni G, et al. Endoscopic clipping of anastomotic leakages in esophagogastric surgery. Endoscopy. 1998;30(5):453–6.
48. Will U, Meyer F, Hartmeier S, et al. Endoscopic treatment of a pseudocystocolonic fistula by band ligation and endoloop application: case report. Gastrointest Endosc. 2004;59(4):581–3.
49. Bohm G, Mossdorf A, Klink C, et al. Treatment algorithm for post-operative upper gastrointestinal fistulas and leaks using combined Vicrylplug and fibrin glue. Endoscopy. 2010;42(7):599–602. PubMed PMID: 20432210.
50. Disibeyaz S, Parlak E, Köksal A, et al. Endoscopic treatment of a large upper gastrointestinal anastomotic leak using a prolene plug and cyanoacrylate. Endoscopy. 2005;37(10):1032–3.
51. van Boeckel PG, Dua KS, Weusten BL, et al. Fully covered self-expandable metal stents (SEMS), partially covered SEMS and selfexpandable plastic stents for the treatment of benign esophageal ruptures and anastomotic leaks. BMC Gastroenterol. 2012;29(2):12:19.
52. Trecca A, Gaj F, Gagliardi G. Our experience with endoscopic repair of large colonoscopic perforations and review of the literature. Tech Coloproctol. 2008;12(4):315–21.
53. Cheriyan D, Enns R. Over-the-scope clip in the management of GI defects. Gastrointest Endosc. 2014;80(4):623–5.
54. Baron TH, Song LM, Ross A, et al. Use of an over-the-scope clipping device: multicenter retrospective results of the first U.S. experience (with videos). Gastrointest Endosc. 2012;76(1):202–8.
55. Mangiavillano B, Morandi E, Masci E. Accidental endoscopic piercing of the tongue with an Ovesco clip. Endoscopy. 2012;44(S 02):E221.
56. Voermans RP, Le Moine O, von Renteln D, et al. Efficacy of endoscopic closure of acute perforations of the gastrointestinal tract. Clin Gastroenterol Hepatol. 2012;10(6):603–8.
57. Alastal Y, Hammad TA, Nawras M, et al. Acute cholangitis following biliary obstruction after duodenal OTSC placement in a case of large chronic duodenocutaneous fistula. Case Rep Gastrointest Med. 2015;2015:647806.

58. Kim M, Jeon SW, Cho KB, et al. Predictive risk factors of perforation in gastric endoscopic submucosal dissection for early gastric cancer: a large, multicenter study. Surg Endosc. 2013;27(4):1372–8.
59. Samalavicius NE, Kazanavicius D, Lunevicius R, et al. Incidence, risk, management, and outcomes of iatrogenic full-thickness large bowel injury associated with 56,882 colonoscopies in 14 Lithuanian hospitals. Surg Endosc. 2013;27(8):1628–35.
60. Technology Committee ASGE, Kantsevoy SV, Adler DG, Conway JD, et al. Endoscopic mucosal resection and endoscopic submucosal dissection. Gastrointest Endosc. 2008;68(1):11–8. Review.
61. Kirschniak A, Kratt T, Stüker D, et al. A new endoscopic over-the-scope clip system for treatment of lesions and bleeding in the GI tract: first clinical experiences. Gastrointest Endosc. 2007;66(1):162–7.
62. Repici A, Arezzo A, De Caro G, et al. Clinical experience with a new endoscopic over-the-scope clip system for use in the GI tract. Dig Liver Dis. 2009;41(6):406–10.
63. Seebach L, Bauerfeind P, Gubler C. "Sparing the surgeon": clinical experience with over-the-scope clips for gastrointestinal perforation. Endoscopy. 2010;42(12):1108–11. PubMed PMID: 21120779.
64. Sandmann M, Heike M, Faehndrich M. Application of the OTSC system for the closure of fistulas, anastomosal leakages and perforations within the gastrointestinal tract. Z Gastroenterol. 2011;49(8):981–5.
65. Gubler C, Bauerfeind P. Endoscopic closure of iatrogenic gastrointestinal tract perforations with the over-the-scope clip. Digestion. 2012;85(4):302–7.
66. Hagel AF, Naegel A, Lindner AS, et al. Over-the-scope clip application yields a high rate of closure in gastrointestinal perforations and may reduce emergency surgery. J Gastrointest Surg. 2012;16(11):2132–8.
67. Nishiyama N, Mori H, Kobara H, et al. Efficacy and safety of over-the- scope clip: including complications after endoscopic submucosal dissection. World J Gastroenterol. 2013;19(18):2752–60.
68. Schlag C, Wilhelm D, von Delius S, et al. EndoResect study: endoscopic full-thickness resection of gastric subepithelial tumors. Endoscopy. 2013;45(1):4–11.
69. Changela K, Virk MA, Patel N, et al. Role of over the scope clips in the management of iatrogenic gastrointestinal perforations. World J Gastroenterol. 2014;20(32):11460–2.
70. Haito-Chavez Y, Law JK, Kratt T, et al. International multicenter experience with an over-the-scope clipping device for endoscopic management of GI defects (with video). Gastrointest Endosc. 2014;80(4):610–22.
71. Farnik H, Driller M, Kratt T, et al. Indication for 'Over the scope' (OTS)-clip vs. covered self-expanding metal stent (cSEMS) is unequal in upper gastrointestinal leakage: results from a retrospective head-to-head comparison. PLoS One. 2015;10(1):e0117483.
72. Paspatis GA, Dumonceau JM, Barthet M, et al. Diagnosis and management of iatrogenic endoscopic perforations: European Society of Gastrointestinal Endoscopy (ESGE) Position Statement. Endoscopy. 2014;46(8):693–711. Review.
73. Griffith PS, Birch DW, Sharma AM, et al. Managing complications associated with laparoscopic Roux-en-Y gastric bypass for morbid obesity. Can J Surg. 2012;55(5):329–36. Review.
74. Fullum TM, Aluka KJ, Turner PL. Decreasing anastomotic and staple line leaks after laparoscopic Roux-en-Y gastric bypass. Surg Endosc. 2009;23(6):1403–8.
75. Sakuramoto S, Kikuchi S, Futawatari N, et al. Laparoscopy-assisted pancreas- and spleen-preserving total gastrectomy for gastric cancer as compared with open total gastrectomy. Surg Endosc. 2009;23(11):2416–23.
76. Kim SG, Lee YJ, Ha WS, et al. LATG with extracorporeal esophagojejunostomy: is this minimal invasive surgery for gastric cancer? J Laparoendosc Adv Surg Tech A. 2008;18(4):572–8.
77. Kim MG, Kim BS, Kim TH, et al. The effects of laparoscopic assisted total gastrectomy on surgical outcomes in the treatment of gastric cancer. J Korean Surg Soc. 2011;80(4):245–50.
78. Smith JD, Paty PB, Guillem JG, et al. Anastomotic leak is not associated with oncologic outcome in patients undergoing low anterior resection for rectal cancer. Ann Surg. 2012;256(6):1034–8.

79. Mirnezami A, Mirnezami R, Chandrakumaran K, et al. Increased local recurrence and reduced survival from colorectal cancer following anastomotic leak: systematic review and meta-analysis. Ann Surg. 2011;253(5):890–9.
80. Schecter WP, Hirshberg A, Chang DS, et al. Enteric fistulas: principles of management. J Am Coll Surg. 2009;209(4):484–91. Review.
81. Parodi A, Repici A, Pedroni A, et al. Endoscopic management of GI perforations with a new over-the-scope clip device (with videos). Gastrointest Endosc. 2010;72(4):881–6.
82. Pohl J, Borgulya M, Lorenz D, et al. Endoscopic closure of postoperative esophageal leaks with a novel over-the-scope clip system. Endoscopy. 2010;42(9):757–9.
83. Albert JG, Friedrich-Rust M, Woeste G, et al. Benefit of a clipping device in use in intestinal bleeding and intestinal leakage. Gastrointest Endosc. 2011;74(2):389–97.
84. Manta R, Manno M, Bertani H, et al. Endoscopic treatment of gastrointestinal fistulas using an over-the-scope clip (OTSC) device: case series from a tertiary referral center. Endoscopy. 2011;43(6):545–8.
85. Surace M, Mercky P, Demarquay JF, et al. Endoscopic management of GI fistulae with the over-the-scope clip system (with video). Gastrointest Endosc. 2011;74(6):1416–9.
86. Arezzo A, Verra M, Reddavid R, et al. Efficacy of the over-the-scope clip (OTSC) for treatment of colorectal postsurgical leaks and fistulas. Surg Endosc. 2012;26(11):3330–3.
87. Dişibeyaz S, Köksal AŞ, Parlak E, et al. Endoscopic closure of gastrointestinal defects with an over-the-scope clip device. A case series and review of the literature. Clin Res Hepatol Gastroenterol. 2012;36(6):614–21. Review.
88. Galizia G, Napolitano V, Castellano P, et al. The Over-The-Scope-Clip (OTSC) system is effective in the treatment of chronic esophagojejunal anastomotic leakage. J Gastrointest Surg. 2012;16(8):1585–9.
89. Mennigen R, Colombo-Benkmann M, Senninger N, et al. Endoscopic closure of postoperative gastrointestinal leakages and fistulas with the Over-the-Scope Clip (OTSC). J Gastrointest Surg. 2013;17(6):1058–65.
90. Winder JS, Kulaylat AN, Schubart JR, et al. Management of non-acute gastrointestinal defects using the over-the-scope clips (OTSCs): a retrospective single-institution experience. Surg Endosc. 2015;28. [Epub ahead of print].
91. Law R, Wong Kee Song LM, Irani S, et al. Immediate technical and delayed clinical outcome of fistula closure using an over-the-scope clip device. Surg Endosc. 2015;29(7):1781–6.
92. Weiland T, Fehlker M, Gottwald T, et al. Performance of the OTSC System in the endoscopic closure of gastrointestinal fistulae--a meta-analysis. Minim Invasive Ther Allied Technol. 2012;21(4):249–58.
93. Mangiavillano B, Pisani A, Viaggi P, et al. Endoscopic sealing of a rectovesical fistula with a combination of an over the scope clip and cyano-acrylate injection. J Gastrointest Oncol. 2010;1(2):122–4. PubMed PMID: 22811817.
94. Schurr MO, Baur FE, Krautwald M, Fehlker M, Wehrmann M, Gottwald T, Prosst RL. Endoscopic full-thickness resection and clip defect closure in the colon with the new FTRD system: experimental study. Surg Endosc. 2015;29:2434–41. PMID: 25318369. doi:10.1007/s00464-014-3923-x.
95. Schurr MO, Baur F, Ho CN, Anhoeck G, Kratt T, Gottwald T. Endoluminal full-thickness resection of GI lesions: a new device and technique. Minim Invasive Ther Allied Technol. 2011;20:189–92. PMID: 21574825. doi:10.3109/13645706.2011.582119.
96. von Renteln D, Kratt T, Rösch T, Denzer UW, Schachschal G. Endoscopic full-thickness resection in the colon by using a clipand-cut technique: an animal study. Gastrointest Endosc. 2011;74:1108–14. PMID: 21944313. doi:10.1016/j.gie.2011.07.003.
97. von Renteln D, Rösch T, Kratt T, Denzer UW, El-Masry M, Schachschal G. Endoscopic full-thickness resection of submucosal gastric tumors. Dig Dis Sci. 2012;57:1298–303. PMID: 22370915. doi:10.1007/s10620-012-2039-1.
98. Schmidt A, Damm M, Caca K. Endoscopic full-thickness resection using a novel over-the-scope device. Gastroenterology. 2014;147:740–2.e2. PMID: 25083605. doi:10.1053/j.gastro.2014.07.045.

99. Valli PV, Kaufmann M, Vrugt B, Bauerfeind P. Endoscopic resection of a diverticulum-arisen colonic adenoma using a fullthickness resection device. Gastroenterology. 2014;147:969–71.
100. Schmidt A, Bauerfeind P, Gubler C, Damm M, Bauder M, Caca K. Endoscopic full-thickness resection in the colorectum with a novel over-the-scope device: first experience. Endoscopy. 2015;47:719–25. doi:10.1055/s-0034-1391781. Epub 2015 Mar 12.
101. Lagoussis P, Soriani P, Tontini GE, Neumann H, Pastorelli L, de Nucci G, Vecchi M. Over-the-scope clip-assisted endoscopic full-thickness resection after incomplete resection of rectal adenocarcinoma. Endoscopy. 2016;48 Suppl 1:E59–60. doi:10.1055/s-0042-100197. Epub 2016 Feb 18.
102. Klare P, Burlefinger R, Neu B, Bajbouj M, Specht K, Schmid RM, von Delius S. Over-the-scope clip-assisted endoscopic full-thickness resection after incomplete resection of a rectal neuroendocrine tumor. Endoscopy. 2015;47(Suppl 1 UCTN):E47–8. doi: 10.1055/s-0034-1391301. Epub 2015 Feb.
103. Saito Y, Uraoka T, Yamaguchi Y, et al. A prospective, multicenter study of 1111 colorectal endoscopic submucosal dissections (with video). Gastrointest Endosc. 2010;72:1217–25.
104. Schmidt A, Meier B, Caca K. Endoscopic full-thickness resection: current status. World J Gastroenterol. 2015;21:9273–85.

Radiofrequency Ablation of Pancreatic Mass

3

Roberto Girelli, Frigerio Isabella, Alessandro Giardino, Paolo Regi, Filippo Scopelliti, and Giovanni Butturini

3.1 Introduction

Pancreatic ductal carcinoma is the fourth cause of death for cancer in Western countries. The high mortality rate is due to the incidence of metastatic or unresectable disease at the time of diagnosis because of the lack of specific symptoms. Advanced pancreatic cancer has a poor prognosis with a median survival range of 9–15 months for locally advanced pancreatic cancer and 6 months for metastatic disease [1]. Although the associated increase in risk is small, the development of pancreatic cancer is strictly linked to cigarette smoking [2–4].

An increased body mass index is also associated with an increased risk [5–7] as well as occupational exposure to chemicals, such as beta-naphthylamine and benzidine [8]. A familial history of PDAC or recent onset of diabetes may play a key role and requires clinical surveillance for these subjects [3, 9–13]. An excess of pancreatic cancer is also seen in families harboring breast cancer susceptibility gene 2 mutations (*BRCA2)* [14, 15]. Specific mutations in the *PALB2* gene have recently been identified as possibly increasing susceptibility for pancreatic cancer [16]. In 70 % of cases, the tumor is located in the pancreatic head, and symptoms are usually related to the involvement of surrounding structures: the duodenum and common bile duct. For tumors of the body and tail, the diagnosis can be late due to nonspecific symptoms (back pain, abdominal discomfort, dyspepsia), particularly when the disease is advanced and the mass has enough room to expand. Less than 20 % of cases are resectable at the time of diagnosis, and it is well known that radical (R0) resection is the only chance to improve long-term survival. However, even under

R. Girelli (✉)
Hepato-Pancreato-Biliary Unit, Pederzoli Hospital, Peschiera del Garda, Verona, Italy
e-mail: rgirelli@cdcpederzoli.it

F. Isabella • A. Giardino • P. Regi • F. Scopelliti • G. Butturini
Pederzoli Hospital, Peschiera del Garda, Verona, Italy

R. Conigliaro, M. Frazzoni (eds.), *Diagnosis and Endoscopic Management of Digestive Diseases*, DOI 10.1007/978-3-319-42358-6_3

optimal conditions, the median survival of these patients ranges from 15 to 19 months, and the 5-year survival rate is approximately 20 % [17].

The three possible scenarios at time of diagnosis are the following:

- The tumor is small and "well located," and surgical resection is possible (20 % of cases) with high chance of clear margins. Negative margin status (R0 resection), tumor DNA content, tumor size, and the absence of lymph node metastases are the strongest prognostic indicators for long-term patient survival [18–21]. The high rate of metastatic recurrence after radical resection of early-stage disease suggests that pancreatic adenocarcinoma is a systemic disease in most patients by the time of clinical presentation [22].
- The tumor is associated with distant metastases (40 % of cases), and there is no chance for curative treatments. The primary goals of treatment for metastatic pancreatic cancer are palliation of symptoms and control of progression. Systemic chemotherapy is the best therapy when general conditions and performance status are suitable. Life expectancy for these patients does not exceed 8–10 months.
- Locally advanced tumor remains the *unsolved issue*. There is no consensus on a common definition and on the gold standard therapy, and surgical or medical treatment usually depends on surgical team skills and attitude. We generally define it as a tumor involving major vessels close to the gland, where an en bloc resection with arterial reconstruction would be the only chance to remove it (40 % of cases). Chemoradiation is the conventional option for treatment of LAPC. Currently, systemic chemotherapy (CHT) followed by chemoradiation (CHRT) is recommended for patients with a good performance status. Initial systemic chemotherapy can be administered to patients with locally advanced disease when chemoradiation therapy is planned. Emerging data suggest that a period of chemotherapy followed by standard chemoradiation may be more effective than up-front chemoradiation [23–26]. Despite this, unresectable stages are characterized by a very poor prognosis, with a reported median survival of 12–14 months [27]. In these patients, increase of resection rate is possible after neoadjuvant CHT as several authors reported, but results on survival rate are not homogeneous [28–32]. Therefore, new treatment options for unresectable pancreatic cancer should be proposed.

3.2 Radiofrequency Ablation and Pancreatic Carcinoma

The use of RFA in pancreatic cancer has been very limited so far [37–41]. Reported experiences are related to small series (20 patients are the largest cohort) with different stages of disease considered: patients with stage III and IV were treated in the same studies. Technical parameters and devices were not uniform, and the results from the different papers were not homogeneous. Only Spiliotis demonstrated a positive impact on survival (33 months), but it is the only, hardly believable, long-term positive result.

During treatment, one RFA probe is placed in the targeted tissue, and high-frequency alternating current is generated leading to frictional heating above 60 °C up to 100 °C inducing coagulative necrosis [33–35]. Higher temperatures would result in desiccation and subsequent increase in tissue impedance which limits further conduction of electricity into the tissue [36].

Application of RFA to the pancreas presents specific, potential problems related to anatomical aspects (surrounding structures), tumor biology, and peculiar properties of pancreatic parenchyma. The risk of an inadvertent thermal injury of the distal common bile duct, duodenum, transverse colon, and portal vein is not negligible. Moreover, thermal damage of healthy pancreatic tissue may cause severe pancreatitis, pancreatic fistula, or pancreatic ascites, i.e., life-threatening complications.

Beside this, the lack of a gross animal experimental model makes the definition of specific parameters of application for pancreatic cancer unachievable.

3.2.1 Operative Technique

The procedure was performed under general anesthesia. To rule out undetected metastases, accurate exploration of peritoneal cavity was performed by the surgeon and supported by intraoperative ultrasound that excluded liver metastases and confirmed unresectability of the lesion. The gastrocolic ligament was divided and the Kocher maneuver was performed to expose the pancreatic head. A cold wet gauze was placed behind the pancreatic head to protect the inferior vena cava. The area surrounding the ablation was irrigated with cold saline solution, and the duodenum was continuously perfused with cold solution through a gastric tube.

RFA procedure A RITA® System Generator 1500X (AngioDynamics®, USA) was used (Fig. 3.1).

The probe (StarBurst XL multi-array or UniBlate single cool tip) was placed in the center of the lesion under US guidance (Fig. 3.2). The depth, opening, and time were decided according to size, shape, and in vivo coagulative effect which was monitored by intraoperative US (Fig. 3.3). In the case of biliary duct dilation or jaundice, and/or duodenal obstruction, biliary and/or gastric bypass was performed. One soft drain was located close to the insertion site in the mass and a second one when biliary bypass was done. After surgery, patients were screened daily for acute pancreatitis, bleeding, and infection with serum amylase, lipase, blood glucose, calcium, white blood count, hematocrit, hemoglobin, and liver function tests. On postoperative day 1 and 3, serum C-reactive protein and amylase content in the abdominal drain were checked. The latter was removed on day 3 if no criteria for pancreatic fistula were encountered [42]. On day 7 after surgery abdominal US, CT scan, and plasma CA 19.9 were performed. Follow-up consisted in clinical examination, CT scan or MRI, and CA 19.9 value every 3 months.

In our study the main outcome measures included 30-day morbidity and mortality.

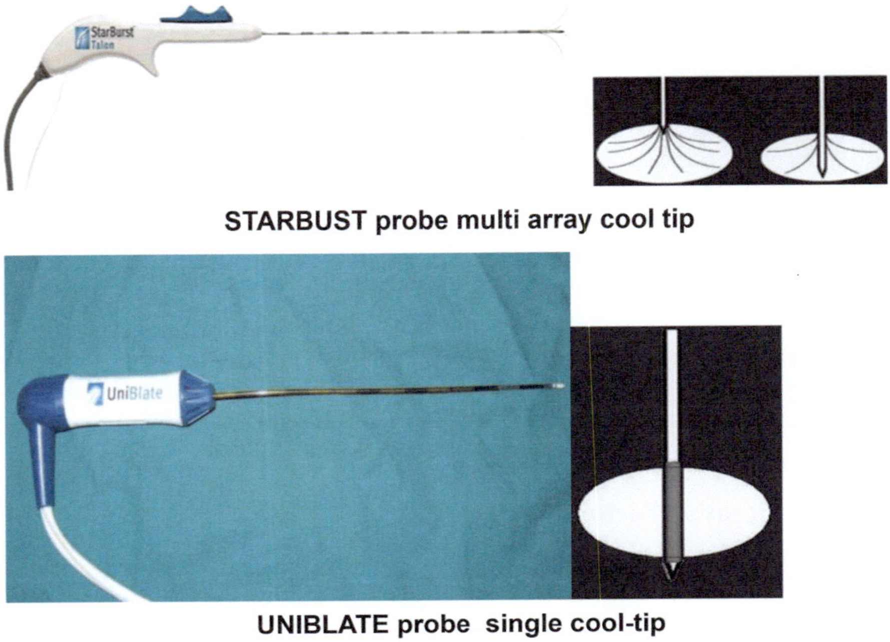

Fig. 3.1 Technical equipment – shape and size of ablated area

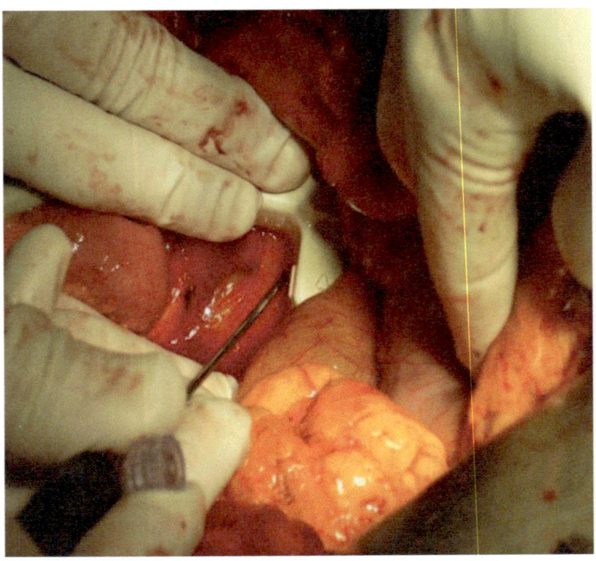

Fig. 3.2 Intraoperative US-guided probe placement

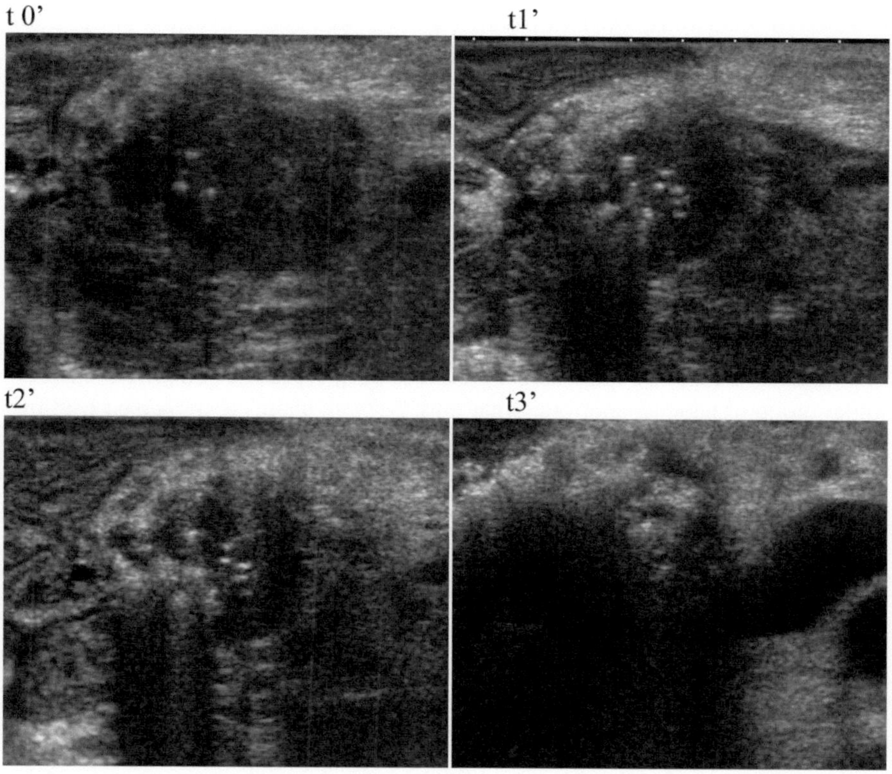

Fig. 3.3 Intraoperative US monitoring at different timing after delivery of the energy: gas bubble production in the tumor mass

Table 3.1 Inclusion and exclusion criteria for pancreatic cancer RFA

Inclusion criteria	Exclusion criteria
Age between 18 and 80 years	Age <18 or >80 years
Specific consent obtained	Contraindications to laparotomy
Solid neoplasia of pancreatic head, body, or tail	Multiple pancreatic lesions
Preoperative cytology positive for pancreatic carcinoma	Stage IV disease
Preoperative staging suggestive for unresectable mass (stage III)	Intraoperative finding of unexpected distant metastasis

3.3 The Pilot Study

After approval from the local medical committee, we carried out a pilot study with satisfactory results: 50 patients corresponding to the inclusion criteria (Table 3.1) were treated in a 20-month period before or after a combination of chemo and chemoradiotherapy. Morbidity and mortality rate was 26 % and 2 %, respectively.

After an interim analysis of the first 25 patients, because of the pilot nature of the study and the lack of specific parameters of application for pancreatic cancer, we decided to decrease the RFA temperature from 105 to 90 °C in the following 25 patients. The overall complication rate significantly decreased to 8 % [43].

After these preliminary results, we felt confident to propose the procedure to our patients as an alternative treatment to stage III PDAC in a multimodal setting. We slightly changed our target and started to consider RFA as a treatment option that could modify the natural history of the disease. RFA should be considered a cytoreductive treatment, which provides direct and rapid necrosis of the mass. This debulking effect on tumor volume may induce the acceptance of a higher perioperative risk when compared to bypass operations alone [44]. We prolonged follow-up of the initial group of patients and found that most of them attended at planned controls. Therefore, we decided to review our results when 100 patients had been treated. In this group of patients treated with a new multimodal therapy, RFA associated to chemo and radiotherapy, the median OS and DSS were 20 and 23 months, respectively, and confirmed the preliminary data of the previous pilot study [45]

3.4 Single-Center Overall Experience

Between February 2007 and December 2014, 200 patients were treated with RFA in our department. All patients had preoperative diagnosis of stage III pancreatic carcinoma confirmed by contrast US, abdominal CT scan, and/or MRCP, all histologically proven by fine-needle aspiration. All demographics data are listed in Table 3.2. The male/female ratio was 112/88 with a mean age of 64 years. The tumor was located in the pancreatic head/uncinate process in 145 cases and in the body/tail in 55 cases. Median tumor size was 35 mm (IQR 34–48). Medium serum CA 19.9 at admission was 110 (IQR 28–479), with mean hospital stay of 10.7 days.

Thirty-nine percent of patients received RFA as up-front treatment when surgical palliation was needed or due to the lack of diagnosis or under staging. The remaining 61 % underwent neoadjuvant chemo or radiochemotherapy.

During RFA operation, associated surgery was performed in 45 % of patients: 49 % single bypass (biliary or gastric), 43 % double bypass, one cholecystectomy, and one pseudocyst-jejunostomy.

Table 3.2 Demographics data

M/F	112/88
Median age	64 years
Tumor site head/body-tail	145/55
Tumor size median (IQR)	35 mm (30–48)
Mean hospital stay	10.7 days
Ca19.9 median (IQR)	110 (28–479)

3.4.1 Complications

Postoperative course was uneventful in 76 % of cases; overall, complication rate was 24 % with systemic complications in 2 % of cases and abdominal complications in 23 % of patients: 12 % RFA-related and 11 % related to associated surgery. All complications are listed in Table 3.3. Mortality rate was 2 %. Four patients died: one for hepatic insufficiency, one for septic shock due to duodenal perforation, and two for massive duodenal bleeding. Reoperation rate was 3 % and in all cases for associated surgery-related complications.

Considering the postoperative complications, duodenal injuries had a main impact on clinical course with different events:

- *Asymptomatic mucosal burn*, requiring conservative medical treatment and endoscopic monitoring at 7 and 30 days.
- *Penetrating ulcer with massive bleeding*: this is the result of an overtreatment of a tumor infiltrating the duodenum. In this case endoscopic treatment could be ineffective, and emergency surgery should be considered.

The whole tumor ablation should be avoided in order to prevent the diffusion of high temperatures to surrounding tissues as the pancreas itself, major vessels, the common bile duct, and the duodenum: a spared peripheral rim is the "safety margin" to prevent thermal damage.

The retrospective analysis on survival confirmed the data previously achieved in 100 patients with a median survival of 19 months (Fig. 3.4) and a progression-free survival of 13 months (Fig. 3.5). Moreover, the results do not seem to depend on the rate of the ablated area. In other words, the benefit on survival is not strictly correlated to the amount of coagulative necrosis we achieved, as already demonstrated for liver cancer. Therefore, we could do a limited ablation with virtually unchanged results but decreasing the risk of complications.

Table 3.3 Type of complications

RFA related 12 %	Acute pancreatitis
	Pancreatic fistula
	Portal or mesenteric thrombosis
	Duodenal injuries
	Intra-abdominal bleeding (site of probe insertion)
Surgery associated related 11 %	Abdominal bleeding
	Biliary or gastric anastomosis leak
	Fluid collection/abscess
	Upper GI dysfunction (delayed gastric emptying, stress ulcer)

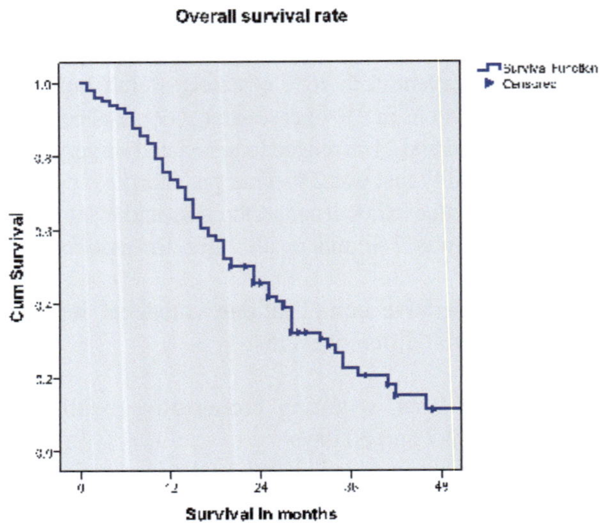

Fig. 3.4 Overall survival rate on 200 patients

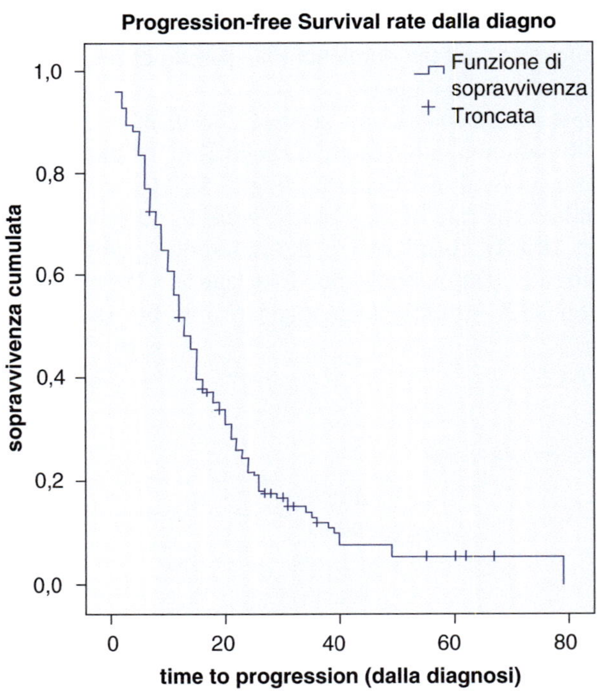

Fig. 3.5 Progression-free survival on 200 patients

On the basis of these observations, we modified the parameters of application as follows:

- *Temperature never above 80° C.*
- *RFA limited to "the core" of the tumor.*
- *Use of the single cool-tip needle UniBlate.*
- *Stay away from the duodenum – at least 10 mm.*

After these last technical changes, we pointed out a significant reduction of morbidity rate from 25 to 13 % and mortality, from 2 to 0 %.

Our preliminary results on survival suggest that, although pancreatic cancer is considered a systemic disease since the very early stages, the local cytoreductive treatment is able to modify its natural course, regardless of the size of the ablated area.

But what is the possible explanation of these surprising and encouraging results?

3.5 Immunomodulatory Effects of RFA

It has been proposed that tumor destruction due to radiofrequency ablation takes two steps: firstly, a direct damage proportional to the applied energy, tumor biology, and its microenvironment and, secondly, an indirect damage after the energy application. The latter represents the progression of tissue damage, which can arise from immunity stimulation due to the ablation [46].

As a matter of fact, the evidence of spontaneous regression of secondary untreated lesions after the ablation of the primary tumor site can lead to the evidence of immunity stimulation by the treatment [47–50].

It is indeed well known that, when a temperature higher than 60 °C is applied, in the treated area, multiple changes occur: enzymes inactivation, protein denaturation, and coagulative necrosis. The events mentioned above can modify the membrane permeability with cytolysis and metabolite accumulation. All the modifications can actively extend for days, also weeks, after the thermal application [34, 35].

Ablation site can be divided into three zones: the central zone where the highest temperature produces coagulative necrosis, the transition zone where sublethal hyperthermia produces cell apoptosis, and the peripheral zone which is excluded from direct temperature damage [51].

Many papers have studied the transition zone, considered as the primary site where inflammatory processes stimulate the immunity system [52, 53]. Murine models and in vivo studies showed the increase of HSP-70 (heat shock protein) after thermal ablation in the transition zone up to 5 days after the treatment [54–57].

HSP-70 is a heterogeneous family of extracellular proteins induced by stress. Calderwood et al. described their role in the intracellular signaling processes and immunity stimulation [75].

Thermal stress increases tissue HSPs and facilitates its permeability through cell membrane into interstitial space [58–62]. Stress-induced proteins can be also produced by neurons, monocytes, macrophages, B-lymphocytes, and tumor cells [63–69]. The main activity is to trigger the innate immunity response by releasing multiple cytokines and stimulation of adaptive immunity by its ability to enhance the peptide ligands. Moreover, the complex HSP peptide, when released by tumor apoptotic cell, links with antigen-presenting cells (APCs), represented by dendritic cells population, promoting the antigen presentation [70–78].

Furthermore, it has been extensively demonstrated a cytotoxic activity after thermal damage.

Multiple studies clearly show the evidence of immunity cells stimulation (like dendritic cells, B- and T-subsets) [79].

Other evidences attribute a power to increase the production of multiple pro-inflammatory cytokines like TNF-α, IL-6, IL-8, IL-10, HGF, and VEGF [80–86].

Fietta et al. underlined the importance of another factor: the lymphocytes T regulators (Tregs) [87]. T regulators are crucial to modulate the immunity response in order to control inflammatory reactions, compared to normal immunity response. Fietta et al. proved that, after RFA ablation, Tregs remain inactivated up to 30 days [87].

In conclusion, RFA stimulates immune activity through different mechanisms: enhancement of antigen presentation by increasing the activity of dendritic cells, stimulation of antitumor response by increasing cytotoxic activity, and suppression of negative modulation decreasing the Treg subset.

The immune stimulation might be particularly effective in pancreatic cancer where the lack of dendritic cells, the limited number of natural apoptosis, and the chemoresistance significantly restrict the immunogenic potential of the tumor. These peculiarities make the pancreatic cancer the "ideal candidate" for thermal ablation [88].

3.6 Control of an Aggressive Disease

Among the "unexpected events" occurred in this study, downstaging of unresectable tumor was definitely at the top of the list: in our series, downstaging rate was 8 %, a value which does not justify the procedure with neoadjuvant intent. However, in many cases we observed *prolonged disease stability rather than a significant mass reduction*: the mass was usually slightly reduced in size at imaging and often associated to a better performance status and negative tumor markers (when previously expressed). This could suggest that "to convert an aggressive entity into a chronic disease" is a realistic goal. The previous considerations allow us to assume that the disease might have a low aggressiveness resulting in less tissue viability. From pathological data, RFA does not seem to have an impact on downstaging rate, but, when this is achieved, it is nearly complete.

When downstaging is not achieved, preliminary data show good control of the disease with an encouraging progression-free survival (13 months).

3.6.1 Imaging and Pathology After RFA

The intraoperative evaluation of RFA effects is challenging [89]. Local effects can be better checked 1 month after the procedure through abdominal CT scan, perfusion CT scan (Fig. 3.6), and contrast enhancement ultrasound (CEUS) (Fig. 3.7).

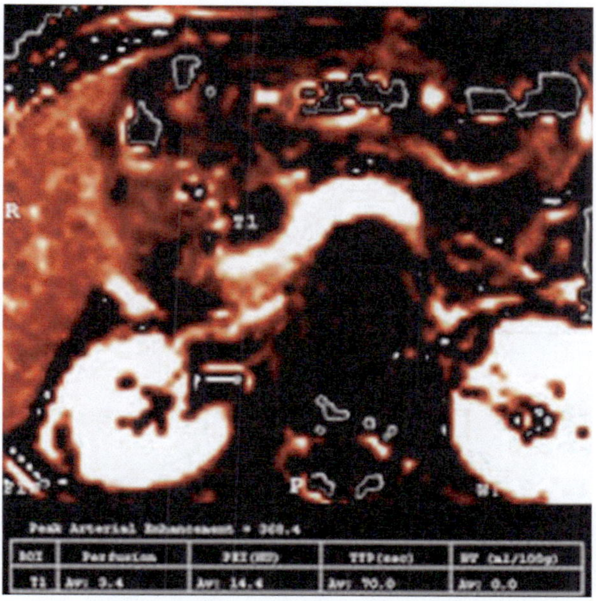

Fig. 3.6 Perfusion CT scan of the ablated area (in T1 the blood flow is zero)

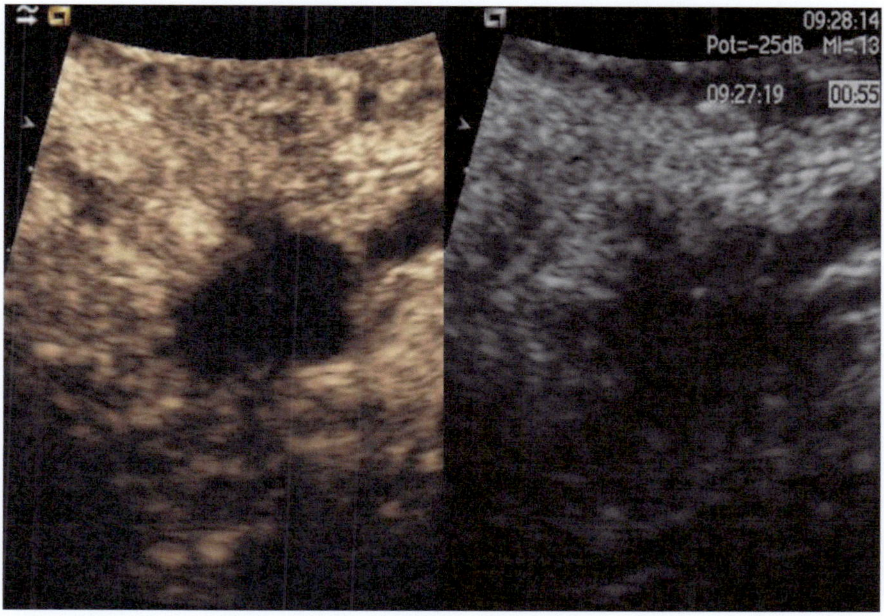

Fig. 3.7 CEUS after tumor ablation: no contrast enhancement in the ablated area

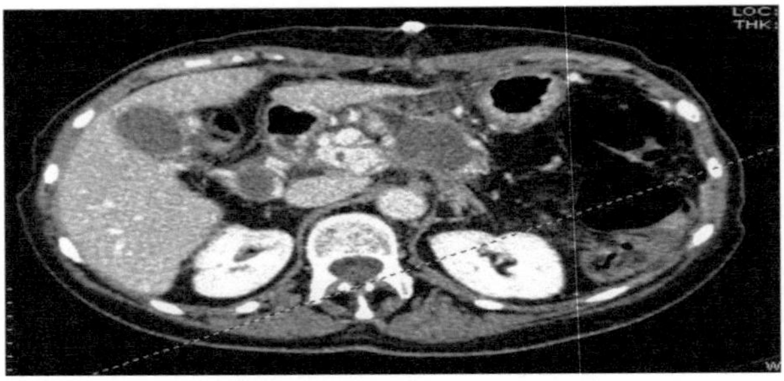

Fig. 3.8 One month CT scan images: well-defined, nonenhancing area corresponding to ablation site in the body-tail of the pancreas

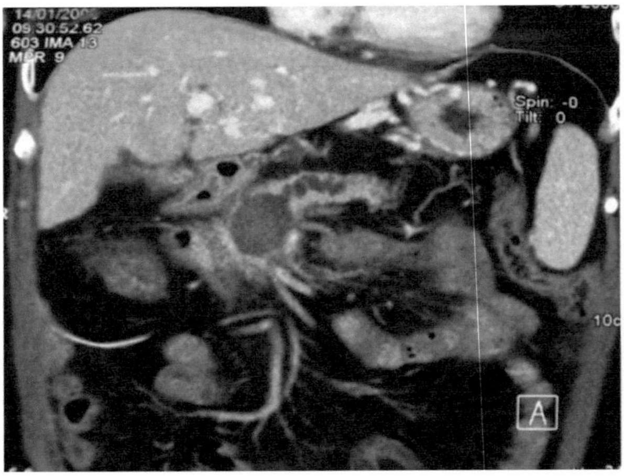

Fig. 3.9 CT 1 month after RFA: hypodense area in the head of the pancreas

The ablation appears like a well-defined, hypodense area with lack of perfusion at CT scan (Figs. 3.8 and 3.9).

The comparison between preoperative and postoperative CT scan images allows checking the size and the rate of coagulative necrosis (Fig. 3.10). However, the quantification of residual neoplastic tissue around the ablated area is still an unsolved problem: does the absence of vascular supply mean the absence of vital neoplastic cells? The answer may come from the histological data in our patients who underwent resection after RFA: only a few neoplastic foci in most cases (Fig. 3.11) and complete tumor regression in one case were detected (Fig. 3.12). Comparison of pre- and post-RFA CA 19.9 serum levels may also help in the assessment of ablative results.

3.7 Timing of the Procedure

The right timing of RFA, up-front or after neoadjuvant CHT, has been a matter of debate. We retrospectively analyzed 57 patients affected by stage III PDC who received short-term chemotherapy between February 2007 and June 2010

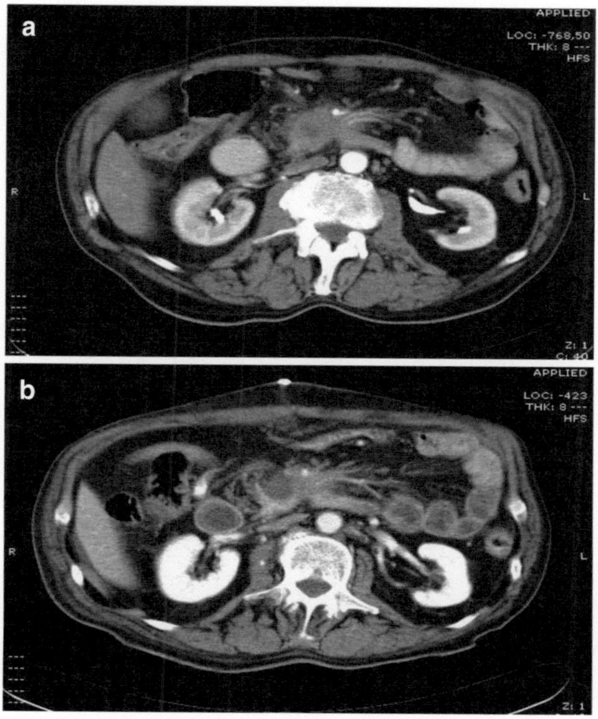

Fig. 3.10 (**a**) Preoperative CT scan: locally advanced pancreatic cancer (3 cm) of the uncinate process and (**b**) ablation area with adequate safety margins – CT scan after 1 month

[90]. Among 57 treated cases, 29 patients had a minimum follow-up of 12 months. We compared their survival data with those from a similar group of patients affected by LAC, observed in the same period, who underwent RFA as up-front therapy, and we saw that there was no difference in survival associated with the timing of RFA (Fig. 3.13).We can therefore propose RFA as an up-front treatment with no fear of neglecting a *neoadjuvant* treatment.

3.8 Clinical Trials

We will keep offering RFA to our patients as one of the possible treatment modalities for stage III disease. The retrospective, preliminary results achieved in our series need to be validated, and therefore a prospective, randomized, controlled trial is ongoing. At the same time, we are carrying out an immunology study protocol with the aim to find out specific immunomodulatory effects after thermal ablation and their role in disease control. Immunity effects of RFA in pancreatic cancer have never been investigated.

As mentioned above, the complication rate is the "Achilles heel" of the surgical ablation. Therefore, on the way to decrease the risks of the procedure, the choice of a minimally invasive approach is strongly encouraged.

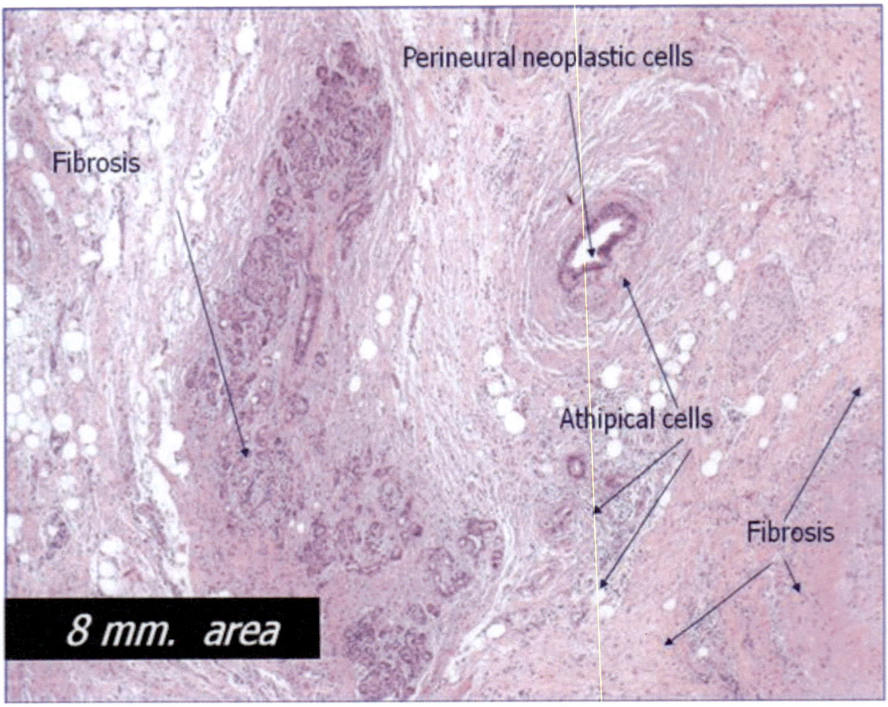

Fig. 3.11 Histological specimen of resected tumor after ablation: within the 2 cm macroscopic tumoral area, 8 mm neoplastic focus, and few microaggregates of atypical cells in a large amount of fibrotic tissue

3.9 Endoscopic Ultrasound-Guided Ablation

Endoscopic ultrasound (EUS) is a well-known procedure that was introduced in clinical practice more than 30 years ago. In the early 1990s, linear-array echoendoscopes equipped with a working channel safely guiding a needle into a target lesion have been introduced. By means of this technique, therapeutic interventions such as drainage of fluid collections and of obstructed pancreatic and biliary ducts, celiac plexus neurolysis, ablation of cyst neoplasms of the pancreas, biliary and gastroenteric anastomoses, injection of antitumor agents inside the tumor, and radiofrequency and cryothermal ablation of solid neoplasms are currently performed.

Radiofrequency thermal ablation (RFA) of solid tumors is widely applied for unresectable tumors, with surgical or percutaneous approaches, in several organs. However, in pancreatic neoplasms the procedure is not yet commonly adopted. RFA for locally advanced pancreatic cancer has been largely applied during laparotomy in retrospective reports demonstrating feasibility, safety, and benefits on overall survival.

Potential advantages of RFA of pancreatic neoplasms under EUS guidance are a less invasive approach, a more accurate identification of the target lesion due to the

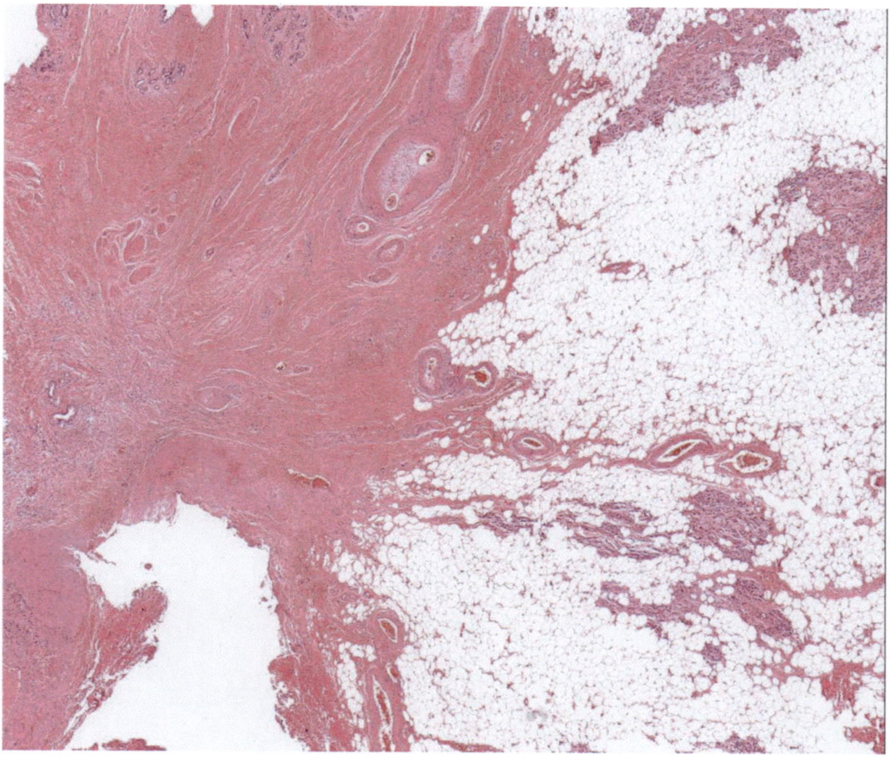

Fig. 3.12 Histological specimen of a resected tumor after ablation: reparative fibrosis without stromal architecture, no cancer cells

high-resolution images, and the short distance between the device and the neoplasm as compared to percutaneous approach.

The RFA with EUS approach (EUS-RFA) of pancreatic lesions in humans was carried out after several attempts in animal models. In 1999 Goldberg et al. [91] reported EUS-RFA in the pancreas of 13 pigs using a modified EUS 19-gauge needle electrode with a 1–1.5 cm tip. No major complications occurred but the ablated area in the pancreas was less than 1 cm size. Only one pig developed pancreatitis. In 2008 Carrara et al. [92] found a good correlation between the size of the ablated area and the duration of ablation in the pancreas of 14 pigs using a flexible bipolar ablation probe combining RFA and cryogenic cooling with carbon dioxide. Two pigs developed necrotizing pancreatitis. It was shown that the same device produced similar effects in the liver and spleen of 19 pigs [93]. A different device was tested in 2009 by Varadarajulu et al. [94]. An umbrella-shaped electrode array introduced through the lumen of a 19-gauge EUS-FNA needle was used to ablate the liver of 5 pigs. No major complications after the procedure have been reported with a mean area of coagulation necrosis at histopathology of 2.6 cm. This method presented the limit of a very large necrotic area for the application in the pancreas and the

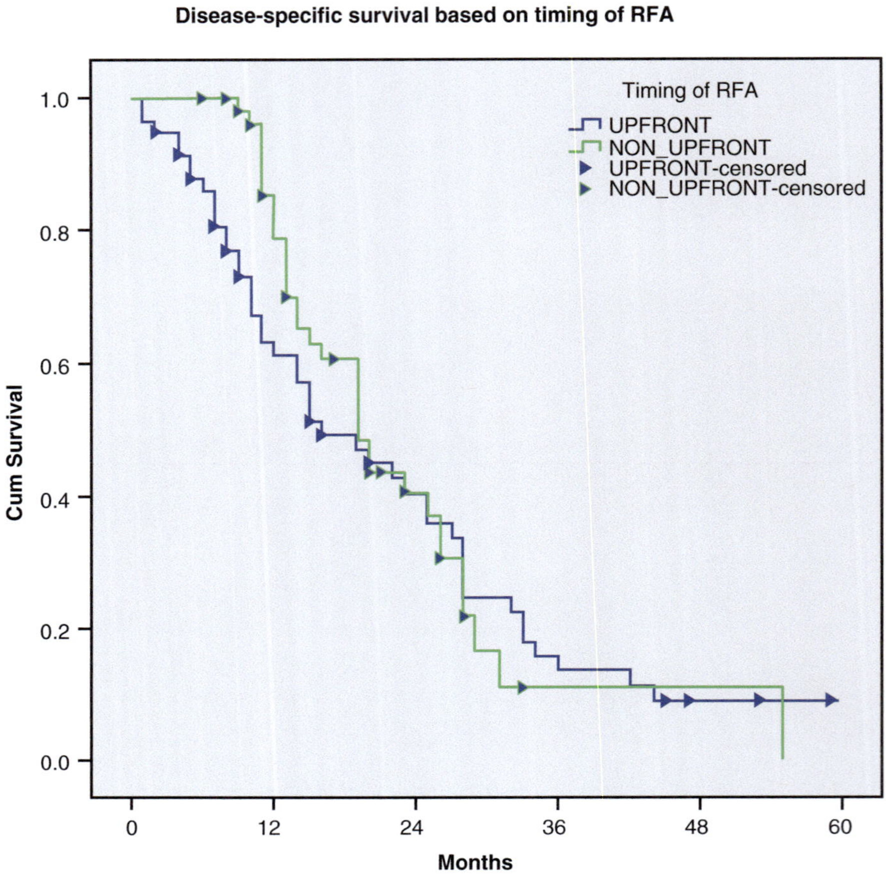

Fig. 3.13 Survival in two groups of patients: up-front RFA vs RFA after chemo/radiotherapy, no difference depending on the timing of the procedure

difficulty in determining the exact position of all the hooks of the umbrella-shaped electrode that lie on a different plane of the probe. In 2012, Gaidhane et al. [95] reported results of RFA of five porcine pancreas using the Habib EUS-RFA 1 Fr wire monopolar probe introduced through the lumen of a 19-gauge EUS-FNA needle: no major complications and moderate pancreatitis in one case were observed. In 2014, Sethi et al. [96] also tested the same device in mediastinal lymph nodes of 18 pigs: no complications occurred and a mean of 17.6 ± 10.3 % of the respected lymph node areas was ablated. Moreover, in 2012 Kim et al. [97] presented a 18-gauge monopolar endoscopic RFA probe tested in the body and tail of 10 porcine pancreas: administration of 50 W for 5 min produced a mean diameter of ablated pancreatic tissue of 23 ± 6.9 mm. In this report, no major complications were described. All these animal model studies demonstrated the feasibility and safety of EUS-RFA in pancreatic tissue with all the electrodes used; the further step was to perform this method in patients with pancreatic neoplasms unfit for surgery.

In 2012, Arcidiacono et al. [98] reported a prospective study on 22 patients affected by locally advanced pancreatic cancer using the abovementioned flexible bipolar ablation probe combining RFA and cryogenic cooling with carbon dioxide (ERBE®) with an electric active part of 1.8 mm of diameter and 20 mm length.. Ablation parameters were 18 W for RF power, cooling pressure of 650 psi, and the application time depended on the size of the lesion (mean time 107 ± 86 s). The procedure was feasible in 16 out of 22 patients (72.8 %), and unsuccessful placement of the probe inside the tumor occurred in 6 cases and was due to stiffness of the gastrointestinal wall and of the tumor due to desmoplastic reaction, tumor infiltration, or fibrosis in patients who had already undergone radiation therapy. No early severe complications have been reported (mild abdominal pain in three cases, one minor duodenal bleeding, and increase in serum amylase in three cases). Four patients experienced late complications. In one case, hemobilia and jaundice were effectively treated by ERCP and biliary stent. A patient presented with jaundice and was successfully treated with ERCP and biliary stent. Another patient presented with duodenal stricture 1 month after the procedure, and the last patient developed an asymptomatic peripancreatic fluid collection. In conclusion, EUS-guided cryothermal ablation was feasible and safe but not applicable in 6 out of 22 patients, probably because the probe was not sharp enough to penetrate in such a stiff tissue as many pancreatic masses are.

The monopolar Habib EUS-RFA catheter (Emcision) with RITA 1500X or ERBE ICC200 RF generators has been used by Pai et al.[99] to treat eight patients. Six of them had mucinous cystic neoplasms of the pancreas and two had pancreatic neuroendocrine tumors (PNETs). No adverse events have been reported. Mild abdominal pain, resolved within 3 days, was the only adverse event. In two cases a complete resolution of the cyst was observed; in the other four, reduction in cyst size was obtained. With regard to the two patients with PNETs, a central necrosis with a change in vascularity was described after treatment. Despite the positive results of this method, the efficacy of RFA of cystic neoplasm and neuroendocrine tumors of the pancreas has not previously been demonstrated, differently from pancreatic cancer, and then, larger series are needed to propose RFA for the treatment of these neoplasms.

The last abovementioned RFA probe is a monopolar 18-gauge RFA electrode 140 cm long (STARmed®), with a sharp conical 1 cm tip for energy delivery and an internal cooling system connected via a pump to an external cold (0 °C) saline solution source (Fig. 3.14). The VIVA RF generator (STARmed®) has variable wattage settings. This system has been tested in two reports. In the first one, Lakhtakia et al. (2015) [100] ablated three patients affected by insulinomas who refused surgery or were considered unfit for surgery. No post-procedure complications were reported. In all the three cases, a rapid relief of insulinoma-related symptoms and a biochemical improvement were obtained, and the patients remained symptom-free at 11–12-month follow-up. In the second report by Song et al. (2015) [101], six patients with stage III or IV pancreatic cancer were treated. No post-procedure complication was described. At short-term follow-up, in only one case, CT scan showed necrosis with air bubbles in the tumor without infection or perforation; long-term follow-up was

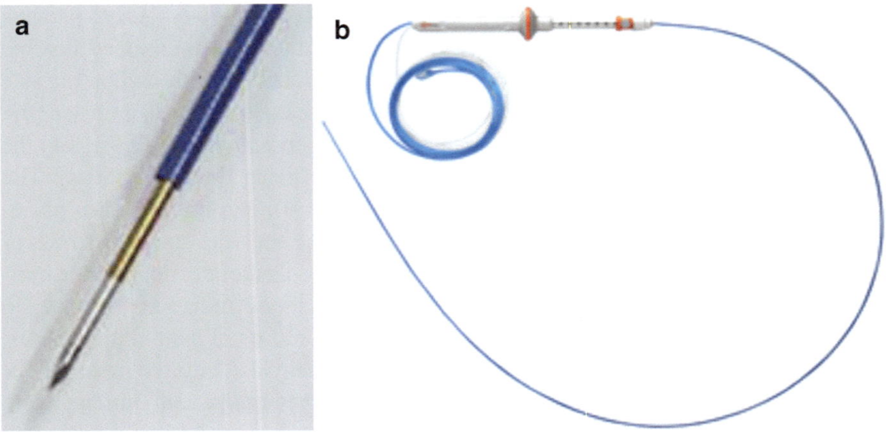

Fig. 3.14 (**a**) The exposed 10 mm tip: sharp, conical, and echogenic. (**b**) EUS-RFA electrode: 18-gauge needle covered with sheath, electrode handle, and catheters for cooling system

not reported. In our opinion, considering the reported studies, this last device resulted the most effective and reliable because of the similarity to a normal FNA needle and because no failures in insertion of the probe into the tumor were described. We recently started a feasibility and safety study of EUS-RFA using this device in five patients with stage III pancreatic adenocarcinoma; the first two cases have been performed with no postoperative complications or adverse events. No follow-up data are available because the procedures have been done very recently.

The endoscopic approach presents several advantages compared to surgery. Firstly, the procedure is less invasive. In fact, the complications related to laparoscopy or laparotomy can be avoided. Moreover, patients unfit for surgery can be safely treated. The insertion of the needle starts through the duodenal or gastric wall: a thermic damage of the hollow viscus wall should be avoided. The post-procedure hospital stay is definitely shorter, and the patients can resume oncological treatments earlier. The EUS-RFA is potentially repeatable with a less relevant impact than a more invasive approach like surgery. In the near future, endoscopic ultrasound may allow tumor local stadiation, cytological diagnosis, and RFA treatment during the same procedure. For all these reasons, this technique appears as a very promising approach for the minimally invasive ablative treatment of locally advanced pancreatic neoplasms.

Conclusions

RFA in LAPC is feasible and safe and may be a new option in a multimodal treatment protocol including chemo and radiotherapy. Its application allows wide and rapid coagulative necrosis with a single application leading to the destruction of a significant part of the tumor. The partial ablation and the increased temperature at the periphery of the treated area induce antitumor immunity by increasing antigen presentation and enhancing antitumor activity. The immunomodulation plays a crucial role in the disease control through a local and systemic response caused by the ablation. These mechanisms can explain preliminary, encouraging results on survival despite pancreatic cancer is commonly considered a systemic disease. Aiming to confirm the retrospective results achieved in our large series, a prospective randomized, controlled trial is ongoing. In order to reduce the risks related to surgical RFA, a minimally invasive approach should be encouraged, and EUS-RFA appears to be the most promising method. As a matter of fact, the endoscopic application of RFA comprises several advantages: it allows a highly precise placement of the needle, permits the control of gastric and duodenal wall during the procedure, is repeatable, can be performed with a short hospital stay, and requires a brief discontinuation of oncological treatments.

References

1. Vincent A, Herman J, Schulick R, Hruban RH, Goggins M. Pancreatic cancer. Lancet. 2011;378:607–20.
2. Lynch SM, Vrieling A, Lubin JH, et al. Cigarette smoking and pancreatic cancer: a pooled analysis from the pancreatic cancer cohort consortium. Am J Epidemiol. 2009;170:403–13.
3. Raimondi S, Maisonneuve R, Lowenfels AB. Epidemiology of pancreatic cancer: an overview. Nat Rev Gastroenterol Hepatol. 2009;6:699–708.
4. Vrieling A, Bueno-de-Mesquita HB, et al. Cigarette smoking, environmental tobacco smoke exposure and pancreatic cancer risk on the European prospective investigation into cancer and nutrition. Int J Cancer. 2010;126:2394–403.
5. Larsson SC, Orsini N, Wolk A. Body mass index and pancreatic cancer risk: a meta-analysis of prospective studies. Int J Cancer. 2007;120:1993–8.
6. Li D, Morris JS, Liu J, et al. Body mass index and risk, age of onset, and survival in patients with pancreatic cancer. JAMA. 2009;301:2553–62.
7. Patel AV, Rodriguez C, Bernstein L, et al. Obesity, recreational physical activity, and risk of pancreatic cancer in a large U.S. Cohort. Cancer Epidemiol Biomarkers Prev. 2005;14:459–66.
8. Mancuso TF, el-Attar AA. Cohort study of workers exposed to beta naphthylamine and benzidine. J Occup Med. 1967;9:277–85.
9. Gupta S, Vittinghoff E, Bertenthal D, et al. New-onset diabetes and pancreatic cancer. Clin Gastroenterol Hepatol. 2006;4:1366–72.
10. Mekan SF, Safa MM, Komrokji RS, et al. Is hyperglycemia a prognostic factor in pancreatic cancer? [abstract]. J Clin Oncol. 2006;24 Suppl 1 Abstract 14076. *J Natl Compr Canc Netw*.
11. Chari ST, Leibson CL, Rabe KG, et al. Probability of pancreatic cancer following diabetes: a population-based study. Gastroenterology. 2005;129:504–11.
12. Wang W, Chen S, Brune KA, et al. PancPRO: risk assessment for individuals with a family history of pancreatic cancer. J Clin Oncol. 2007;25:1417–22.
13. Lynch HT, Smyrk T, Kern SE, et al. Familial pancreatic cancer: a review. Semin Oncol. 1996;23:251–75.
14. Hahn SA, Greenhalf B, Ellis I, et al. BRCA2 germline mutations in familial pancreatic carcinoma. J Natl Cancer Inst. 2003;95:214–21.
15. Ferrone CR, Levine DA, Tang LH, et al. BRCA germline mutations in Jewish patients with pancreatic adenocarcinoma. J Clin Oncol. 2009;27:433–8.
16. Slater EP, Langer P, Niemczyk E, et al. PALB2 mutations in European familial pancreatic cancer families. Clin Genet. 2010;78(5):490–4.
17. Yeo CJ, Abrams RA, Grochow LB, et al. Pancreaticoduodenectomy for pancreatic adenocarcinoma: postoperative adjuvant chemoradiation improves survival. A prospective, single institution experience. Ann Surg. 1997;225:621–33.

18. Allison DC, Piantadosi S, Hruban RH, et al. DNA content and other factors associated with ten year survival after resection of pancreatic carcinoma. J Surg Oncol. 1998;67:151–9.
19. Sohn TA, Yeo CJ, Cameron JL, et al. Resected adenocarcinoma of the pancreas-616 patients: results, outcomes, and prognostic indicators. J Gastrointest Surg. 2000;4:567–79.
20. Howard TJ, Krug JE, Yu J, et al. A margin-negative R0 resection accomplished with minimal postoperative complications is the surgeon's contribution to long-term survival in pancreatic cancer. J Gastrointest Surg. 2006;10:1338–45.
21. Zervos EE, Rosemurgy AS, Al-Saif O, Durkin AJ. Surgical management of early-stage pancreatic cancer. Cancer Control. 2004;11:23–31.
22. Raut CP, Tsen JF, Sun CC, Wang H, Wolff RA, Crane CH, et al. Impact of resection status on pattern of failure and survival after pancreaticoduodenectomy for pancreatic adenocarcinoma. Ann Surg. 2007;246:52–60.
23. Huguet F, Andre T, Hammel P, et al. Impact of chemoradiotherapy after disease control with chemotherapy in locally advanced pancreatic adenocarcinoma in GERCOR phase II and III studies. J Clin Oncol. 2007;25:326–31.
24. Krishnan S, Rana V, Janjan NA, et al. Induction chemotherapy selects patients with locally advanced, unresectable pancreatic cancer for optimal benefit from consolidative chemoradiation therapy. Cancer. 2007;110:47–55.
25. Huguet F, Girard N, Seblain-El Guerche C, et al. Chemoradiotherapy in the management of locally advanced pancreatic carcinoma. J Clin Oncol. 2009;27:2269–77.
26. Ko AH, Quivey JM, Venook AP, et al. A phase II study of fixed-dose rate gemcitabine plus low dose cisplatin followed by consolidative chemoradiation for locally advanced pancreatic cancer. Int J Radiat Oncol Biol Phys. 2007;68:809–16.
27. Gillen S, Schuster T, Meyer Zum Büschenfelde C, Friess H, Kleeff J. Preoperative/neoadjuvant therapy in pancreatic cancer: a systematic review and meta-analysis of response and resection percentages. PLoS Med. 2010;7(4):e1000267. Review.
28. Strobel O, Berens V, Hinz U, Hartwig W, Hackert T, Bergmann F, Debus J, Jäger D, Büchler MW, Werner J. Resection after neoadjuvant therapy for locally advanced, "unresectable" pancreatic cancer. Surgery. 2012;152(3 Suppl 1):S33–42. doi:10.1016/j.surg.2012.05.029. Epub 2012 Jul 6.
29. Andriulli A, Festa V, Botteri E, Valvano MR, Koch M, Bassi C, Maisonneuve P, Sebastiano PD. Neoadjuvant/preoperative gemcitabine for patients with localized pancreatic cancer: a meta-analysis of prospective studies. Ann Surg Oncol. 2012;19(5):1644–62. doi:10.1245/s10434-011-2110-8. Epub 2011 Oct 20.
30. Sahora K, Kuehrer I, Eisenhut A, Akan B, Koellblinger C, Goetzinger P, Teleky B, Jakesz R, Peck-Radosavljevic M, Ba'ssalamah A, Zielinski C, Gnant M. NeoGemOx: gemcitabine and oxaliplatin as neoadjuvant treatment for locally advanced, nonmetastasized pancreatic cancer. Surgery. 2011;149(3):311–20. doi:10.1016/j.surg.2010.07.048.Epub2010Sep.
31. Laurence JM, Tran PD, Morarji K, Eslick GD, Lam VW, Sandroussi C. A systematic review and meta-analysis of survival and surgical outcomes following neoadjuvant chemoradiotherapy for pancreatic cancer. J Gastrointest Surg. 2011;15(11):2059–69. doi:10.1007/s11605-011-1659-7. Epub 2011 Sep 13.
32. Barugola G, Partelli S, Crippa S, Capelli P, D'Onofrio M, Pederzoli P, Falconi M. Outcomes after resection of locally advanced or borderline resectable pancreatic cancer after neoadjuvant therapy. Am J Surg. 2012;203(2):132–9.
33. Siperstein E, Gitomirski A. History and technological aspects of radiofrequency thermoablation. Cancer J. 2000;6(4):5293–303.
34. Pereira PL. Actual role of radiofrequency ablation of liver metastases. Eur Radiol. 2007;17(8):2062–70.
35. Clasen S, Krober SM, Kosan B, et al. Pathomorphologic evaluation of pulmonary radiofrequency ablation: proof of cell death is characterized by DNA fragmentation and apoptotic bodies. Cancer. 2008;113(11):3121–9.
36. Wright S, Sampson LA, Warner TF, Mahvi DM, Lee FT. Radiofrequency versus microwave ablation in a hepatic porcine model. Radiology. 2005;236(1):132–9.

37. Siriwardena AK. Radiofrequency ablation for locally advanced cancer of the pancreas. J Oncol Pract. 2006;7:1–4.
38. Hadjicostas P, Malakounides N, Varianos C, Kitiris E, Lerni F, Symeonides P. Radiofrequency ablation in pancreatic cancer. HPB. 2006;8:61–4.
39. Spiliotis JD, Datsis AC, Michalopoulos NV, Kekelos SP, Vaxevanidou A, Rogdakis AG, et al. Radiofrequency ablation combined with palliative surgery may prolong survival of patients with advanced cancer of the pancreas. Langenbecks Arch Surg. 2007;392:55–60.
40. Matsui Y, Nakagawa A, Kamiyama Y, Yamamoto K, Kubo N, Nakase Y. Selective thermocoagulation of unresectable pancreatic cancers by using radiofrequency capacitive heating. Pancreas. 2000;20:14–20.
41. Varshney S, Sewkani A, Sharma S, Kapoor S, Naik S, Sharma A, Patel K. Radiofrequency ablation of unresectable pancreatic carcinoma: feasibility, efficacy and safety. J Oncol Pract. 2006;11:7(1).
42. Molinari E, Bassi C, Salvia R, Butturini G, Crippa S, Talamini G, et al. Amylase value in drains after pancreatic resection as predictive factor of postoperative pancreatic fistula: results of a prospective study in 137 patients. Ann Surg. 2007;246:281–7.
43. Girelli R, Frigerio I, Salvia R, Barbi E, Tinazzi Martini P, Bassi C. Feasibility and safety of radiofrequency ablation for locally advanced pancreatic cancer. Br J Surg. 2010;97:220–5.
44. Koninger J, Wente MN, Muller MW, Gutt CN, Friess H, Buchler MW. Surgical palliation in patients with pancreatic cancer. Langenbecks Arch Surg. 2007;392:13–21.
45. Girelli R, Frigerio I, Giardino A, Regi P, Gobbo S, Malleo G, Salvia R, Bassi C. Results of 100 pancreatic radiofrequency ablations in the context of a multimodal strategy for stage III ductal adenocarcinoma. Langenbecks Arch Surg. 2013;398(1):63–9.
46. Nikfarjam M, Muralidharan V, Christophi C. Mechanisms of focal heat destruction of liver tumors. J Surg Res. 2005;127:208.
47. Gravante G, Sconocchia G, Ong SL, Dennison AR, Lloyd DM. Immunoregulatory effects of liver ablation therapies for the treatment of primary and metastatic liver malignancies. Liver Int. 2009;29(1):18–24.
48. Soanes WA, Ablin RJ, Gonder MJ. Remission of metastatic lesions following cryosurgery in prostatic cancer: immunologic considerations. J Urol. 1970;104(1):154–9.
49. Ablin RJ, Soanes WA, Gonder MJ. Elution of in vivo bound antiprostatic epithelial antibodies following multiple cryotherapy of carcinoma of prostate. Urology. 1973;2(3):276–9.
50. Sanchez-Ortiz RF, Tannir N, Ahrar K, Wood CG. Spontaneous regression of pulmonary metastases from renal cell carcinoma after radio frequency ablation of the primary tumor: an in situ tumor vaccine? J Urol. 2003;170(1):178–9.
51. Chu KF, et al. Thermal ablation of tumours: biological mechanisms and advances in therapy. Nat Rev Cancer. 2014;14(3):199–208.
52. Neil Bhardwaj, John Dormer, Fateh Ahmad, Andrew D. Strickland, Gianpiero Gravante, Ian Beckingham, Kevin West, Ashley R. Dennison, David M. Lloyd. Heat shock protein 70 expression following hepatic radiofrequency ablation is affected by adjacent vasculature. J Surg Res. 2012;173(2):249–57.
53. Frich L, Bjornland K, Pettersen S, Clausen OP, Gladhaug IP. Increased activity of matrix metalloproteinase 2 and 9 after hepatic radiofrequency ablation. J Surg Res. 2006;135:297–304.
54. Rai R, Richardson C, Flecknell P, Robertson H, Burt A, Manas DM. Study of apoptosis and heat shock protein (HSP) expression in hepatocytes following radiofrequency ablation (RFA). J Surg Res. 2005;129:147–51.
55. Rea IM, McNerlan S, Pockley AG. Serum heat shock protein and anti-heat shock protein antibody levels in aging. Exp Gerontol. 2001;36:341–52.
56. Schueller G, Kettenbach J, Sedivy R, Bergmeister H, Stift A, Fried J, Gnant M, Lammer J. Expression of heat shock proteins in human hepatocellular carcinoma after radiofrequency ablation in an animal model. Oncol Rep. 2004;12:495–9.
57. Schueller G, Kettenbach J, Sedivy R, Stift A, Friedl J, Gnant M, Lammer J. Heat shock protein expression induced by percutaneous radiofrequency ablation of hepatocellular carcinoma in vivo. Int J Oncol. 2004;24:609–13.

58. Stuart K. Calderwood, Salamatu S. Mambula, Phillip J. Gray, Jr. Extracellular heat shock proteins in cell signaling and immunity. Ann N Y Acad Sci. 2007;1113:28–39. C 2007 New York Academy of Sciences.
59. Beere HM. 'The stress of dying': the role of heat shock proteins in the regulation of apoptosis. J Cell Sci. 2004;117:2641–51.
60. Tytell M, Greenberg SG, Lasek RJ. Heat shock-like protein is transferred from glia to axon. Brain Res. 1986;363:161–4.
61. Hightower LE, Guidon Jr PT. Selective release from cultured mammalian cells of heat-shock (stress) proteins that resemble glia-axon transfer proteins. J Cell Physiol. 1989;138:257–66.
62. Mambula SS, Calderwood SK. Heat shock protein 70 is secreted from tumor cells by a nonclassical pathway involving lysosomal endosomes. J Immunol. 2006;177:7849–57.
63. Robinson MB, et al. Extracellular heat shock protein 70: a critical component for motoneuron survival. J Neurosci. 2005;25:9735–45.
64. Clayton A, et al. Induction of heat shock proteins in B-cell exosomes. J Cell Sci. 2005;118:3631–8.
65. Davies EL, et al. Heat shock proteins form part of a danger signal cascade in response to lipopolysaccharide and GroEL. Clin Exp Immunol. 2006;145:183–9.
66. Hunter-Lavin C, et al. Hsp70 release from peripheral blood mononuclear cells. Biochem Biophys Res Commun. 2004;324:511–7.
67. Campisi J, Fleshner M. Role of extracellular HSP72 in acute stressinduced potentiation of innate immunity in active rats. J Appl Physiol. 2003;94:43–52.
68. Mambula SS, Calderwood SK. Heat induced release of Hsp70 from prostate carcinoma cells involves both active secretion and passive release from necrotic cells. Int J Hyperthermia. 2006;22:575–85.
69. Todryk S, et al. Heat shock protein 70 induced during tumor cell killing induces Th1 cytokines and targets immature dendritic cell precursors to enhance antigen uptake. J Immunol. 1999;163:1398–408.
70. Mackenzie A, et al. Rapid secretion of interleukin-1beta by microvesicle shedding. Immunity. 2001;15:825–35.
71. Baraldi PG, Di Virgilio F, Romagnoli R. Agonists and antagonists acting at P2'7 receptor. Curr Top Med Chem. 2004;4:1707–17.
72. Srivastava PK. Heat shock protein-based novel immunotherapies. Drug News Perspect. 2000;13:517–22.
73. Srivastava PK, Amato RJ. Heat shock proteins: the 'Swiss Army Knife' vaccines against cancers and infectious agents. Vaccine. 2001;19:2590–7.
74. Calderwood SK, Theriault JR, Gong J. Message in a bottle: role of the 70 kilodalton heat shock protein family in anti-tumor immunity. Eur J Immunol. 2005;35:2518–27.
75. Asea A, et al. HSP70 stimulates cytokine production through a CD14-dependant pathway, demonstrating its dual role as a chaperone and cytokine. Nat Med. 2000;6:435–42.
76. Asea A, et al. Novel signal transduction pathway utilized by extracellular HSP70: role of toll-like receptor (TLR) 2 and TLR4. J Biol Chem. 2002;277:15028–34.
77. Noessner E, et al. Tumor-derived heat shock protein 70 peptide complexes are cross-presented by human dendritic cells. J Immunol. 2002;169:5424–32.
78. Singh-Jasuja H, et al. Cross-presentation of glycoprotein 96-associated antigens on major histocompatibility complex class I molecules requires receptor-mediated endocytosis. J Exp Med. 2000;191:1965–74.
79. Dressel R, Lubbers M, Walter L, Herr W, Gunther E. Enhanced susceptibility to cytotoxic T lymphocytes without increase of MHC class I antigen expression after conditional overexpression of heat shock protein 70 in target cells. Eur J Immunol. 1999;29:3925.
80. Widenmayer M, Shebzukhov Y, Haen SP, Schmidt D, Clasen S, Boss Am Kuprash DV, Nedospanov SA, Stenzl A, Aebert H, Wernet D, Stevanovic S, Pereira P, Rammensee HG, Gouttefangeas C. Analysis of tumor antigen-specific T cell and antibodies in cancer patients treated with radiofrequency ablation. Int J Cancer. 2011;128:2653–62.

81. Wissniowski TT, Hansler J, Neureiter D, Frieser M, Schaber S, Esslinger B, Voll R, Strobel D, Hahn EG, Schuppan D. Activation of tumor-specific T lymphocytes by radio-frequency ablation of the VX2 hepatoma in rabbits. Cancer Res. 2003;63:6496–500.
82. Zerbini A, Pilli M, Penna A, Pelosi G, Schianchi C, Molinari A, Schivazappa S, Zibera C, Fagnoni FF, Ferrari C, Missale G. Radiofrequency thermal ablation of hepatocellular carcinoma liver nodules can activate and enhance tumor-specific T-cell responses. Cancer Res. 2006;66:1139–46.
83. Napoletano C, Taurino F, Biffoni M, De Majo A, Coscarella G, Bellati F, Rahimi H, Pauselli S, Pellicciotta I, Burchell JM, Gaspari LA, Ercoli L, et al. RFA strongly modulates the immune system and antitumor immune responses in metastatic liver patients. Int J Oncol. 2008;32:481–90.
84. Hansler J, Wissniowski TT, Schuppan D, Witte A, Bernatik T, Hahn EG, Strobel D. Activation and dramatically increased cytolytic activity of tumor specific T lymphocytes after radiofrequency ablation in patients with hepatocellular carcinoma and colorectal liver metastases. World J Gastroenterol. 2006;12:3716–21.
85. Chen T, Guo J, et al. Heat shock protein 70, released from heat stressed tumor cells, initiates antitumor immunity by inducing tumor cell chemokine production and activating dendritic cells via TLR4 pathway. J Immunol. 2009;182:1449–59.
86. Harris HE, Andersson U. The nuclear protein HMGB1 as a proinflammatory mediator. Eur J Immunol. 2004;34:1503–12.
87. Fietta AM, Morosini M, et al. Systemic inflammatory response and downmodulation of peripheral CD25Foxp3 T-regulatory cells in patients undergoing radiofrequency thermal ablation or lung cancer. Hum Immunol. 2009;70(7):477–86.
88. Rovere-Querini P, Manfredi A. Tumour destruction and in situ delivery of antigen presenting cells promote anti-neoplastic immune responses: implications for the immunotherapy of pancreatic cancer. J Oncol Pract. 2004;5(4):308–14.
89. D'Onofrio M, Barbi E, Girelli R, Martone E, et al. Radiofrequency ablation of locally advanced pancreatic adenocarcinoma: an overview. World J Gastroenterol. 2010;16(28):3478–83.
90. Frigerio I, Girelli R, Giardino A, Regi P, Salvia R, Bassi C. Short term chemotherapy followed by radiofrequency ablation in stage III pancreatic cancer: results from a single center. J HBP Cancer. 2013;20:574–7.
91. Goldberg SN, Mallery S, Gazelle GS, Brugge WR. EUS-guided radiofrequency ablation in the pancreas: results in a porcine model. Gastrointest Endosc. 1999;50(3):392–401. doi:10.1053/ge.1999.v50.98847.
92. Carrara S, Arcidiacono PG, Albarello L, Addis A, Enderle MD, Boemo C, Campagnol M, Ambrosi A, Doglioni C, Testoni PA. Endoscopic ultrasound-guided application of a new hybrid cryotherm probe in porcine pancreas: a preliminary study. Endoscopy. 2008;40(4):321–6. doi:10.1055/s-2007-995595.
93. Carrara S, Arcidiacono PG, Albarello L, Addis A, Enderle MD, Boemo C, Neugebauer A, Campagnol M, Doglioni C, Testoni PA. Endoscopic ultrasound-guided application of a new internally gas-cooled radiofrequency ablation probe in the liver and spleen of an animal model: a preliminary study. Endoscopy. 2008;40(9):759–63. doi:10.1055/s-2008-1077520.
94. Varadarajulu S, Jhala NC, Drelichman ER. EUS-guided radiofrequency ablation with a prototype electrode array system in an animal model (with video). Gastrointest Endosc. 2009;70(2):372–6. doi:10.1016/j.gie.2009.03.008.
95. Gaidhane M, Smith I, Ellen K, Gatesman J, Habib N, Foley P, Moskaluk C, Kahaleh M. Endoscopic Ultrasound-Guided Radiofrequency Ablation (EUS-RFA) of the pancreas in a Porcine model. Gastroenterol Res Pract. 2012;2012:431451. doi:10.1155/2012/431451. PubMed PMID: 23049547, PubMed Central PMCID: PMC3459266.
96. Sethi A, Ellrichmann M, Dhar S, Hadeler KG, Kahle E, Seehusen F, Klapper W, Habib N, Fritscher-Ravens A. Endoscopic ultrasound-guided lymph node ablation with a novel radiofrequency ablation probe: feasibility study in an acute porcine model. Endoscopy. 2014;46(5):411–5. doi:10.1055/s-0034-1364933.

97. Kim HJ, Seo DW, Hassanuddin A, Kim SH, Chae HJ, Jang JW, Park do H, Lee SS, Lee SK, Kim MH. EUS-guided radiofrequency ablation of the porcine pancreas. Gastrointest Endosc. 2012;76(5):1039–43. doi:10.1016/j.gie.2012.07.015.
98. Arcidiacono PG, Carrara S, Reni M, Petrone MC, Cappio S, Balzano G, Boemo C, Cereda S, Nicoletti R, Enderle MD, Neugebauer A, von Renteln D, Eickhoff A, Testoni PA. Feasibility and safety of EUS-guided cryothermal ablation in patients with locally advanced pancreatic cancer. Gastrointest Endosc. 2012;76(6):1142–51. doi:10.1016/j.gie.2012.08.006.
99. Pai M, Habib N, Senturk H, Lakhtakia S, Reddy N, Cicinnati VR, Kaba I, Beckebaum S, Drymousis P, Kahaleh M, Brugge W. Endoscopic ultrasound guided radiofrequency ablation, for pancreatic cystic neoplasms and neuroendocrine tumors. World J Gastrointest Surg. 2015;7(4):52–9. doi:10.4240/wjgs.v7.i4.52. PubMed PMID: 25914783, PubMed Central PMCID: PMC4390891.
100. Lakhtakia S, Ramchandani M, Galasso D, Gupta R, Venugopal S, Kalpala R, Reddy DN. EUS-guided radiofrequency ablation for management of pancreatic insulinoma by using a novel needle electrode (with videos). Gastrointest Endosc. 2015. doi:10.1016/j.gie.2015.08.085.
101. Song TJ, Seo DW, Lakhtakia S, Reddy N, Oh DW, Park DH, Lee SS, Lee SK, Kim MH. Initial experience of EUS-guided radiofrequency ablation of unresectable pancreatic cancer. Gastrointest Endosc. 2015. doi:10.1016/j.gie.2015.08.048.

4 TEM and TAMIS for Large Rectal Neoplasm

Simone Arolfo and Alberto Arezzo

4.1 Introduction

Minimally invasive treatment of large rectal adenomas and early rectal cancer by transanal endoscopic microsurgery (TEM) has become a common procedure during the last 30 years [1]. It has been shown how this technique is much more accurate and effective than traditional transanal excision in terms of clear margins, non-fragmented specimen and recurrence [2]. About 20 % of sessile adenomas of the rectum preoperatively assessed as benign are actually malignant. This is evidently more frequent among those biopsied as high-grade dysplasia (HGD). Fortunately it has been shown that 'en bloc' excision of up to T1sm1 cancer is oncologically radical, with a low recurrence rate. The Paris classification [3] substages T1 cancers, as originally suggested by Haggitt et al. [4] and Kikuchi et al. [5], to define more accurately the risk of recurrence and lymphatic dissemination in pedunculated and sessile lesions, respectively [6]. For pedunculated carcinomas, the classification includes four levels of invasion; level 4 lesions (which extend beyond the polyp stalk but do not invade the muscularis propria) are predictive of negative patient outcome [4]. For sessile lesions, Kikuchi et al. defined the three levels of submucosal invasion, split into superficial (sm1), middle (sm2) and deep (sm3) thirds of the submucosa. The frequency of lymph node metastases is proportional to the degree of depth being 2, 8 and 23 %, respectively [6]. The Paris classification [3], revised in Kyoto in 2008 [7], defines every lesion extended no more than 1 mm in the submucosal layer as 'sm1'. According to these results, the risk can be negligible if a neoplasia is limited to the mucosa. In addition, the risk is also very low in well-differentiated colorectal adenocarcinoma with superficial invasion of the submucosa and no infiltration of lymphatic vessels. If a cancer more advanced than T1sm1 stage is found, radical surgery,

S. Arolfo • A. Arezzo (✉)
General Surgery I, Department of Surgical Sciences, University of Torino,
C.so Dogliotti 14, 10126 Torino, Italy
e-mail: alberto.arezzo@unito.it

R. Conigliaro, M. Frazzoni (eds.), *Diagnosis and Endoscopic Management of Digestive Diseases*, DOI 10.1007/978-3-319-42358-6_4

also named ‘salvage surgery’, consisting of total mesorectal excision (TME), is indicated within 4–8 weeks. The oncological outcomes after salvage surgery, consisting of rectal anterior resection (RAR) or abdominoperineal resection (APR) with TME, are comparable to those of radical surgery performed as a primary treatment [8, 9]. This is supposed to be due to the fact that this two-step procedure respects one of the principles of oncologic appropriateness for rectal cancer treatment that is to maintain the integrity of the mesorectal fascia. Preoperative staging is critical to assess a correct indication to local excision. There are many tools available, even if the global accuracy is unfortunately still low.

4.1.1 Pit Pattern Classification

The idea of observing the surface microstructure of colorectal epithelium dates back to the 1970s, with the use of dissecting microscopes on resected specimens. It was Nishizawa in the early 1980s [10] who showed that normal colonic mucosa, adenoma and adenocarcinoma have their own characteristic surface structures. Already in the 1980s, the development of magnifying fibre colonoscopes enabled the microstructure of the various colorectal lesions to be seen in vivo [11]. Ten years later, the advent of commercially available high-resolution magnifying video colonoscopes stressed the study of the microstructures of colonic lesions [12]. Expectations were that endoscopic pit pattern classification could determine not only the lateral extent but also the depth of a lesion, thus contributing to the indication for local or radical excision. Although it is true that a totally disorganised or a nonstructural pattern seems to correspond to carcinomas with a submucosal invasion, pit pattern analysis failed to become a completely reliable method of pretreatment classification, and it is still routinely used only in Eastern countries. In order to improve the accuracy of diagnosis in vivo, it has been suggested to use natural or electronic chromoendoscopy techniques (narrow band imaging (NBI), Fuji intelligent chromoendoscopy (FICE)) with or without optical or electronic magnification [13]. If these techniques have been used rarely in Western countries so far as they are considered too burdensome for routine endoscopy, the progressive implementation and simplification of electronic chromoendoscopy on the new instruments should lead to a more widespread use of this technique.

4.1.2 Endoscopic Ultrasound (EUS)

In a recent review, Marone [14] reported an overall accuracy of 84 % (range 63 %–96 %) for assessing the tumour penetration depth in the rectal wall. Marusch et al. [15] analysed the diagnostic accuracy of rectal EUS in the clinical staging of 7000 patients with rectal cancer. This allowed the comparison between ultrasonographic T stage (uT) and pathological T stage (pT). The study showed a uT-pT correspondence of 65 %, demonstrating that, in clinical routine, the diagnostic accuracy of transrectal ultrasound in staging rectal carcinoma does not attain some very good results reported in the literature. This is also our experience. To define a correct indication for local excision, it is mandatory to know whether the observed lesion invades the submucosal layer, and if it does, if this goes deeper than 1 mm below the lamina propria. This is probably too much to be asked for any in vivo diagnostic tool. By reviewing our experience of the last 5 years, to be sure that no technology improvement could be responsible for changing the results, we could verify that about one fourth of the lesions preoperatively assessed as ultrasonographic T0 (uT0), i.e. limited to the mucosal layer, were in fact invasive carcinomas.

4.1.3 Biopsy

Although in Eastern countries the routine usage of magnification is assumed to reduce the requirement for biopsies, Western endoscopists tend to base treatment decisions largely on the size and the location of the tumour and on the histology of biopsy specimens, considering the Japanese classification too complex for practical use. Nevertheless, the routine use of biopsy has certain limitations due to superficiality and sampling errors [16]. It has been shown, however, that by applying the revised Vienna classification to biopsy specimens, the risk of finding an invasive carcinoma in the resected lesion can be effectively assessed [17]. Our experience of the last 5 years allows us to define that almost half of those neoplasms that resulted at definitive histology of the specimen invasive cancers had a preoperative biopsy histology of dysplasia, in about 7 % of cases judged as low grade, so that no grade of dysplasia detected at biopsy could be considered an assurance of not having to deal with an invasive cancer in the end.

4.1.4 Lifting Sign

A highly accurate endoscopic sign to evaluate a possible invasion of cancer that affects the radical resection is the no-lifting sign after injection of saline into the submucosa below the polyp. When the lesion does not lift completely it is likely to have already passed the submucosa, preventing complete endoscopic excision of the lesion. Although not ideal, due to the limits of other criteria to assess correct indication for local excision, as exposed above, the lifting sign still remains, at least in Western countries, a routine procedure. As not all the neoplasms that infiltrate the submucosal layer are good indications for local excision, and the risk of deep margin infiltration of the specimen increases, the lifting of the neoplasm does not assure that the endoscopic local excision would be considered curative [18, 19].

4.1.5 Digital Examination

At least in the low- and mid-rectum, digital examination can easily replace the need to inject lifting agents into the submucosa to exclude infiltration of the muscular layer. With similar accuracy, this easy manoeuvre also allows to detect the consistency of the lesion, the distance from the anal verge and the location along the circumference which might help during the dissection manoeuvre, both by endoscopic and by transanal surgery [20–22]

4.2 Technique

TEM is a well-standardised and reproducible operation; herewith a description of the technique is performed at our institution [23].

All patients are asked to commence a low-fibre diet the week before TEM, and a rectal enema is performed 12 and 2 h preoperatively. Intravenous antibiotics, such as a second-generation cephalosporin and metronidazole, are administered before insertion of the proctoscope and continued for 24 h at 12-h intervals. Deep venous thrombosis prophylaxis is not administered.

4.2.1 Equipment

Nowadays there are two platforms available for transanal local excision: the original Richard Wolf (Knittlingen, Germany) TEM equipment and the transanal endoscopic operation (TEO) instrumentation by Karl Storz GmbH (Tuttlingen, Germany). The original Wolf equipment has many technical advantages like stereoscopic vision and peristaltic CO2 inflating pump stabilising pneumorectum and evacuating surgical smoke from the rectum (Fig. 4.1). The main advantage of the TEO instrumentation is its cost effectiveness, as it can be connected to a standard laparoscopic tower. Due to its better practicability, we actually use the TEO system since 2008. TEO instrumentation includes a 7- or 15-cm rectal tube which is 4 cm in diameter and has three working channels (12, 5 and 5 mm) for dedicated or conventional laparoscopic instruments, plus a 5-mm channel dedicated to a 30° 2D optic (Fig. 4.2). The proctoscope is connected to the operating table via a holding arm consisting of three joints and a single screw (Fig. 4.3). The system is used in combination with standard laparoscopic units. Camera imaging is projected on-screen, and insufflation is obtained by a conventional CO2 thermo-insufflator, which is connected to the proctoscope via a Luer Lock connector. The shape of the tip of the proctoscope allows manipulation and suturing of the rectal wall on a 360° surface. Therefore, most patients are kept in a supine position, thereby reducing the need for time-consuming patient repositioning on the operating table.

4.2.2 Positioning of the Patient on the Operating Table

The TEM procedure is traditionally performed under general anaesthesia, although since about 2 years we adopted spinal anaesthesia as a standard with no exclusion

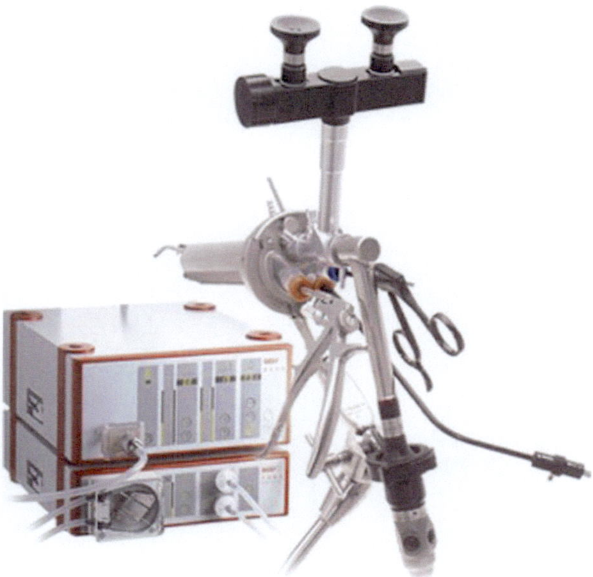

Fig. 4.1 The original transanal endoscopic microsurgery (TEM) instrumentation (R. Wolf)

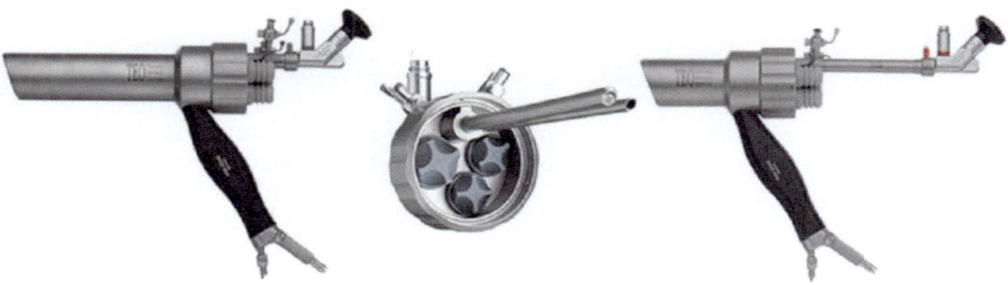

Fig. 4.2 Transanal endoscopic operation (TEO®) instrumentation (K. Storz)

criteria [24]. The patient is placed either prone or supine in order to keep the lesion as close to the 6-o'clock position as possible, even with lateral lesions. Different from the technique originally conceived by Buess, we avoid placing the patient in the lateral decubitus position, as this is extremely difficult and the benefit is minimal. Patients with lateral lesions are usually placed in the supine position, unless the lesion is predominantly located in the right or left upper quadrant (i.e. 12- to 3-o'clock position or 9- to 12-o'clock position). With circumferential lesions, the patient is always positioned prone due to the higher risk of entering the peritoneal cavity and the consequent need to reduce the descent of small bowel loops into the surgical field while repairing the opening itself.

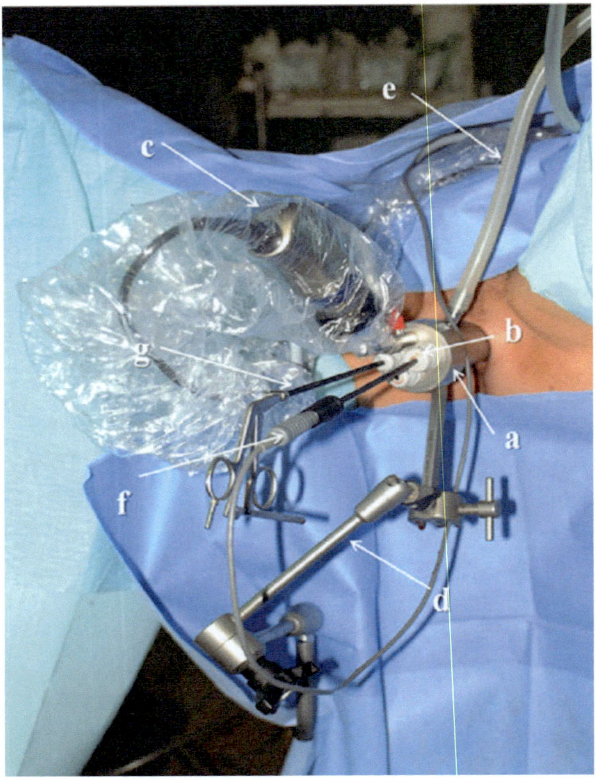

Fig. 4.3 TEO® instrumentation setting: *a* rigid proctoscope; *b* operative channel; *c* camera; *d* Martin arm secured to the operating bed; *e* insufflation cable (CO2); *f* monopolar hook; *g* grasping forceps

4.2.3 Surgical Technique

4.2.3.1 Step 1: Dissection

After insertion of the proctoscope, the lesion is identified, and the proctoscope is fixed in the correct position. However, the position is adjusted throughout the procedure in order to ensure optimal visualisation and access to the margins of the lesion. High-flow carbon dioxide (CO2) insufflation is required, and endoluminal pressure is generally maintained at 8 mmHg, although it might need to be increased up to 16 mmHg. Dissection is usually started at the right lower border of the tumour (Fig. 4.4a). A macroscopic margin of at least 5 mm from the neoplasm needs to be obtained with both benign and malignant lesions. Tumour excision is performed by monopolar hook cautery. In difficult cases, especially if a partial mesorectal excision is recommended for malignancy, ultrasonic shears such as Ultracision ACE™ (Johnson & Johnson Medical, Cincinnati, OH) or an electrothermal radio frequency and bipolar vessel sealing system such as LigaSure™ (Covidien, Tyco, Medtronic, Minneapolis, MN) may be helpful. Dissection is continued circumferentially around the lesion to the perirectal fat (Fig. 4.4b, c). Due to the uncertainty of the preoperative diagnosis and

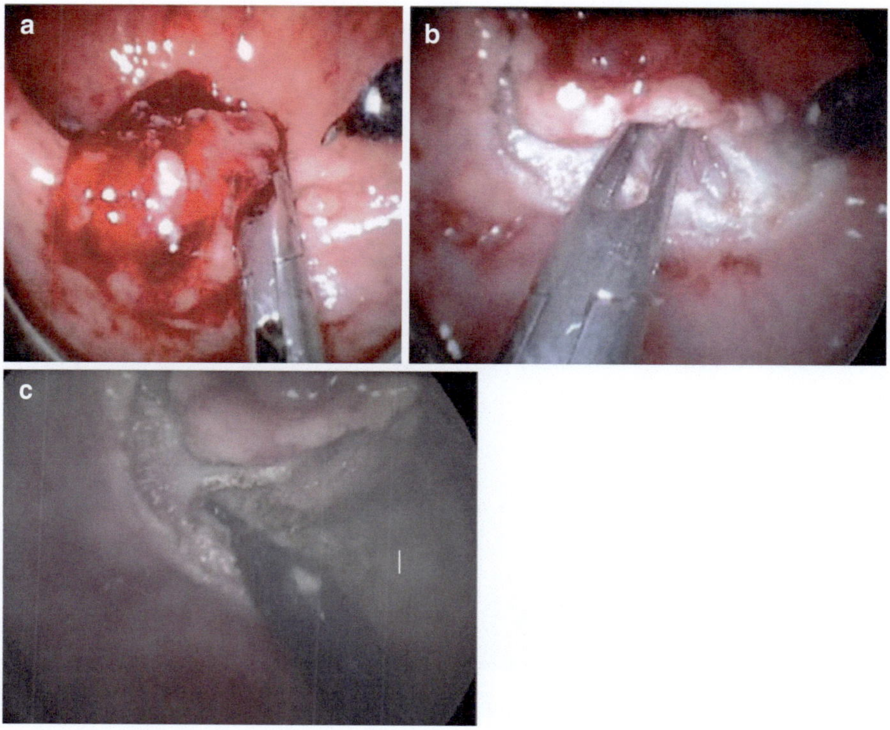

Fig. 4.4 Full-thickness dissection of a rectal lesion. (**a**) Mucosal dotting around the lesion to mark the area to excise; (**b**) mucosal incision; (**c**) full-thickness excision

staging, a full-thickness resection with adequate margins of clearance should always be performed. The specimen is retrieved transanally and pinned on a corkboard before fixation in 10% buffered formalin in order to preserve the margins of the normal mucosa surrounding the tumour. The specimen is analysed by permanent section.

4.2.3.2 Step 2: Wall Defect Suturing

After the parietal defect is disinfected with iodopovidone solution, the rectal wall is always closed with one or more Maxon 3-0 (Covidien, Tyco, Medtronic, Minneapolis, MN) running sutures secured with dedicated silver clips (Richard Wolf, Knittlingen, Germany). These clips serve to anchor the suture in place, since knotting during TEM is challenging. As an alternative, a barbed suture V-Loc™ (Covidien, Tyco, Medtronic, Minneapolis, MN) may also be used, avoiding the need of clips or knotting. If the peritoneum was opened, the defect might be closed as a single layer being careful to include the serosal layer in the stitches or as a two-layer running suture.

At this stage, the endoluminal pressure may be reduced to allow better compliance of the rectal wall. Suturing is performed with particular attention to the integrity of the rectal lumen. Therefore, when suturing large defects, a midline stitch to approximate proximal and distal margins is placed (Fig. 4.5). At the end of the procedure, patency of the rectum is carefully verified through the TEM proctoscope.

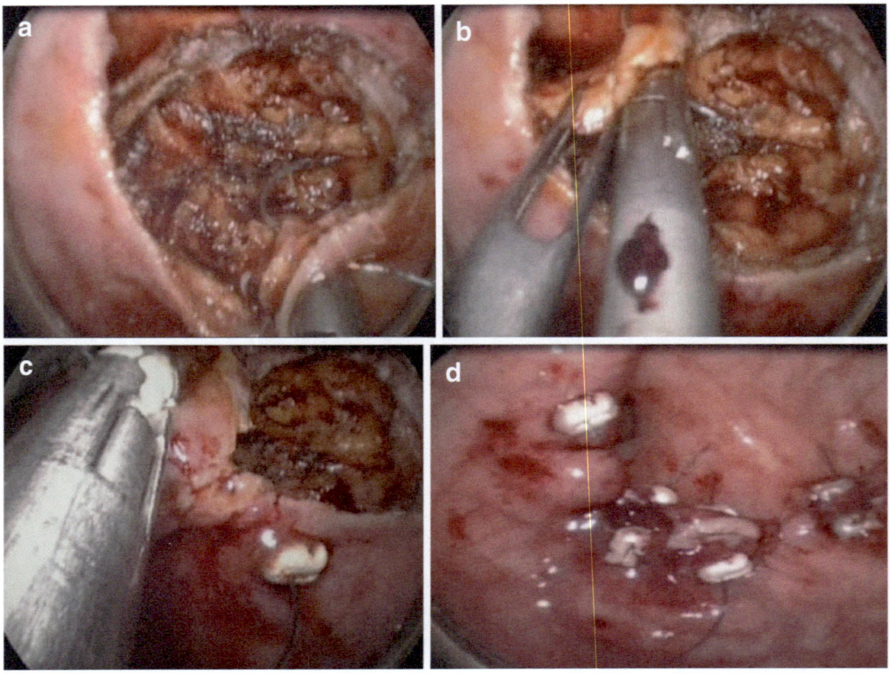

Fig. 4.5 Rectal wall suture. (**a**) Perirectal fat after the excision; (**b**) beginning of the suture; (**c**) silver clip positioning to secure the running suture; (**d**) final aspect

4.2.4 Postoperative Management

Patients are mobilised the same day as surgery. The urinary catheter placed at the time of surgery is removed 24 h after surgery (48 h if the anterior wall was involved). Postoperative analgesia is ensured by intravenous paracetamol for 24 h. Oral intake is allowed the day after flatus is reported.

4.3 TEM Versus ESD

With the advent of endoscopic submucosal dissection (ESD) about 15 years ago, flexible endoscopy permitted a surgical-like technique for en bloc resection of superficial lesions of the digestive tract. First indicated for the upper gastrointestinal tract [25], ESD then was applied to the lower gastrointestinal tract with promising results [26]. Although ESD represents an alternative to endoscopic mucosal resection (EMR) of the colon, its application to the rectum can be compared with TEM, aiming to achieve en bloc R0 excision. A meta-analysis [27] including 11 ESD and 10 TEM series (2,077 patients in total) showed that the en bloc resection rate was 87.8 % (95 % confidence interval [CI] 84.3–90.6) for the ESD patients versus 98.7 %

(95 % CI 97.4–99.3 %) for the TEM patients ($P<0.001$). The R0 resection rate was 74.6 % (95 % CI 70.4–78.4 %) for the ESD patients versus 88.5 % (95 % CI 85.9–90.6 %) for the TEM patients ($P<0.001$). The postoperative complications rate was 8.0 % (95 %, CI 5.4–11.8 %) for the ESD patients versus 8.4 % (95 % CI 5.2–13.4 %) for the TEM patients ($P=0.874$). The recurrence rate was 2.6 % (95 % CI 1.3–5.2 %) for the ESD patients versus 5.2 % (95 % CI 4.0–6.9 %) for the TEM patients ($P=0.068$). Nevertheless, the rate for the overall need of further abdominal treatment, defined as any type of surgery performed through an abdominal access, including both complications and pathology indications, was 8.4 % (95 % CI 4.9–13.9 %) for the ESD patients versus 1.8 % (95 % CI 0.8–3.7 %) for the TEM patients ($P<0.001$). Despite the retrospective nature of the studies included, TEM seems to be able to warrant better oncologic results compared to ESD, with similar complication rate. The major advantage advocated by flexible endoscopists is the avoidance of general anaesthesia for ESD technique. We recently collected data of a series of 50 patients who underwent TEM under spinal anaesthesia showing promising results [24]. No intraoperative complications occurred, and operative time was comparable to the procedure performed under general anaesthesia. The need of opioids in the operating room and in the postoperative time was very low, and median postoperative pain assessed by VAS was 0 (range, 0–3) at 4 h, 0 (range, 0–2) at 8 h, 0 (range, 0–2) at 24 h and 0 (range, 0–1) at 48 h. TEM is safe and feasible under spinal anaesthesia and in selected cases will probably become a 1-day surgery procedure. It should be kept in mind that ESD is a long-lasting procedure (many hours) requiring long-lasting sedation and is probably less comfortable for the patient than a spinal anaesthesia. Moreover, due to the low accuracy of the preoperative staging, a full-thickness R0 resection is advisable, and TEM is probably nowadays the best technique to reach this goal in the rectum.

4.4 TAMIS

Transanal minimally invasive surgery (TAMIS) was introduced as an alternative to TEM in 2010. TAMIS is defined as the use of any multichannel port (single port) transanally, combined with the use of ordinary laparoscopic instruments, a laparoscopic camera lens and a standard laparoscopic CO2 insufflator for the purpose of performing endoluminal or, more recently, extraluminal surgery (Fig. 4.6). A systematic review summarised the existing literature on TAMIS [28]. Since the inception of TAMIS in 2009, 33 retrospective studies and case reports and 3 abstracts have been published, including 390 TAMIS procedures for local excision of rectal neoplasms from 16 countries. The average size of the lesions resected was 3.1 cm, and the mean distance to the anal verge was 7.6 cm. Overall margin positivity rate was 4.36 % and mean operative time was 76 min. Only 9 out of 390 excisions (2.31 %) could not be completed with TAMIS and required conversion to TEM or a laparoscopic abdominal approach. The average length of stay was 2 days; the overall complication rate was 7.4 %. A full-thickness excision was

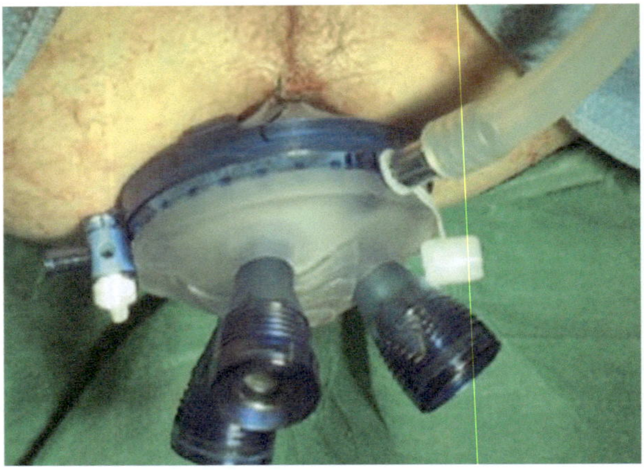

Fig. 4.6 Transanal minimally invasive surgery device (GelPOINT)

performed only in 60.6 % of the publications reviewed; inadvertent peritoneal entry during TAMIS was reported on four cases (1.025 %); in two cases the closure was done transanally. Peritoneal entry during TEM can usually be managed transanally with full-thickness suture closure by experienced operators. A recent publication of a high-experienced group [29] strongly underlines how, in rectal lesions located in the upper rectum, TAMIS was associated with a high risk of complicated peritoneal entry requiring conversion to a rigid platform. Peritoneal entry occurred more frequently during TAMIS (66.7 %) and resulted in critical loss of pneumorectum and collapse of the rectum precluding adequate suture closure. All cases were salvaged by replacing the TAMIS platform with the 12.5-cm-long rigid TEO platform, effectively stenting the rectum open up to the level of the rectal defect, which permitted adequate suture closure of the defect. There is another important limitation of this platform, due to the shape of the single port. With rigid platforms (TEO or TEM), low rectal lesions close to the dentate line can be excised with high precision and stability of the device. The single port used in TAMIS procedure must be placed inside the anal canal, with the proximal edge of the device overcoming the anal sphincter, this way making impossible the access to the lower 5–6 cm of the rectum. Considering both technical limitations, it can be argued that TAMIS is probably a useful and safe technique only for middle rectal lesions, not being able to get access to the lower rectum and not being able to maintain a stable operating field if a peritoneal opening occurs in excising upper rectal lesions (Figs. 4.4 and 4.5).

Furthermore there are many concerns regarding the efficacy of this platform in the most challenging phase of a transanal operation: the suture of the rectal wall. In 2013 we published a pilot study assessing the feasibility and efficacy of TAMIS in an ex vivo model compared to TEM [30]. In a dedicated trainer box for transanal procedures, ten surgeons with no experience in transanal surgery were asked to perform a dissection/suture task using both TAMIS and TEM in randomly allocated order. Dissection and suturing were significantly quicker in the TEM group. In three cases in the TAMIS group, completing the suture was not considered possible, and the procedures were terminated by TEM. Subjective evaluation revealed a better appreciation of TEM in all proposed comparisons: dissection, suturing difficulty, quality of vision and instrument conflicts, concluding that both techniques were comparable for achieving a good dissection, although TAMIS failed to prove effective in suturing the rectal wall.

To overcome this limitation, some authors proposed a robotic TAMIS with the da Vinci system. Hompes et al. [31] showed how robotic TAMIS can be performed using a glove port in a series of 16 patients. Atallah et al. [32] reported a series of 18 robotic TAMIS procedures including complex fistula repair and transanal total mesorectal excision, showing the feasibility of this complex operation. Further research with robotic transanal approaches is necessary to determine whether or not this approach can provide patients' significant benefit.

Last but not least is a consideration about costs. Mark Whiteford, Director of the Colon and Rectal Surgery Unit at the Oregon Clinic, presented during the European Colorectal Congress in 2014 a cost analysis comparing TEM and TAMIS. With a case load of 30 procedures per year, TAMIS is much more expensive (about 11,400–38,000 € per procedure) compared to TEM (about 3600–6600 € per procedure).

Nowadays we can state that local resections performed with TAMIS platform are feasible, but the device has many limitations and is not cost-effective compared to TEM. Randomised controlled trials are needed to really define the real usefulness of TAMIS.

4.5 Extended Indications

Low accuracy of preoperative staging is the biggest issue in properly selecting patients suitable for TEM. T1 tumours invading the rectal wall more than 1 mm in the submucosa (T1 sm2-3) and T2 tumours have a risk of lymph node involvement up to 25 %, which imposes a further TME. TME after full-thickness TEM is a challenging operation, with a significantly higher risk of APR compared to primary TME [33]. After a full-thickness TEM, the primary tumour is completely excised, and the patient has a probability of 75 % or more to have been cured by the transanal procedure alone. So it would be advisable to find a way to warrant the complete 'sterilisation' of the mesorectum, in order to kill metastatic lymph nodes and improve the oncologic outcome of local excisions.

The idea to extend the indication of TEM to T2 tumours by means of a combined neoadjuvant chemoradiotherapy was clearly shown to be effective by Lezoche et al. [34]. In this randomised controlled trial, patients underwent neoadjuvant long-course chemoradiation therapy: 50.4 Gy in 28 fractions associated with a continuous infusion of 5-fluorouracil, 200 mg/m^2/day. Although this schedule showed great efficacy in terms of control of the disease, it is quite uncomfortable for patients, who often are elderly. Moreover, there are concerns regarding the wound healing process after neoadjuvant long-course chemoradiation therapy [35]. We conducted a pilot study to assess short-term outcomes of short-course radiotherapy (25 grays in 5 fractions) followed by TEM after 4–10 weeks for selected T1-T2 N0 extraperitoneal rectal cancers [36]. Unfortunately we had to stop the study after 14 cases for unexpected extremely disappointing results. Although no intraoperative complications occurred, rectal suture dehiscence was observed in seven patients (50 %) at 4 weeks follow-up, associated with an enterocutaneous fistula in the sacral area in two cases. With a median follow-up of 10 months (range: 6–26 months), we observed 1 (7 %) local recurrence at 6 months that was treated with abdominoperineal resection. We concluded that neoadjuvant short-course radiotherapy followed by TEM is burdened by a high rate of painful dehiscence of the suture line and enterocutaneous fistula and should be abandoned.

4.6 Future Perspectives

The possibility to extend the indications of TEM depends on the capability to assess lymph node status, either preoperatively or intraoperatively. We tried to detect positive lymph nodes applying the concept of sentinel lymph node (SLN) biopsy to suspected invasive rectal cancers treated by TEM [37]. Before the beginning of the intervention, indocyanine green solution (ICG) was injected submucosally underneath the lesion, at the four cardinal points. Once the primary neoplasm was excised and the perirectal fat widely exposed from the inside, a dedicated 10-mm near-infrared (NIR) optic was inserted into one of the working channels, and its illumination switched to fluorescence-guided image. NIR fluorescence emitting ICG previously injected designed a map of mesorectal lymphatic vessels and nodes, which were excised and sent to the pathologist for final examination. In all cases, the pathologist confirmed the presence of lymph nodes in the excised tissue and no case showed metastasis. This is only a preliminary report and the technique has to be validated. What makes this technique very interesting is the submucosal injection of the dye and the dissection of the mesorectal fat through the rectal wall. This warrants to maintain the integrity of the mesorectal fascia, allowing further TME if necessary and not jeopardising the oncologic outcome.

Rectal-sparing surgery represents the paradigm of real minimally invasive surgery. Tarantino et al. developed a new technique called endoscopic posterior mesorectal resection (EPMR) [38]. After local excision and histological confirmation of a T1 rectal cancer, distant metastases were excluded by means of abdomino-pelvic computed tomography and chest radiography. The specimens removed by TEM were analysed histologically for radical resection and for risk criteria, and then a rectum-preserving EPMR was performed 4–6 weeks after. With the patient in a prone jackknife position, the retrorectal space was dilated with a distension balloon system through a perineal incision. Using a three-port access, the posterior part of the mesorectum was dissected from the posterior wall of the rectum. Resected tissue was examined histologically with regard to the number of lymph nodes and existence of lymph node metastases. Even if this technique does not allow a complete mesorectal excision, it removes the posterior and lateral fat of the mesorectum, where the majority of lymphatic tissue is located. Authors included in this publication only T1 cancer showing good results in terms of oncological outcome: no recurrences even if only 2 out of 25 patients were node positive. The technique is extremely promising, but further evaluation is mandatory.

A new technique combining both abdominal and transanal approaches to perform a precise TME in low rectal cancers has been recently developed. In transanal total mesorectal excision (TaTME), the rectum is mobilised transanally in a retrograde fashion by means of TEM or TAMIS platforms. A recent meta-analysis [39] including 36 retrospective studies concluded that TaTME is a safe and reproducible technique with excellent results in terms of negative circumferential margin rate (95 %) and negative distal margin rate (99.7 %). For very low tumours located in a narrow pelvis, this technique represents an innovative solution to get a good quality specimen and reduce local recurrences. Further studies are needed to strongly validate the technique and to show a real clinical benefit.

Conclusion

Transanal endoscopic microsurgery represented a revolution in rectal surgery, which opened new unexplored horizons overcoming the purpose the technique was thought for. Rectal-sparing surgery should be the goal in treating early rectal cancer, but only if capable to warrant a radical and curative resection. In order to do this, patients' selection has to be improved and innovative multidisciplinary therapies have to be implemented. While some T1 rectal cancers benefit of a TME, a consistent number of T2 rectal cancers, as high as 75 %, can be safely cured by a simple local excision alone. A consistent improvement in rectal cancer staging will therefore allow a real tailored therapy, contributing to a significant reduction of invasiveness of the treatment.

References

1. Hompes R, Cunningham C. Extending the role of Transanal Endoscopic Microsurgery (TEM) in rectal cancer. Colorectal Dis. 2011;13 Suppl 7:32–6.
2. Moore JS, Cataldo PA, Osler T. Hyman NH Transanal endoscopic microsurgery is more effective than traditional transanal excision for resection of rectal masses. Dis Colon Rectum. 2008;51(7):1026–30.
3. Partecipants in the Paris Workshop, The Paris endoscopic classification of superficial neoplastic lesions: esophagus, stomach and colon. Gastrointest Endosc. 2003;58:S3–S43.
4. Haggitt RC, Glotzbach RE, Soffer EE, Wruble LD. Prognostic factors in colorectal carcinomas arising in adenomas: implications for lesions removed by endoscopic polypectomy. Gastroenterology. 1985;89:328–36.
5. Kikuchi R, Takano M, Takagi K, Fujimoto N, Nozaki R, Fujiyoshi T, Uchida Y. Management of early invasive colorectal cancer: risk of recurrence and clinical guidelines. Dis Colon Rectum. 1995;38:1286–95.
6. Nascimbeni R, Burgart LJ, Nivatvongs S, Larson DR. Risk of lymph node metastasis in T1 carcinoma of the colon and rectum. Dis Colon Rectum. 2002;45:200–6.
7. Kudo S, Lambert R, Allen JI, Fujii H, Fujii T, Kashida H, Matsuda T, Mori M, Saito H, Shimoda T, Tanaka S, Watanabe H, Sung JJ, Feld AD, Inadomi JM, O'Brien MJ, Lieberman DA,

Ransohoff DF, Soetikno RM, Triadafilopoulos G, Zauber A, Teixeira CR, Rey JF, Jaramillo E, Rubio CA, Van Gossum A, Jung M, Vieth M, Jass JR, Hurlstone PD. Nonpolypoid neoplastic lesions of the colorectal mucosa. Gastrointest Endosc. 2008;68:S3–S47.

8. Bach SP, Hill J, Monson JR, et al. A predictive model for local recurrence after transanal endoscopic microsurgery for rectal cancer. Br J Surg. 2009;96:280–90.
9. Hahnloser D, Wolff BG, Larson DW, et al. Immediate radical resection after local excision of rectal cancer: an oncologic compromise? Dis Colon Rectum. 2005;48:429–37.
10. Nishizawa M, Okada T, Sato F, Kariya A, Mayama S, Nakamura K. A clinicopathological study of minute polypoid lesions of the colon based on magnifying fiber-colonoscopy and dissecting microscopy. Endoscopy. 1980;12:124–9.
11. Tada M, Kawai K. Research with the endoscope: new techniques using magnification and chromoscopy. Clin Gastroenterol. 1986;15:417–37.
12. Kudo S, Hirota S, Nakajima T, Hosobe S, Kusaka H, Kobayashi T, et al. Colorectal tumours and pit pattern. J Clin Pathol. 1994;47:880–5.
13. Ko WJ, An P, Ko KH, Hahm KB, Hong SP, Cho JY. Image quality analysis of various gastrointestinal endoscopes: Why image quality is a prerequisite for proper diagnostic and therapeutic endoscopy. Clin Endosc. 2015;48(5):374–9.
14. Marone P, de Bellis M, D'Angelo V, Delrio P, Passananti V, Di Girolamo E, Rossi GB, Rega D, Tracey MC, Tempesta AM. Role of endoscopic ultrasonography in the loco-regional staging of patients with rectal cancer. World J Gastrointest Endosc. 2015;7(7):688–701.
15. Marusch F, Ptok H, Sahm M, Schmidt U, Ridwelski K, Gastinger I, Lippert H. Endorectal ultrasound in rectal carcinoma--do the literature results really correspond to the realities of routine clinical care? Endoscopy. 2011;43:425–31.
16. Morino M, Risio M, Bach S, Beets-Tan R, Bujko K, Panis Y, Quirke P, Rembacken B, Rullier E, Saito Y, Young-Fadok T, Allaix ME, European Association for Endoscopic Surgery, European Society of Coloproctology. . Early rectal cancer: the European Association for Endoscopic Surgery (EAES) clinical consensus conference. Surg Endosc. 2015;29(4):755–73.
17. Tominaga K, Fujinuma S, Endo T, Saida Y, Takahashi K, Maetani I. Efficacy of the revised Vienna classification for diagnosing colorectal epithelial neoplasias. World J Gastroenterol. 2009;15:2351–6.
18. Jung M. The 'difficult' polyp: pitfalls for endoscopic removal. Dig Dis. 2012;30 Suppl 2:74–80.
19. Park W, Kim B, Park SJ, Cheon JH, Kim TI, Kim WH, Hong SP. Conventional endoscopic features are not sufficient to differentiate small, early colorectal cancer. World J Gastroenterol. 2014;20(21):6586–93.
20. Brown G, Davies S, Williams GT, Bourne MW, Newcombe RG, Radcliffe AG, Blethyn J, Dallimore NS, Rees BI, Phillips CJ, Maughan TS. Effectiveness of preoperative staging in rectal cancer: digital rectal examination, endorectal ultrasound or magnetic resonance imaging? Br J Cancer. 2004;91:23–9.
21. Rafaelson SR, Kronberg O, Fenger C. Digital rectal examination and transrectal ultrasonography in staging of rectal cancer. A prospective, blind study. Acta Radiol. 1994;35:300–4.
22. Thumbe V, Iqbal M, Bhalerao S. Accuracy of digital rectal examination in the estimation of height of rectal lesions. Tech Coloproctol. 2007;11:111–3.
23. Allaix ME, Arezzo A, Arolfo S, Caldart M, Rebecchi F, Morino M. Transanal endoscopic microsurgery for rectal neoplasms. How I Do It. J Gastrointest Surg. 2013;17(3):586–92.
24. Arezzo A, Cortese G, Arolfo S, Bullano A, Passera R, Galietti E, Morino M. Transanal Endoscopic Operation (TEO®) under spinal anaesthesia. Br J Surg. 2016;103(7):916–20.
25. Ohkuwa M, Hosokawa K, Boku N, et al. New endoscopic treatment for intramucosal gastric tumors using an insulated-tip diathermic knife. Endoscopy. 2001;33:221–6.
26. Tamegai Y, Saito Y, Masaki N, et al. Endoscopic submucosal dissection: a safe technique for colorectal tumors. Endoscopy. 2007;39:418–22.
27. Arezzo A, Passera R, Saito Y, Sakamoto T, Kobayashi N, Sakamoto N, Yoshida N, Naito Y, Fujishiro M, Niimi K, Ohya T, Ohata K, Okamura S, Iizuka S, Takeuchi Y, Uedo N, Fusaroli P, Bonino MA, Verra M, Morino M. Systematic review and meta-analysis of endoscopic submu-

cosal dissection versus transanal endoscopic microsurgery for large noninvasive rectal lesions. Surg Endosc. 2014;28(2):427–38.
28. Martin-Perez B, Andrade-Ribeiro GD, Hunter L, Atallah S. A systematic review of Transanal Minimally Invasive Surgery (TAMIS) from 2010 to 2013. Tech Coloproctol. 2014;18:775–88.
29. Molina G, Bordeianou L, Shellito P, Sylla P. Transanal endoscopic resection with peritoneal entry: a word of caution. Surg Endosc. 2016;30(5):1816–25. doi:10.1007/s00464-015-4452-y.
30. Rimonda R, Arezzo A, Arolfo S, Alessandro Salvai A, Morino M. TransAnal Minimally Invasive Surgery (TAMIS) with SILS™ Port versus Transanal Endoscopic Microsurgery (TEM): a comparative experimental study. Surg Endosc. 2013;27:3762–8.
31. Hompes R, Rauh SM, Ris F, Tuynman JB, Mortensen NJ. Robotic transanal minimally invasive surgery for local excision of rectal neoplasms. Br J Surg. 2014;101:578–81.
32. Atallah S, Martin-Perez B, Parra-Davila E, deBeche-Adams T, Nassif G, Albert M, Larach S. Robotic transanal surgery for local excision of rectal neoplasia, transanal total mesorectal excision, and repair of complex fistulae: clinical experience with the first 18 cases at a single institution. Tech Coloproctol. 2015;19:401–10.
33. Morino M, Allaix ME, Arolfo S, Arezzo A. Previous transanal endoscopic microsurgery for rectal cancer represents a risk factor for an increased abdominoperineal resection rate. Surg Endosc. 2013;27:3315–21.
34. Lezoche E, Baldarelli M, Lezoche G, et al. Randomized clinical trial of endoluminal locoregional resection versus laparoscopic total mesorectal excision for T2 rectal cancer after neoadjuvant therapy. Br J Surg. 2012;99:1211–8.
35. Marks JH, Valsdottir EB, DeNittis A, et al. Transanal endoscopic microsurgery for the treatment of rectal cancer: comparison of wound complication rates with and without neoadjuvant radiation therapy. Surg Endosc. 2009;23:1081–7.
36. Arezzo A, Arolfo S, Allaix ME, Munoz F, Cassoni P, Monagheddu C, Ricardi U, Ciccone G. Morino M Results of neoadjuvant short-course radiation therapy followed by transanal endoscopic microsurgery for t1-t2 n0 extraperitoneal rectal cancer. Int J Radiat Oncol Biol Phys. 2015;92(2):299–306.
37. Arezzo A, Arolfo S, Mistrangelo M, Mussa B, Cassoni P, Morino M. Transrectal sentinel lymph node biopsy for early rectal cancer during transanal endoscopic microsurgery. Minim Invasive Ther Allied Technol. 2014;23(1):17–20.
38. Tarantino I, Hetzer FH, Warschkow R, Zünd M, Stein HJ, Zerz A. Local excision and endoscopic posterior mesorectal resection versus low anterior resection in T1 rectal cancer. Br J Surg. 2008;95(3):375–80.
39. Simillis C, Hompes R, Penna M, Rasheed S, Tekkis PP. A systematic review of transanal total mesorectal excision. Is this the future of rectal cancer surgery? Colorectal Dis. 2016;18(1): 19–36. doi:10.1111/codi.13151.

5 Unusual Applications of Metal Stents in Gastrointestinal Tract

Angelo Caruso and Andrea Parodi

5.1 Introduction

Much progress has been made since Coyas deployed the first esophageal stent in a patient with a malignant esophageal stricture in 1955 [1]. Over time, many steps have been taken in the search for the most suitable material for gastrointestinal endoprosthesis: the first stents were rigid, made of materials such as rubber, ivory, sandalwood, and polyvinyl. In most cases they were "homemade."

Self-expandable metallic stents (SEMS) have been the main turning point, ensuring a widespread of these devices in the gastroenterological field, initially for the treatment of malignant esophageal strictures, subsequently of colon cancer obstruction and then in a wide variety of clinical scenarios.

SEMS consist of a mesh of braided metal wires that are assembled in a tubelike structure. They are available in different lengths and calibers, and they can be with or without coating. Physical properties of materials, texture, and shape determine the radial and longitudinal force exerted by SEMS when released. Therefore, the technical characteristics of stents must be known in order to use the most appropriate device in the various clinical situations.

The first alloy used in the construction of SEMS was stainless steel, with different percentages of iron, chromium, and molybdenum; the latter helps to stabilize the crystal structure and to determine the physical characteristics. The final process of electropolishing removes most of the elements from the metal surface leaving a high concentration of chromium; after exposure to air and sterilization, a layer of a

A. Caruso (✉)
Digestive Endoscopy Unit, Baggiovara Hospital, Modena, Italy

New Civil Hospital -Baggiovara, Viale Giardini 1355, 41100 Modena, Italy
e-mail: angelocaruso@hotmail.it

A. Parodi
Department of Gastroenterology and Digestive Endoscopy, Ospedale Galliera, Genoa, Italy

R. Conigliaro, M. Frazzoni (eds.), *Diagnosis and Endoscopic Management of Digestive Diseases*, DOI 10.1007/978-3-319-42358-6_5

few nanometers in thickness stabilizes the surface and prevents oxidation. Surface defects and trace elements can cause changes in protein and affect cellular reactions. Other materials used in the construction of stents are titanium and nitinol (nickel-titanium alloy). Titanium is a metallic element well known for its resistance to corrosion (almost as much as platinum) and for its high strength/weight ratio. It is lightweight and tough, with a low density (40 % of that of steel). When it is in the pure state, it is quite ductile, shiny, white metal. Titanium is as strong as steel but 45 % lighter. Titanium is also used as an alloy. Nitinol is instead a superelastic alloy composed of nickel-titanium, which belongs to the category of "shape memory" metals (Shape Memory Alloys, SMA). In particular, the term shape memory alloys indicates a broad class of metal alloys, discovered fairly recently, which are able to recover a macroscopic preset form, thanks to the simple change of temperature. When an SMA is below its transformation temperature, it can be deformed quite easily; however, if we heat the material above the transformation temperature, it takes over a change in the crystal structure which causes the return to the original form and develops considerable force. Moreover, they have other characteristics, such as the superelastic behavior, which has multiplied the possibilities of use and the ability to generate high forces in the recovery phase of the shape. Greater flexibility and more accurate positioning in angled segments are favored by the introduction of a heart of platinum within the nitinol wire: this material is called platinol. Another alloy called elgiloy used in the manufacture of SEMS is constituted by cobalt-chromium-nickel which gives a combination of high strength, ductility, with good mechanical properties.

The presence of coating is of great interest and determines the possibility of application of SEMS in particular clinical situations: in fact, uncovered SEMS have a greater gripping at the level of the visceral wall, but they cannot generally be removed and over time are likely to experience neoplastic or granulation tissue ingrowth within the stent meshes, with subsequent obstruction. On the other hand, fully covered SEMS are at increased risk of migration, given the reduced gripping, but can be removed and are less likely to encounter ingrowth. Moreover, they can be useful in the presence of visceral wall perforation or fistula. Partially covered SEMS are also available: they have a complete coating at the level of the body and bare ends. This type of SEMS has theoretically a lower risk of migration compared to completely coated ones and allows to exploit the cover at the level of the body, for example, to treat a defect in the gastrointestinal wall.

Currently the most widely used coating materials are polyethylene terephthalate (PET), polytetrafluoroethylene (PTFE), and polyurethane (PU, used only in few cases). PET is a polymer composed of long chains of glycol and terephthalic acid: its good expansion force derives from high dissociation energy of covalent bonds of the polymer chains. It has a high surface energy and a weaving disposed in the longitudinal or transversal space which gives elasticity. PTFE is composed of carbon chains saturated with fluorine: the final structure is somewhat rigid and chemically stable. This explains some of the characteristics of this polymer, such as the low coefficient of friction, the high melting point, and the low surface energy. These physical properties are correlated with some biological behaviors, such as small tissue reaction. PU, unlike PET and PTFE, can be rigid or soft according to its composition. Compared to the past, polyurethanes have been abandoned by their low biodegradability; current ones have a higher biodegradability. The key features are the porosity of the material, the expansion about six times the diameter in closing, and the high surface energy.

SEMS also differ in the delivery system: currently available stents are mounted on systems that can be introduced into the working channel of the endoscope (through-the-scope, TTS) or on larger diameter catheters that go directly on guidewire (over-the-wire, OTW) and which cannot be introduced into the working channel of the endoscope. Both devices are constituted by a system of coaxial tubes in which the stent is loaded around a catheter that carries the guidewire, forced inside a shorter carrier catheter. Once this is retracted, SEMS is released from the distal end. Some systems allow instead of releasing the stent starting from the proximal flare. Another delivery system consists of a catheter on which the stent is maintained fixed with a braided suture. The prosthesis is gradually released by pulling a ring connected to the wire that allows to unravel the suture (Ultraflex esophageal or colonic stents, Boston Scientific, Natick, Massachusetts). Therefore, also the characteristics of delivery systems must be carefully considered in relation to the seat and to the characteristics of the target lesion.

Currently, SEMS with particular technical characteristics are available on the market, such as anti-reflux valves and anti-migration systems. Such devices may be used to make a more tailored endoscopic therapeutic approach to the patient.

Finally we must remember that nonmetallic stents are also available: biodegradable stents (ELLA-CS, Trebes, Czech Republic) and self-expanding plastic stents (SEPS, Polyflex, Boston Scientific, Natick, Massachusetts). These latter have found wide application in the treatment of benign esophageal strictures as an alternative to SEMS.

Enteral SEMS are a nonsurgical alternative for the palliative treatment of malignant esophageal and colonic strictures. In this chapter, we will discuss the role of SEMS in some particular clinical situations in the upper and lower digestive tract, taking into account also benign disorders, gastrointestinal perforations, and anastomotic leakages after surgery.

5.2 Unusual Application of Stents in Upper GI Tract

5.2.1 Upper Malignant Esophageal Strictures

The tumors of the cervical esophagus account for approximately 10 % of esophageal cancers, and they are commonly considered difficult to manage. The use of SEMS in the palliation of dysphagia in inoperable patients is particularly controversial because frequently stents may evoke an unbearable foreign body sensation in the pharynx. In addition, more rarely, they can cause dangerous complications such as aspiration of the bolus in the larynx, perforation or esophagotracheal fistula, or proximal migration with airway obstruction.

In 1999 Conio et al. described the use of SEMS in the palliation of dysphagia in six patients with squamocellular upper esophageal cancer. Stents were deployed within 2 cm of the cricopharyngeal muscle, under simultaneous endoscopic and fluoroscopic control. Dysphagia improved significantly in all patients. Four patients had tumor ingrowth, and three of them were successfully treated by placing a second SEMS. No patient complained of globus sensation [2]. Macdondald et al. reported 22 patients with malignant strictures of cervical esophagus treated with SEMS, which was correctly placed in 93 % of cases, among them 82 % reported no foreign body sensation [3]. Other authors reported similar results [4, 5]. A more recent study by Parker et al. compared a large group of patients with cervical esophageal cancer and a matched control group of patients with distal esophageal cancer. They found no differences in terms of clinical success, survival rate, and complication rate between the two groups [6]. Also in a large study by Verschuur et al., 104 patients with primary esophageal carcinoma or recurrent cancer after gastric tube interposition within 8 cm distance distal of the UES were treated with SEMS [7]. Twenty-four (23 %) patients also had a tracheoesophageal fistula. Technical success was 96 %, with significant improvement of dysphagia in all treated patients and fistula sealing was achieved in 79 % of cases. However, major complications (aspiration pneumonia, hemorrhage, fistula, and perforation) occurred in 21 % of patients. Persistent globus sensation was reported by 8 % of patients; however, none of them required stent retrieval [7]. In conclusion, while lacking large prospective randomized trials, the use of SEMS in the treatment of stenosis of the cervical esophagus is considered to be useful and safe in expert hands.

Though the use of large-diameter SEMS in the treatment of cervical esophageal strictures [8] has been described, we recommend the use of small caliber stents, possibly with a small proximal flare. Several SEMS were designed with specific features for this purpose [9]. The body of the stent should not exceed 16 mm in size. Smaller sizes are recommended in patients who have undergone radiation therapy, due to an increased risk of esophagotracheal fistula. Furthermore, the stent should be completely covered, in order to easily remove, in the event the patient develops a feeling of foreign body.

5.2.2 Benign Esophageal Strictures

Although the use of SEMS in the treatment of malignant esophageal strictures is considered effective, their use in benign refractory stenosis has number of issues. Benign strictures can be caused by gastroesophageal reflux disease, caustic ingestion, radiation therapy, and sclerotherapy, or they can occur on surgical anastomosis. If despite repeated sessions of dilation with bougies or balloon, dysphagia persists; SEMS become a therapeutic option. Since this is a benign disease, the stent used should be removable after obtaining the degree of expansion desired, so the choice should fall on covered or partially covered SEMS [10, 11]. Partially covered SEMS guarantee better gripping to the esophageal wall and have a lower risk of distal migration. However, studies available in the literature demonstrate a high rate of complications with this type of stent. In particular, the most feared complication is the appearance of ingrowth of granulation tissue at the level of bare heads of the endoprosthesis [12]. In these cases, it is possible to place a fully covered SEMS inside the previous one: in this way it is possible to remove both stents after 10–14 days, because the pressure exerted by the coated stent determines necrosis of the granulation tissue [13]. As previously indicated, also self-expanding plastic stents/biodegradable stents have been widely indicated for the treatment in refractory benign esophageal strictures [14]. In a recent pooled analysis of 232 patients with refractory benign esophageal strictures treated with self-expandable stent placement, technical and clinical success resulted to be quite disappointing. Fully covered SEMS were correctly deployed in 85 % of patients, but only 14.1 % experienced a significant clinical improvement of dysphagia [15]. Also with biodegradable stents and self-expanding plastic stents, authors reported poor rate of technical and clinical success (67 %, 25 % and 77 %, 12 %, respectively) [15]. In the same study, the overall rate of severe complications was 17.7 %. Among 85 subjects treated with SEMS, five patients had severe retrosternal pain, two severe nausea and vomiting, two aspiration pneumonia, and one arrhythmia [15]. SEMS migration occurred in 31.8 % of patients treated with fully covered stents, while tissue ingrowth occurred only in 3.5 % of patients. Stent removal was planned after 4–12 weeks and was successfully achieved in 97.6 % of cases [15]. In the light of these data, we believe the treatment of benign stenosis with covered or partially covered SEMS should be considered only in those patients who are refractory to dilation and who are unfit for surgery (Fig. 5.1).

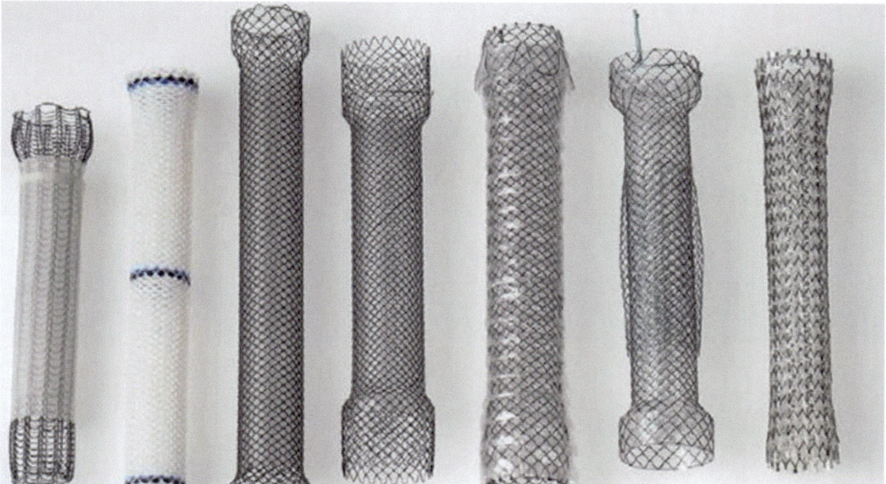

Fig. 5.1 Panorama of esophageal stent. From the *left* to the *right*: Partially covered stent (Ultraflex), Polyflex stent, Partially covered stent (Evolution), Fully covered stent (SX-Ella), fully covered stent (Niti-S antimigration), fully covered stent (Alimaxx-E stent)

5.2.3 Benign Esophageal Leakages or Fistula

Benign esophageal leakages or fistula are frequently encountered and require urgent intervention to the high risk of sepsis and the high mortality rate. Anastomotic leakage may occur in up to 10 % of patients undergoing esophageal resection. Also iatrogenic perforation or Boerhaave syndrome have been successfully treated with SEMS. As shown in Fig. 5.2, the placement of covered or partially covered SEMS constitutes an indication to treat an esophageal fistula resulting in a valid alternative to surgery, favoring the healing of the defect in the esophageal wall, the control of sepsis, and a more rapid intake of an oral diet. A recent meta-analysis of Dasari et al. reported data on 117 patients from 12 studies [16]. Technical and clinical successes were 96.5 % and 86.2 %, respectively. Stent migration occurred in 11 % of treated patients. However, five patients had a perforation induced by stent, two of them due to erosion of the wall of the aorta [16]. Endoscopic reintervention and surgical intervention were needed in 5 % and 15 % of cases, respectively [16]. In the same meta-analysis, the authors also considered patients treated with SEPS: the data show that they have a higher incidence of migration and need more frequent endoscopic reoperation, while the need for a surgical intervention does not seem to significantly differ from that of SEMS [16]. The use of SEMS in the treatment of a defect in the esophageal wall must be always taken into account: the choice of the stent must take account of the greater risk of migration in the absence of stenosis. We believe the choice should fall on large-diameter partially covered SEMS. The removal must be programmed within 4–6 weeks, in order to minimize the risk of ingrowth. Also in this scenario, the stent-in-stent technique should be considered in case of embedment [13]. It is also

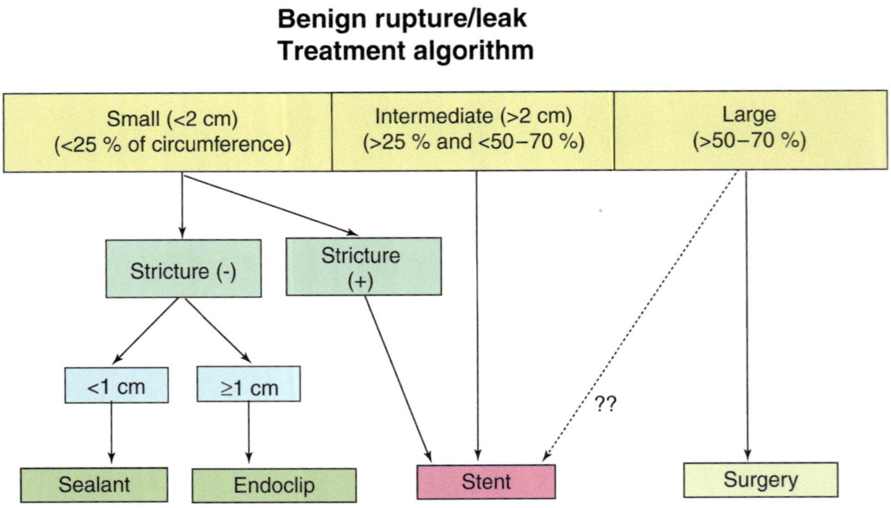

Fig. 5.2 Diagram indications to apply stents in esophageal fistula or rupture (Esophageal perforation In: Tham T, Collins J and Soetikno R, eds. *Gastrointestinal Emergencies* Oxford: Blackwell Publishing Ltd 2008)

necessary to remember that any periesophageal collection must be drained, and the patient must always be treated with broad-spectrum antibiotics.

5.2.4 Variceal Bleeding

Active bleeding from esophageal varices is considered a major cause of mortality in patients with decompensated liver cirrhosis. Treatment is currently based on vaso-active drugs, band ligation or sclerosis, and antibiotic therapy; however, they can fail in 10–15 % of patients. Tamponade balloon or the positioning of TIPSS may be proposed in these cases, however in clinical practice, TIPSS is not readily available quickly. Over the past 10 years, many cases of patients with refractory variceal bleeding treated with SEMS with excellent results have been described in literature, so that the 2015 Baveno Workshop on portal hypertension has proposed the placement of SEMS as a possible therapeutic option, awaiting further confirmations from clinical trials [17]. A review by Changela et al. showed data about 103 cases of patients treated with fully covered SEMS: Technical success rate was 97 %, with a bleeding control achieved in 96 % of treated patients. All SEMS were successfully removed after 4–14 days. Stent migration occurred in about 21 % of patients [18]. A more recent systematic review with meta-analysis took into account data on 13 studies [19]. The pooled estimate rates were 0.12 (95 % CI = 0.07–0.21) for variceal bleeding mortality and 0.18 (95 % CI = 0.11–0.29) for failure to control bleeding with SEMS [19]. The available data suggest that a proportion of less than 40 % of patients with refractory variceal bleeding dies 1 month after placement of SEMS. Therefore SEMS could be considered as a bridge therapy in selected patients undergoing other interventions such as TIPSS or liver transplantation. The choice must fall on a completely covered and large-diameter stent. The removal must be scheduled within 2 weeks, making it easier to prevent the removal of the device, reducing the risk of injury and variceal rebleeding.

5.2.5 Esophageal Achalasia

Therapeutic interventions for endoscopic esophageal achalasia include pneumatic dilation, intrasphincteric injection of botulinum toxin, and most recently the peroral endoscopic myotomy (POEM). The rate of clinical remission obtained with pneumatic dilatation, however, dramatically decreases over time from 20 to 60 % in 10 years. Temporary placement of large-diameter SEMS at the level of the cardia has been proposed as a possible therapeutic intervention in patients with achalasia. The rationale of their use is linked to the possibility to perform a gradual and prolonged dilation at the level of the lower esophageal sphincter, which, compared to traditional pneumatic dilation, should secure better long-term results.

In a study by Ying-Sheng, 90 patients with achalasia have been treated with different size SEMS: 20, 25, and 30 mm. Partially covered SEMS have been deployed across the esophageal cardia, and they were left in place for 4–5 days, before being removed. Technical success was achieved in all patients; however, best results were obtained with larger-diameter SEMS: the treatment failure rate was lower in patients treated with 30 mm SEMS (13 %) compared to the other groups [20]. SEMS migration occurred more frequently in patients receiving 20 and 25 mm SEMS. Moreover, patients were followed up to 10 years and larger-diameter SEMS showed better long-term results [20]. Similar results have been reported also in other studies [21–23]. In another study comparing SEMS and pneumatic dilation, a temporary, 30-mm diameter SEMS was associated with a better long-term clinical efficacy in the treatment of patients with achalasia [22]. Similar better long-term outcomes have been shown in another study comparing removable SEMS and botulinum toxin injection [23]. While these data are promising, studies from Western countries are lacking, and SEMS dedicated to achalasia are not widespread used.

5.2.6 Staple Line Leaks Postlaparoscopic Sleeve Gastrectomy

The use of SEMS deserves a special mention in the treatment of staple line dehiscence after laparoscopic sleeve gastrectomy. This is the most feared complication of this surgery, providing greater morbidity. Its incidence varies depending on the series but seems to have decreased over time from 2.5 % to 1.1 % [24]. However other authors reported higher incidence of leakages up to 20 %, also in experienced hands [25]. Leakage typically develops at the esophagogastric junction and proximal stomach, near the angle of His. The cause of leakage is to be attributed to an altered healing process of the suture line, which depends on many risk factors, such as ischemia due to the devascularization of gastric wall. An increased intraluminal pressure of gastric tube has also been invoked as another mechanism involved in staple line leaks, especially if the gastric tube is little distensible or if there is a stricture of the sleeve [26]. Although it is not accepted by all, in recent years, several authors have proposed the use of fully covered SEMS in the treatment of this type of fistula with variable results [27, 28]. Only the leakages located at the esophagogastric junction or the proximal portion of gastric tube are susceptible to such treatment. SEMS migration is the most frequent complication, occurring in up to 30 % of cases. Therefore these SEMS should be as wide and as long as possible, in order to prevent dislocation. Many authors remove them after 6–8 weeks to ensure complete healing of the fistula. Recently covered SEMS with a large diameter and length have been introduced on the market, dedicated to the treatment of staple line leaks postlaparoscopic sleeve gastrectomy (Megastent, Taewoong Medical co, South Korea). It is a completely coated prosthesis with a large diameter (24–28 mm) and varying in length from 15 to 23 cm. This stent has two large flares in the proximal and distal part, ensuring an optimal gripping. Moreover, given its length, the proximal and distal ends can be opened upstream of the leak in the esophagus and in the duodenal bulb, respectively. This allows to reset the high pressure within the gastric tube, promoting the healing of the fistula. A recent case series by Galloro et al. showed that Megastent was effective in four patients with staple leaks, allowing rapid resumption of enteral nutrition and early discharge [26] (Fig. 5.3).

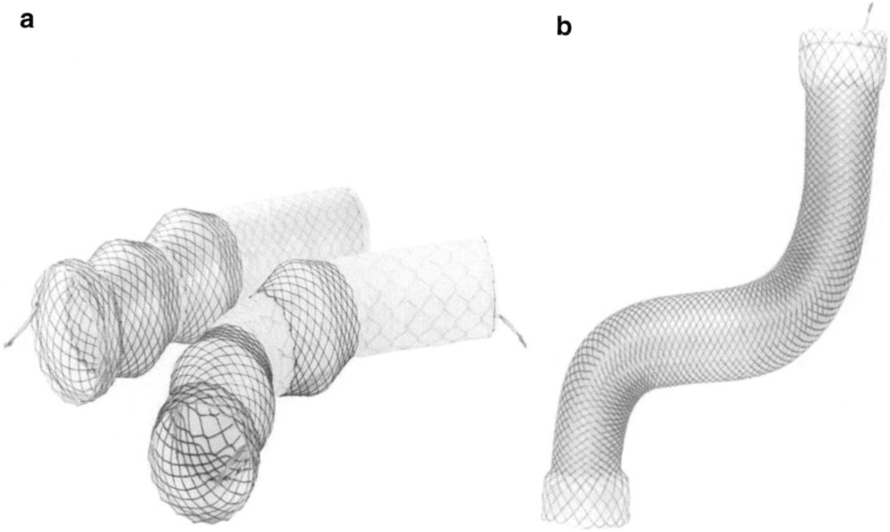

Fig. 5.3 Stent used to treat staple line leaks postlaparoscopic sleeve gastrectomy (**a** Betastent, Taewoong; **b** Megastent, Taewoong) (www.stent.net)

5.3 Unusual Application of Stents in Low GI Tract

Placement of SEMS within the low GI tract is an advanced endoscopic technique used to treat a variety of condition including obstruction, fistula, and perforation.

The most common indication for low GI tract stenting is the colon malignant obstruction. There are two major indications for colonic stenting in patients with colorectal cancer: palliation of advanced disease and preoperative decompression. In the latter case, placement of a stent can convert a surgical procedure from an emergent two-step procedure (including a colostomy) into an elective one-step resection with a primary anastomosis, which can be performed laparoscopically [29].

Large-bowel obstruction caused by advanced colon cancer occurs in three-fourths of all malignant colonic obstruction. The management of this severe clinical condition remains controversial.

The majority of colon cancer causing obstruction are localized to the left side of the colon, with the sigmoid colon being the most common location. Extrinsic colon cancer (in particular pelvic tumors) can infiltrate the colonic wall and may cause a lumen obstruction or a colonic compression. Malignant colonic obstruction may be treated by using conventional surgery with resection or diversion procedures, but patients presenting with malignant obstruction often are poor surgical candidates. Patients treated with a diverting colostomy frequently retain the stoma indefinitely because of the discovery of metastatic disease [30]. Urgent surgical intervention in this setting is associated with a mortality rate of 10 % and morbidity up to 40 % [31]. The most important endoscopic alternative to the urgent surgical management of malignant colonic obstruction is the placement of SEMS.

Over the last decade, many articles have been published on the subject of colonic stenting for malignant colonic obstruction, including randomized controlled trials (RCTs) and systematic reviews. However, the definitive role of self-expandable metal stents (SEMS) in the treatment of malignant colonic obstruction has not yet been clarified, and a collaborative approach to patient management, including surgeons and endoscopists, is recommended to guide patient care [31].

5.3.1 Self-Expanding Metallic Stents for Malignant Obstruction

Endoscopic placement of colorectal stents is an effective alternative to surgical decompression for colonic obstruction. In a pooled analysis of 54 trials, reporting on 1198 patients with malignant colorectal obstruction, SEMS placement achieved clinical success in 91 % [32]. In the most current review of 88 articles incorporating the results of SEMS placement in 1785 patients for malignant colonic obstruction, clinical success was achieved at a median rate of 92 % [33]. Serious complications, including colon perforations, were reported in 5 % of patients in each of these two papers.

Two precautions emerge from these studies. First, stricture dilation before or immediately after stent placement results in a five- to sixfold higher rate of perforation (10 %–18 %) and should generally be avoided [32]. Second, covered stents may have inferior outcomes compared with uncovered stents because of a significantly higher migration rate (31 % vs. 3 %) [33].

Although excellent right-side colonic SEMS placement outcomes have been reported from expert centers, data are more limited than for left-side colonic SEMS placement.

5.3.2 Colonic SEMS as a Bridge to Surgery

In patients with malignant colonic obstruction who are candidates for surgical resection, placement of a colonic SEMS allows colonic decompression without the morbidity and mortality of urgent surgery.

The most recent systematic review and meta-analysis evaluated the efficacy and safety of colonic stenting as a bridge to surgery ($n = 195$) compared with emergency surgery ($n = 187$). All seven RCTs that focused on the postoperative outcome of SEMS and emergency surgery were included in this meta-analysis. The mean technical success rate of colonic stent placement was 76.9 % (range 46.7 %–100 %). There was no statistically significant difference in the postoperative mortality comparing SEMS as bridge to surgery (10.7 %) and emergency surgery (12.4 %). The meta-analysis showed a lower overall morbidity (33.1 % vs. 53.9 %, $P = 0.03$), a higher successful primary anastomosis rate (67.2 % vs. 55.1 %, $P < 0.01$), and a lower permanent stoma rate (9 % vs. 27.4 %, $P < 0.01$) in the SEMS group [34].

According to these results, SEMS placement are related to significantly lower complication rates and shorter hospital stays, better health-related quality of life, and reduced costs.

Moreover, the relief of symptoms provided by SEMS placement allows additional time to stabilize the patient, address underlying comorbid medical illnesses, perform a thorough staging evaluation of the cancer, and offer the opportunity to provide neoadjuvant therapy in patients with rectal cancer. In this way, colorectal stent placement serves as a favorable "bridge to surgery." For those patients who appear to be surgical candidates but later are found to have widely metastatic disease, the SEMS can be left in place as palliative therapy and a potentially permanent colostomy avoided [35]

Oncological Outcomes Potential concerns have been found about impaired oncological results after SEMS treatment in the bridge to surgery group patient, particularly following colon stent perforation. The outcome of long-term follow-up comparing SEMS as a bridge to elective surgery versus acute resection was analyzed by three RCTs [36–38]. Although the study groups were small (15–26 patients in the stent arms), all trials report higher oncologic disease recurrence rates in the SEMS group. However, no difference in survival was seen in the SEMS group compared with the surgery group in the three trials [36–38].

The use of SEMS and the occurrence of tumor stenting perforation were identified to correlate with worse overall survival. The outcome data of the "Dutch Stent-In 2" trial showed a significantly higher overall recurrence disease rate in the SEMS group between the two arms (42 % in the surgical group vs. 25 % in the SEMS group), which was even higher in the subgroup of patients who experienced stent-related perforation (83 %) [38]. The oncological risks of SEMS placement should be balanced against the operative risks of emergency surgery. Because there is no reduction in postoperative mortality and stenting seems to impact on the oncological safety, the use of SEMS as a bridge to surgery could not be recommended as a standard treatment for potentially curable patients. However, placement of SEMS is considered an alternative option in patients at high surgical risk.

Risk factors as increasing age and an ASA score $\geq$ III are associated with adverse outcomes following elective as well as emergency surgery in colorectal cancer. Therefore, the use of SEMS as a bridge to elective surgery may be considered the preferred alternative treatment option in patients potentially unfit for surgery: older than 70 years and/or with an ASA score $\geq$ III [39].

5.3.3 Colonic SEMS as Palliative Therapy

Colonic SEMS can also provide effective palliation for patients with malignant colonic obstruction who are recognized at initial evaluation to be poor operative candidates. Follow-up data of colonic SEMS placement for palliation are favorable; the median rate of clinical success was 90 %–93 %, and the median rate of reobstruction ranges from 12 % to 16 % [32, 33] Patients who underwent to colonic SEMS placement as palliative therapy, compared with surgery, had lower medical complications, shorter hospitalization, reduced number of colostomy [40, 41], more prompt initiation of chemotherapy [42], and a trend toward decreased mortality [43].

In recognition of these findings, recent reviews support endoscopic placement of colonic SEMS as an effective approach to palliation of patients with stage IV colon cancer obstruction.

Colonic SEMS also may serve for palliation of rectal cancer. Hünerbein et al. achieved initial technical success in 33 out of 34 patients (97 %) but suggested that stent placement is contraindicated for low rectal cancer (5 cm from anal verge) because of tenesmus and patient's incontinence [44].

According to the results of two meta-analyses [45, 46], colon SEMS are related to a significant lower 30-day mortality (4% vs. 11 %, SEMS vs. surgery, respectively), a shorter hospitalization (10 vs. 19 days), and a lower intensive care unit (ICU) admission (0.8 % vs. 18.0 %) while permitting a shorter time to initiation of chemotherapy (16 vs. 33 days). Surgical stoma formation was significantly lower after palliative SEMS compared with emergency surgery (13 % vs. 54 %).

No significant difference in overall morbidity between the stent group (34 %) and the surgery group (38 %) has been observed. Early complications did occur more often in the surgery group, while higher late complications were more frequent in the SEMS group. The most frequent stent-related complications in the SEMS palliative group included colon perforation (10 %), stent migration (9 %), and reobstruction (18 %) [45, 46].

Together, these analyses demonstrate that SEMS placement provides cost-effective relief of malignant colonic obstruction with an acceptable rate of complications in a broad population of patients.

Chemotherapy without anti-angiogenic agents (bevacizumab) is not associated with an increased risk of colon stent perforation. Patients who have undergone palliative stenting can be safely treated with chemotherapy without anti-angiogenic agents [47].

Retrospective series found an increased risk of stent-related colon perforation (17–50 %) in patients treated with angiogenesis inhibitor [48]. A meta-analysis found the treatment with anti-angiogenic agents as a risk factor of increased colon perforation during colon stenting: 12.5 % of colon perforation rate was observed in patients treated with bevacizumab compared to 7.0 % of colon perforation registered in patients treated with standard chemotherapy [47]. Considered the high risk of colon perforation identified in this subgroup of patient, the use of SEMS as palliative treatment is not recommended if an anti-angiogenic therapy is being administered [47].

5.3.4 SEMS in Benign Colorectal Diseases

There are two major applications of SEMS in this field: benign colorectal obstruction and colorectal fistula.

Colorectal obstruction could be associated to diverticulitis, post-actinc stricture, IBD-related stricture, postsurgical anastomotic stricture. Management of benign colorectal obstructive disease is a challenging effort. Endoscopic balloon dilation is the most used and simplest therapeutic choice, but it is associated with a high recurrence rate, and refractoriness is observed in more than 20 % of cases [49]. Results concerning the long-term obstruction symptom relief in patients with benign colon obstructive disease have been obtained in heterogeneous series, and there is some controversy about efficacy and safety [50–54]. Stents have not been so commonly studied in patients with benign colorectal obstruction. Few and controversial data are available on the application of SEMS in Crohn's disease (CD) strictures. Clinical success ranges from 45 % to 80 % in published series involving patients with postsurgical strictures mostly [55]. Loras et al. found an overall efficacy of 64.7 % after a follow-up of 60 weeks. Patient's refractory to balloon endoscopic treatment or cases in which balloon dilations were unsuitable have been included in this series. The results showed that this technique may offer an alternative to endoscopic treatment considered the limited minor complications (distal migration in 52 % of cases). Authors conclude that placement of FCSEMS in CD strictures maintained over a period of 4 weeks is a safe and effective treatment for strictures refractory to endoscopic dilatations; the length and location of stricture are important considerations for the correct choice of the stent [55].

Keranen et al.'s series included patients with diverticular colon obstruction (n = 10) remarking a high major complication rate with colon perforation observed in three out of ten patients. High colon perforation rates were found in other series in which diverticular strictures were treated with SEMS: Small AJ et al. noted two cases of colon perforation out of 14 patients treated with SEMS [51, 55].

The application of SEMS in diverticular disease is complicated by high perforation rate in both palliative and bridge to surgery cases. This may be due to persisting sepsis or inflammatory activity making the bowel friable and susceptible to local damage. According to these results, the use of SEMS for obstruction caused by diverticulitis has not been recommended because of concern for high perforation rate.

The best results on the applications of FCSEMS in benign colorectal strictures have been reached in colorectal anastomotic stenosis. Caruso et al. showed an early clinical success in the absence of endoscopic or surgical reintervention in all cases. Prolonged clinical success (median follow-up of 21 months) was reached in 56 % cases. Complications consisted of spontaneous stent migration only and occurred in 19 % of cases. The multivariate analysis of this retrospective series showed a lower stent migration rate (19 %) when large-diameter stents (i.e., 24–26 mm) were used, in turn favoring clinical success. According to these data, FCSEMS can represent effective and safe treatment for anastomotic colorectal strictures, and large stents are warranted for better results [56]. Similarly, Vanbiervliet et al. [57] found a recurrence rate in half (53 %) of patients treated with SEMS for postsurgical colon stricture obstruction in long-term follow-up and high stent migration rate (63 %) occurred.

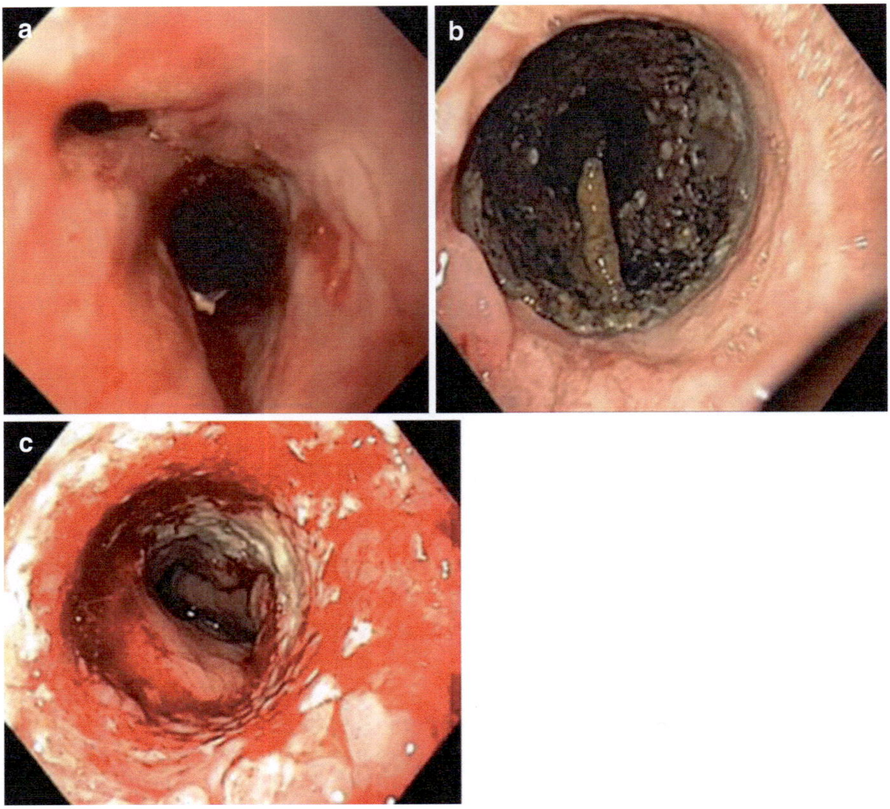

Fig. 5.4 Example of fistula closure using SEMS. (**a**) Fistula across a colorectal anastomotic rhyme. (**b**) FCSEMS has been positioned across the anastomosis. (**c**) Fistula healing after stent retrieval

In small case series, SEMS have been applied as nonsurgical therapeutic option to heal a colorectal fistula [51, 58]. Mostly data deal with the use of SEMS in anastomotic leak (Figs. 5.4 and 5.5). Authors have used both covered and uncovered SEMS registering the absence of migration in all cases and an overall long-term clinical efficacy of 73 %.

In our center, few cases with good results have been treated using biodegradable stents in alternative to FCSEMS when a postsurgical fistula is associated to the anastomotic stricture; in this pattern, biodegradable stent helps to heal fistula, thanks to the overgrowth tissue stimulation, and stenosis should be treated, thanks to the intrinsic high radial force of biodegradable stent (Fig. 5.6).

Likewise biodegradable stents, uncovered stents induce hyperplastic and overgrowth tissue reaction permitting fistula closure, but uncovered stents are very difficult to be removed endoscopically. FCSEMS can be safely removed endoscopically but are complicated by migration in 30 %–60 % of cases.

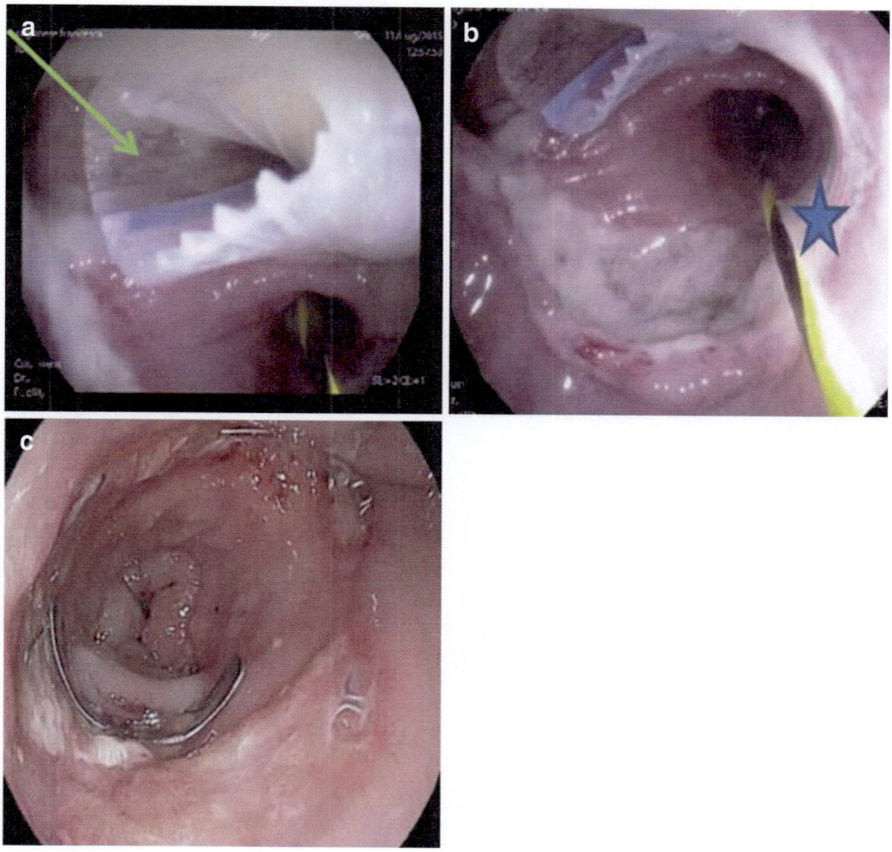

Fig. 5.5 Postsurgical colon dehiscence. (**a**) Penrose tube drainage (*arrow*) is located through the anastomotic dehiscence in the colon lumen. (**b**) Through a guidewire (*star*), a colon SEMS is placed across the anastomosis. (**c**) Anastomotic healing after 6 months of follow-up: an OTSC (over-the-scope clip) has been released in the site of dehiscence at the same time of stent placement to improve the possibility of anastomotic healing

The absence of migration in the series cited above [58] is uncommon, and the long-term management of patients treated with SEMS concerning the undefined long-time uncovered stent placement is unclear.

Covered SEMS have several potential advantages over uncovered or plastic stents.

The overgrowth of mucosal hyperplastic reaction in uncovered and partially covered SEMS facilitate the impaction of the stent with difficulties in removal; therefore, these types of stents are less ideal for the treatment of benign strictures [55]. Owing to their flexibility, FCSEMS are easier to insert and deploy, and retrieval is easier owing to absent overgrowth tissue.

Experiences from different centers with a larger number of patients are needed, before any definitive conclusion or clinical application can be accepted.

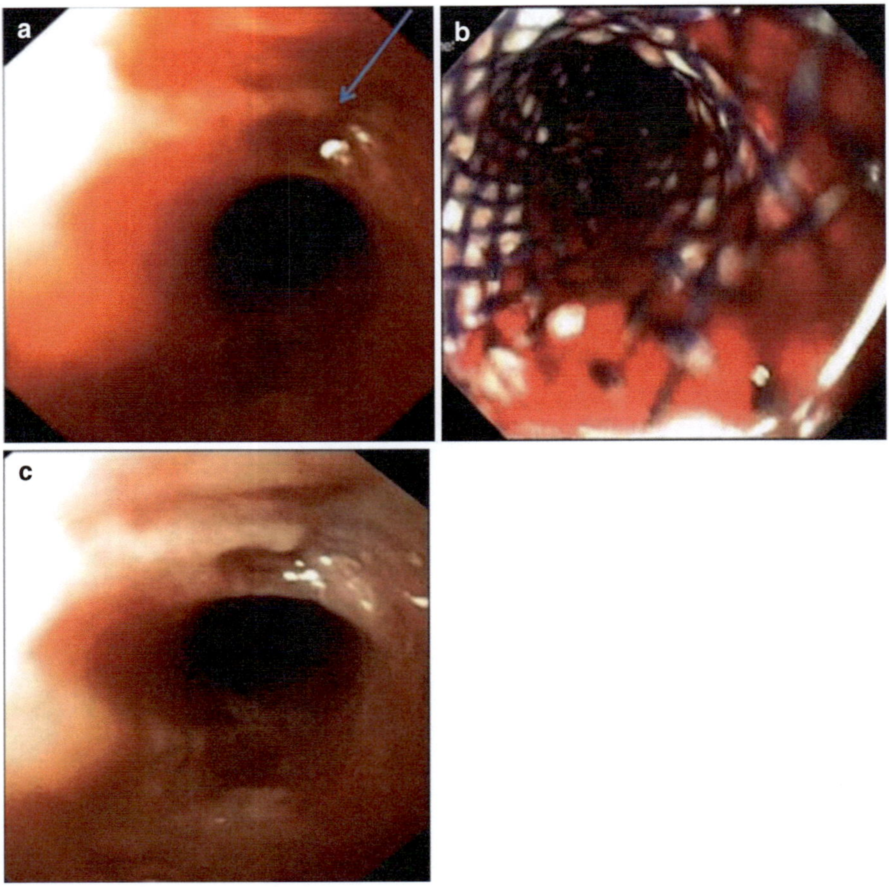

Fig. 5.6 Biodegradable stent applied in anastomotic postsurgical stricture associated to fistula: (**a**) *Arrow* shows fistula in the colon anastomotic stricture. (**b**) Biodegradable stent is released. (**c**) Results after 5 months of follow-up: fistula is closed and anastomotic colon orifice has a larger diameter

References

1. Coyas A. Palliative intubation in carcinoma of oesophagus. Lancet. 1955;269(6891):647–9.
2. Conio M, Caroli-Bosc F, Demarquay JF, Sorbi D, Maes B, Delmont J, Dumas R. Self-expanding metal stents in the palliation of neoplasms of the cervical esophagus. Hepatogastroenterology. 1999;46(25):272–7.
3. Macdonald S, Edwards RD, Moss JG. Patient tolerance of cervical esophageal metallic stents. J Vasc Interv Radiol. 2000;11(7):891–8.
4. Eleftheriadis E, Kotzampassi K. Endoprosthesis implantation at the pharyngo-esophageal level: problems, limitations and challenges. World J Gastroenterol. 2006;12:2103–8.
5. Gallo A, Pagliuca G, de Vincentiis M, Martellucci S, Iallonardi E, Fanello G, Cereatti F, Fiocca F. Endoscopic treatment of benign and malignant strictures of the cervical esophagus and hypopharynx. Ann Otol Rhinol Laryngol. 2012;121(2):104–9.

6. Parker RK, White RE, Topazian M, Chepkwony R, Dawsey S, Enders F. Stents for proximal esophageal cancer: a case–control study. Gastrointest Endosc. 2011;73(6):1098–105.
7. Verschuur EM, Kuipers EJ, Siersema PD. Esophageal stents for malignant strictures close to the upper esophageal sphincter. Gastrointest Endosc. 2007;66(6):1082–90.
8. Bassi M, Luigiano C, Fabbri C, Ferrara F, Ghersi S, Alibrandi A, Fuccio L, Virgilio C, Patelli M, Zanello M, Cennamo V. Large diameter fully covered self-expanding metal stent placement for palliation of proximal malignant esophageal strictures. Dis Esophagus. 2015;28(6):579–84.
9. Conio M, Blanchi S, Filiberti R, Repici A, Barbieri M, Bilardi C, Siersema PD. A modified self-expanding Niti-S stent for the management of benign hypopharyngeal strictures. Gastrointest Endosc. 2007;65(4):714–20.
10. Wadhwa RP, Kozarek RA, France RE, et al. Use of self-expandable metallic stents in benign GI diseases. Gastrointest Endosc. 2003;58(2):207–12.
11. Song HY, Jung HY, Park SI, et al. Covered retrievable expandable nitinol stents in patients with benign esophageal strictures: initial experience. Radiology. 2000;217(2):551–7.
12. Cheng YS, Li MH, Chen WX, Chen NW, Zhuang QX, Shang KZ. Temporary partially-covered metal stent insertion in benign esophageal stricture. World J Gastroenterol. 2003;9(10):2359–61.
13. Hirdes MM, Siersema PD, Houben MH, Weusten BL, Vleggaar FP. Stent-in-stent technique for removal of embedded esophageal self-expanding metal stents. Am J Gastroenterol. 2011;106(2):286–93.
14. Siersema PD. Stenting for benign esophageal strictures. Endoscopy. 2009;41(4):363–73.
15. van Halsema EE, van Hooft JE. Clinical outcomes of self-expandable stent placement for benign esophageal diseases: a pooled analysis of the literature. World J Gastrointest Endosc. 2015;7(2):135–53.
16. Dasari BV, Neely D, Kennedy A, Spence G, Rice P, Mackle E, Epanomeritakis E. The role of esophageal stents in the management of esophageal anastomotic leaks and benign esophageal perforations. Ann Surg. 2014;259(5):852–60.
17. de Franchis R, Baveno VI. Faculty. Expanding consensus in portal hypertension: report of the baveno VI consensus workshop: stratifying risk and individualizing care for portal hypertension. J Hepatol. 2015;63(3):743–52.
18. Changela K, Ona MA, Anand S, Duddempudi S. Self-Expanding Metal Stent (SEMS): an innovative rescue therapy for refractory acute variceal bleeding. Endosc Int Open. 2014;2(4):E244–51.
19. Marot A, Trépo E, Doerig C, Moreno C, Moradpour D, Deltenre P. Systematic review with meta-analysis: self-expanding metal stents in patients with cirrhosis and severe or refractory oesophageal variceal bleeding. Aliment Pharmacol Ther. 2015;42(11–12):1250–60.
20. Cheng YS, Ma F, Li YD, Chen NW, Chen WX, Zhao JG, Wu CG. Temporary self-expanding metallic stents for achalasia: a prospective study with a long-term follow-up. World J Gastroenterol. 2010;16(40):5111–7.
21. Zhao JG, Li YD, Cheng YS, Li MH, Chen NW, Chen WX, Shang KZ. Long-term safety and outcome of a temporary self-expanding metallic stent for achalasia: a prospective study with a 13-year single-center experience. Eur Radiol. 2009;19(8):1973–80.
22. Li YD, Cheng YS, Li MH, Chen NW, Chen WX, Zhao JG. Temporary self-expanding metallic stents and pneumatic dilation for the treatment of achalasia: a prospective study with a long-term follow-up. Dis Esophagus. 2010;23(5):361–7.
23. Cai XB, Dai YM, Wan XJ, Zeng Y, Liu F, Wang D, Zhou H. Comparison between botulinum injection and removable covered self-expanding metal stents for the treatment of achalasia. Dig Dis Sci. 2013;58(7):1960–6.
24. Gagner M. Decreased incidence of leaks after sleeve gastrectomy and improved treatments. Surg Obes Relat Dis. 2014;10:611–2.
25. Clinical Issues Committee of the American Society for Metabolic and Bariatric Surgery. Updated position statement on sleeve gastrectomy as a bariatric procedure. Surg Obes Relat Dis. 2010;6:1–5.
26. Galloro G, Ruggiero S, Russo T, Telesca DA, Musella M, Milone M, Manta R. Staple-line leak after sleeve gastrectomy in obese patients: a hot topic in bariatric surgery. World J Gastrointest Endosc. 2015;7(9):843–6.

27. Murino A, Arvanitakis M, Le Moine O, Blero D, Devière J, Eisendrath P. Effectiveness of endoscopic management using self-expandable metal stents in a large cohort of patients with post-bariatric leaks. Obes Surg. 2015;25(9):1569–76.
28. Alazmi W, Al-Sabah S, Ali DA, Almazeedi S. Treating sleeve gastrectomy leak with endoscopic stenting: the Kuwaiti experience and review of recent literature. Surg Endosc. 2014;28(12):3425–8.
29. van Hooft JE, van Halsema EE, Vanbiervliet G. Self-expandable metal stents for obstructing colonic and extracolonic cancer: European Society of Gastrointestinal Endoscopy (ESGE) Clinical Guideline. Endoscopy. 2014;46(11):990.
30. Frago R, Ramirez E, Millan M, et al. Current management of acute malignant large bowel obstruction: a systematic review. Am J Surg. 2014;207:127–38.
31. ASGE Standards of Practice Committee. Endoscopy in colonic obstruction management. Gastrointest Endosc. 2010;71(4):669–79.
32. Khot UP, Lang AW, Murali K, et al. Systematic review of the efficacy and safety of colorectal stents. Br J Surg. 2002;89:1096–102.
33. Watt A, Faragher I, Griffin T, et al. Self-expanding metallic stents for relieving malignant colorectal obstruction: a systemic review. Ann Surg. 2007;246:24–30.
34. Huang X, Lv B, Zhang S, et al. Preoperative colonic stents versus emergency surgery for acute left-sided malignant colonic obstruction: a meta-analysis. J Gastrointest Surg. 2014;18:584–91.
35. Ho KS, Quah HM, Lim JF, et al. Endoscopic stenting and elective surgery versus emergency surgery for left-sided malignant colonic obstruction:a prospective randomized trial. Int J Colorectal Dis. 2012;27:355–62.
36. Tung KL, Cheung HY, Ng LW, et al. Endo-laparoscopic approach versus conventional open surgery in the treatment of obstructing left-sided colon cancer: long-term follow-up of a randomized trial. Asian J Endosc Surg. 2013;6:78–81.
37. Alcantara M, Serra-Aracil X, Falco J, et al. Prospective, controlled, randomized study of intraoperative colonic lavage versus stent placement in obstructive left-sided colonic cancer. World J Surg. 2011;35:1904–10.
38. Sloothaak D, van den Berg M, Dijkgraaf M et al. Recurrences after endoscopic stenting as treatment for acute malignant colonic obstruction in the Dutch Stent-In 2 trial. Conference: 21st UEG Week, 12–16 Oct Berlin; 2013.
39. Guo MG, Feng Y, Zheng Q, et al. Comparison of self-expanding metal stents and urgent surgery for left-sided malignant colonic obstruction in elderly patients. Dig Dis Sci. 2011;56:2706–10.
40. Few Law WL, Choi HK, Chu KW. Comparison of stenting with emergency surgery as palliative treatment for obstructing primary left-sided colorectal cancer. Br J Surg. 2003;90:1429–33.
41. Fiori E, Lamazza A, De Cesare A, et al. Palliative management of malignant rectosigmoidal obstruction. Colostomy vs. endoscopic stenting. A randomized prospective trial. Anticancer Res. 2004;24:265–8.
42. Karoui M, Charachon A, Delbaldo C, et al. Stents for palliation of obstructive metastatic colon cancer: impact on management and chemotherapy administration. Arch Surg. 2007;142:619–23.
43. Breitenstein S, Rickenbacher A, Berdajs D, et al. Systemic evaluation of surgical strategies for acute malignant left-sided colonic obstruction. Br J Surg. 2007;94:1451–60.
44. Hünerbein M, Krause M, Moesta KT, et al. Palliation of malignant rectal obstruction with self-expanding metal stents. Surgery. 2005;137:42–7.
45. Liang TW, Sun Y, Wei YC, et al. Palliative treatment of malignant colorectal obstruction caused by advanced malignancy: a self-expanding metallic stent or surgery? a system review and meta-analysis. Surg Today. 2014;44:22–33.
46. Zhao XD, Cai BB, Cao RS, et al. Palliative treatment for incurable malignant colorectal obstructions: a meta-analysis. World J Gastroenterol. 2013;19:5565–74.
47. Van Halsema EE, van Hooft JE, Small AJ, et al. Perforation in colorectal stenting: a meta-analysis and a search for risk factors. Gastrointest Endosc. 2014;79:970–82.

48. Cennamo V, Fuccio L, Mutri V, et al. Does stent placement for advanced colon cancer increase the risk of perforation during bevacizumab based therapy? Clin Gastroenterol Hepatol. 2009;7:1174–6.
49. Suchan KL, Muldner A, Manegold BC. Endoscopic treatment of postoperative colorectal anastomotic strictures. Surg Endosc. 2003;17:1110–3.
50. Forshaw MJ, Sankararajah D, Stewart M, Parker MC. Self-expanding metallic stents in the treatment of benign colorectal disease: indications and outcomes. Colorectal Dis. 2006;8:102–11.
51. Small AJ, Young-Fadok TM, Baron TH. Expandable metal stent placement for benign colorectal obstruction: outcomes for 23 cases. Surg Endosc. 2008;22:454–62.
52. Rayhanabad J, Abbas MA. Long-term outcome of endoscopic colorectal stenting for malignant and benign disease. Am Surg. 2009;75(10):897–900.
53. Dai Y, Chopra SS, Wysocki WM. Treatment of benign colorectal strictures by temporary stenting with self-expanding stents. Int J Colorectal Dis. 2010;25:1475–9.
54. Keranen I, Lepisto A, Udd M, Halttunen J, Kylanpaa L. Outcome of patients after endoluminal stent placement for benign colorectal obstruction. Scand J Gastroenterol. 2010;45:725–31.
55. Loras C, Perez-Roldan F, Gornals JB, et al. Endoscopic treatment with self-expanding metal stents for Crohn's disease strictures. Aliment Pharmacol Ther. 2012;36:833–9.
56. Caruso A, Conigliaro R, Manta R, et al. Fully covered self-expanding metal stents for refractory anastomotic colorectal strictures. Surg Endosc. 2015;29:1175–8.
57. Vanbiervliet G, Bichard P, Demarquay JF, et al. Fully covered self-expanding metal stents for benign colonic strictures. Endoscopy. 2013;45:35–41.
58. Lamazza A, Fiori E, Schillaci A, et al. Treatment of anastomotic stenosis and leakage after colorectal resection for cancer with self expandable metal stents. Am J Surg. 2014;208:465–9.

Endoscopic Suturing Systems

6

Joseph Ramon Armengol-Miro, Joan Dot, Monder Abu-Suboh, Jordi Armengol, Miquel Masachs, and Sergey V. Kantsevoy

Several types of endoscopic suturing systems have been developed for the last two decades. According to the working principles, these devices can be divided into several groups [1].

Suction-based devices [2, 3] (EndoCinch [Bard, Murray Hill, NJ, USA], LSI Solution [Victor, NY, USA], Spiderman [Ethicon Endo Surgery, Cincinnati, OH, USA], Sew-Right [Cook Endoscopy, Winston-Salem, NC, USA]) had a vacuum chamber to aspirate gastrointestinal (GI) tract wall. Then a needle was advanced through the aspirated tissue delivering a suture. The suture later was tightened using extracorporeal knot tying or specially created cinching mechanism. The common problem of suction-based suturing systems was large variability in the depth of suture placement: insufficient suction created only superficial sutures [2]. Excessive suction could cause transmural suture placement with potential damage to organ adjacent to GI tract. None of the suction-based suturing system is currently used in clinical practice in humans.

Second group of suturing systems was based on a working overtube delivering preloaded stitch (NDO plicator [NDO Surgical, Mansfield, MA, USA], Esophyx

J.R. Armengol-Miro, MD (✉) • J. Dot, MD • M. Abu-Suboh, MD • J. Armengol, MD
M. Masachs, MD
World Institute for Digestive Endoscopy (WIDER), Barcelona, Spain

Digestive Endoscopy, Vall D'Hebron University Hospital, Barcelona, Spain
e-mail: jrarmengol@gmail.com

S.V. Kantsevoy, MD, PhD
World Institute for Digestive Endoscopy (WIDER), Barcelona, Spain

Medicine, University of Maryland School of Medicine, Baltimore, MD, USA

Therapeutic Endoscopy Mercy Medical Center Baltimore, Baltimore, MD, USA

R. Conigliaro, M. Frazzoni (eds.), *Diagnosis and Endoscopic Management of Digestive Diseases*, DOI 10.1007/978-3-319-42358-6_6

[EndoGastric Solutions, Redmond, WA, USA]) [4]. These devices were used in retroflex position to create plications tightening the gastroesophageal junction. Although NDO plicator is no longer commercially available, Esophyx device is still, but rarely, used for endoscopic correction of gastroesophageal reflux disease [4].

The third group of suturing systems was developed by Power Medical (now Covidien based at New Haven, CT, USA) and was built as a flexible endoscopic stapling device. Despite the initial success in acute and survival animal experiments and several successful endoscopic procedures in humans, this device is no longer available for clinical use [5–8].

The forth group of endoscopic suturing system was based of delivery of T-tags with attached sutures through a hollow needle [9–11]. The T-tags were placed into opposite edges of the GI tract wall incision and then were cinched together by a special cinching mechanism. Several companies (Olympus Optical LTD [Tokyo, Japan], Cook Endoscopy [Winston-Salem, NC, USA], Ethicon Endo-Surgery Inc [Cincinnati, OH, USA]) have previously developed their own T-tag suturing systems. The common problem with this type of suturing devices was the need for a blind puncture of the GI tract wall, which could cause unpredictable damage to adjacent organs [12]. Only one device of this group (TAS system from Ethicon Endo-Surgery Inc) has been cleared by US Food and Drug Administration for clinical use in humans. However, at the present time, none of these systems is commercially available [1].

The last group of endoscopic suturing devices (G-Prox [USGI Medical, San Clemente, CA], Eagle Claw [Olympus Optical LTD, Tokyo, Japan], OverStitch [Apollo Endosurgery Inc, Austin, TX, USA]) is based on the use of a curved needle and most closely resembles surgical suturing technique [13–17]. Eagle claw was successfully used in numerous animal experiments but has never been available for human use [13–15]. G-Prox system has large outer diameter and cannot be inserted through the biopsy channel of commercially available endoscopes [18]. It requires a special delivery system and currently mostly used in bariatric patients for revision of dilated gastrojejunal anastomosis postprevious gastric bypass and other endoscopic bariatric procedures [19, 20].

OverStitch endoscopic suturing device (Fig. 6.1) is commercially available for clinical use in humans since 2011 [1]. The device assembly and use are straightforward and easy: [1, 16] it is front-loaded on double-channel gastroscope (Olympus 2 T160 or Olympus 2 T180) and inserted into GI tract. When the endoscope reaches the site requiring endoscopic suturing, the suturing arm caring the needle with attached suture is opened and then closed driving the needle through the first edge of the sutured tissue. Then the needle is grasped with a needle holder, the suturing arm is opened releasing the tissue, and the needle is reloaded back onto the suturing arm. The suturing arm is closed again delivering the needle through the second edge of the sutured tissue. At this point the needle can be released from the suturing arm to become a T-bar. Then a special mechanism is deployed bringing together and cinching both edges of the sutured tissue to complete a separate stitch. However, instead of releasing the needle, the needle can be reloaded back onto the suturing

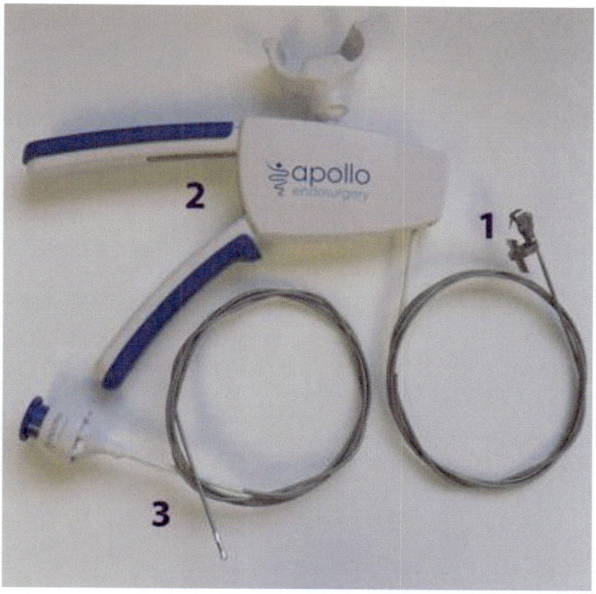

Fig. 6.1 OverStitch endoscopic suturing device consists of a curved suturing arm on end plate (*1*) accentuated by a handle (*2*) and a needle holder (*3*)

arm to continue the creation of a continuous suturing line of necessary length. After completion of each stitch (separate or continuous), a new needle with attached suture can be again loaded onto the suturing arm to create the next stitch. The OverStitch can be reloaded with a new needle unlimited number of times without the need to remove the suturing device from a patient.

OverStitch endoscopic suturing device has been successfully used for numerous clinical indications:

Closure of GI tract fistulas [21, 22]
Fixation of internal stents to prevent stent migration (Fig. 6.2) [23–25]
Repair of dilated gastrojejunal anastomosis postprevious gastric bypass (Fig. 6.3) and primary bariatric procedures for treatment of obesity
Facilitation of endoscopic submucosal dissection with a suture-pulley technique [26, 27]
Repair of inadvertent iatrogenic GI tract perforations [28–32]
Closure of large mucosal defect (Figs. 6.4 and 6.5) postendoscopic mucosal resection or endoscopic submucosal dissection (ESD) [33]
Closure of GI tract wall defects postfull-thickness resection of GI tract lesions (Fig. 6.6) [34–38]

In conclusion, several types of endoscopic devices have been developed for endoscopic suturing inside the GI tract. OverStitch is the most widely used endoscopic suturing device allowing the creation of endoscopic sutures, closely

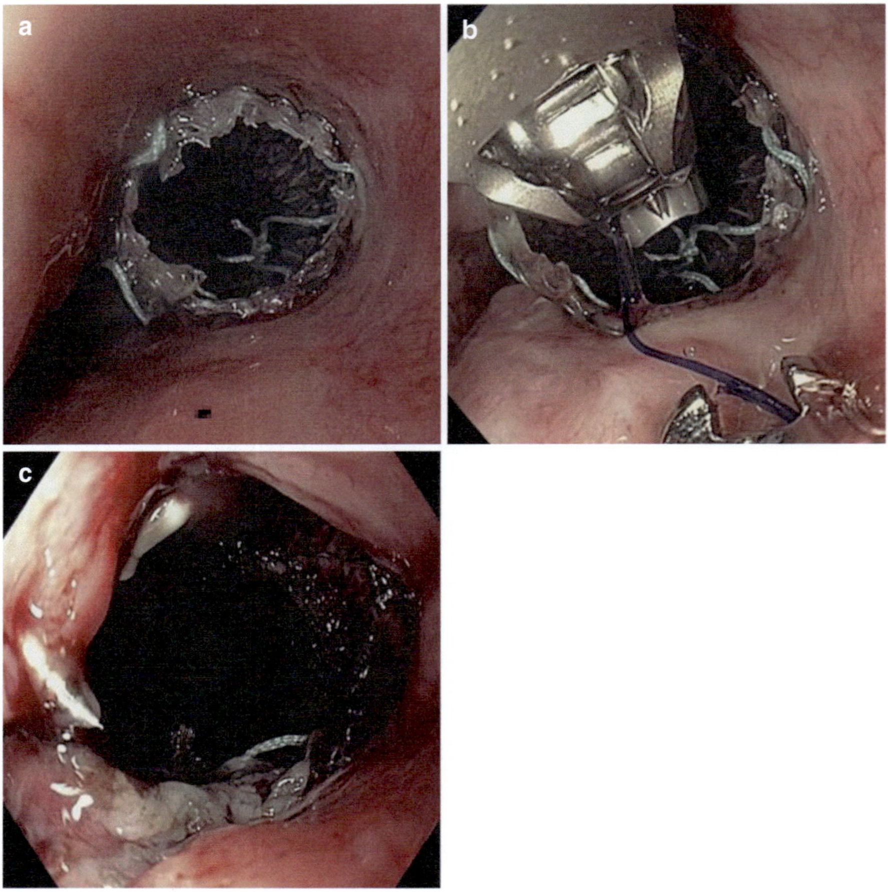

Fig. 6.2 Fixation of internal stent with OverStitch endoscopic suturing device. (**a**) A fully covered self-expending metal stent is placed proximal in the esophagus. (**b**) OverStitch endoscopic suturing device has been advanced into the esophagus to perform stent fixation toward the esophageal wall. (**c**) The stent has been sutured to esophageal wall with OverStitch endoscopic suturing device to prevent stent migration

resembling surgical suturing. The indications for endoscopic suturing continue to expand positioning the OverStitch as a very valuable tool for therapeutic endoscopy.

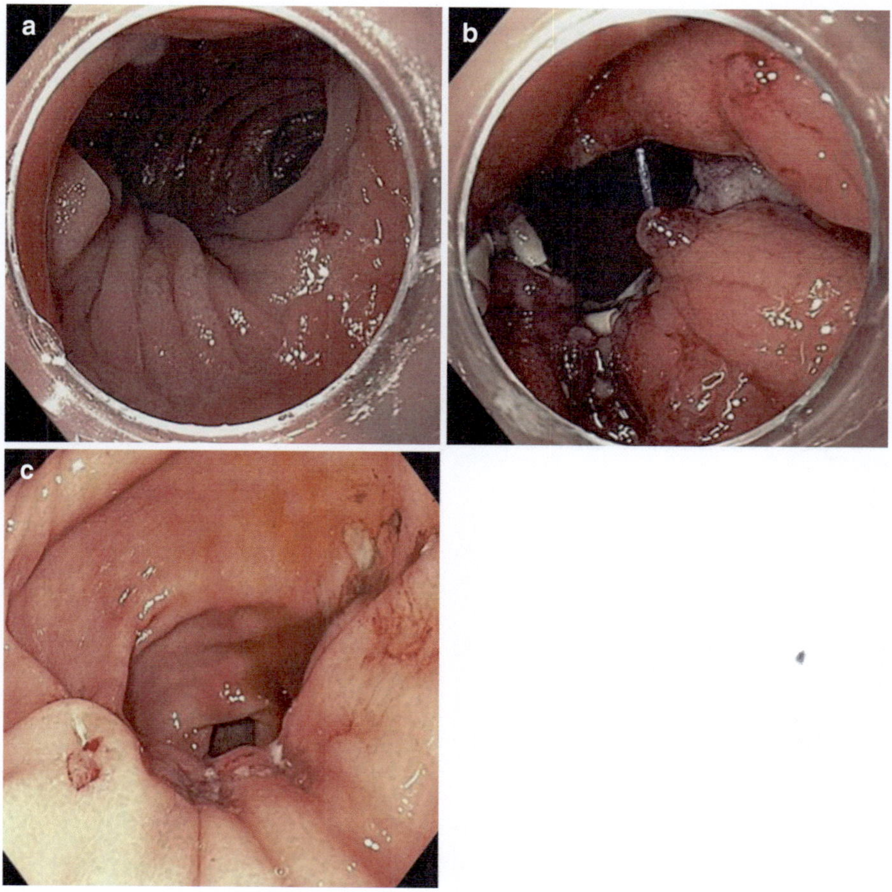

Fig. 6.3 Endoscopic correction of dilated gastrojejunal anastomosis. (**a**) Dilated gastrojejunal anastomosis postprevious gastric bypass. (**b**) Dilated anastomosis has been narrowed with separate stitches to 1 cm in diameter using OverStitch endoscopic suturing device

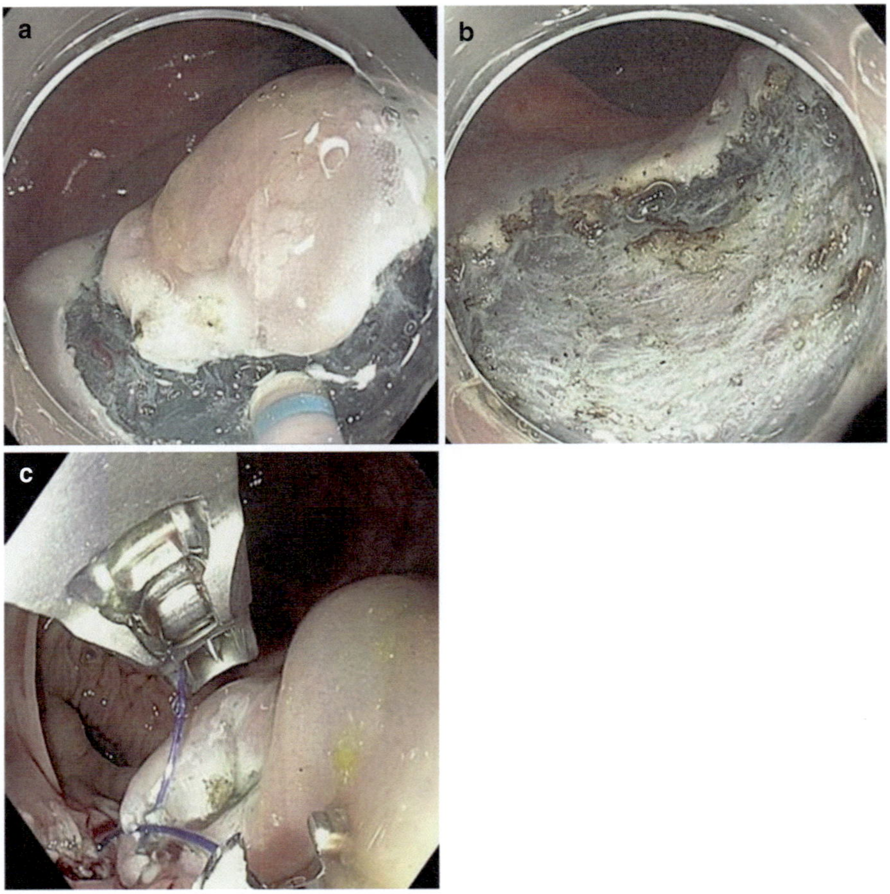

Fig. 6.4 Endoscopic suturing closure of mucosal defect postgastric ESD. (**a**) Large mucosal defect post-ESD in the antrum of the stomach. (**b**) Endoscopic suture has been advanced through both edges of mucosal incision at the right corner of mucosal defect post-ESD. (**c**) Mucosal defect post-ESD has been closed with continuous suturing line using OverStitch endoscopic suturing system

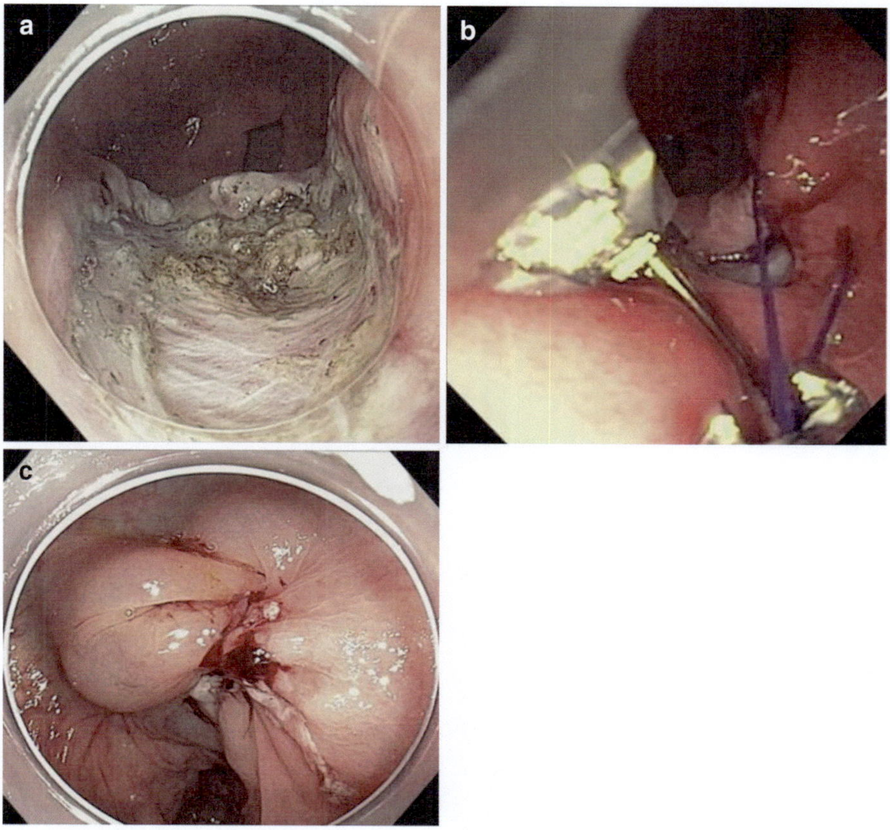

Fig. 6.5 Endoscopic suturing closure of mucosal defect postcolonic ESD. (**a**) ESD of a large and flat ascending colon polyp has been started with a dual knife. (**b**) Large mucosal defect postcompletion of ESD in ascending colon. (**c**) OverStitch endoscopic suturing device has been advanced into ascending colon for suturing closure of the mucosal defect post-ESD. (**d**) Mucosal defect has been completely closed with continuous suturing line using OverStitch endoscopic suturing system

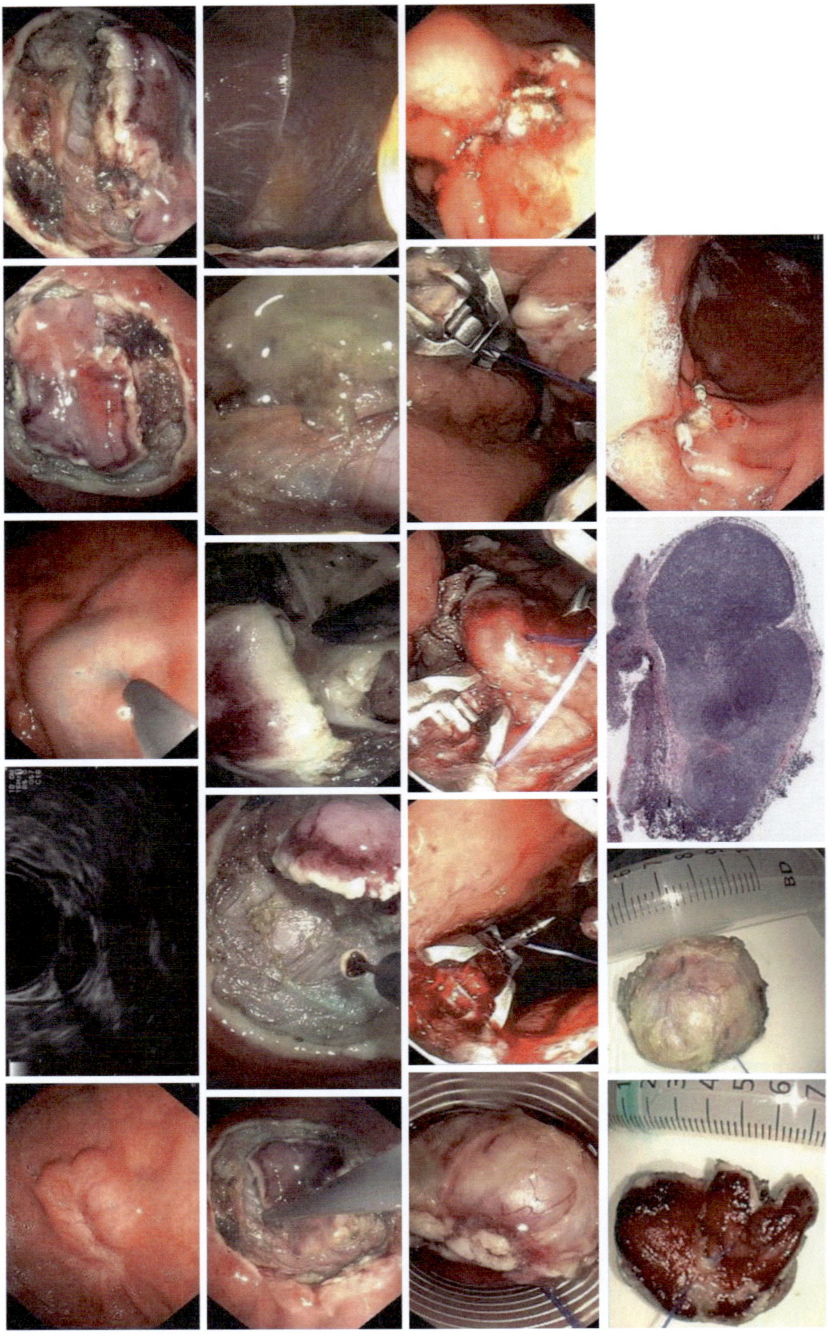

Fig. 6.6 Closure of GI tract wall defect postfull-thickness resection of gastric stromal tumor

References

1. Kantsevoy SV. Endoscopic suturing devices. In: Testoni PA, Arcidiacono PG, Mariani A, editors. Endoscopic management of gastrointestinal cancer and precancerous conditions. Turin: Edizoni Minerva Medica; 2015. p. 249–55.
2. Schwartz MP, Schreinemakers JR, Smout AJ. Four-year follow-up of endoscopic gastroplication for the treatment of gastroesophageal reflux disease. World J Gastrointest Pharmacol Ther. 2013;4:120–6.
3. Chen YK. Endoscopic suturing devices for treatment of GERD: too little, too late? Gastrointest Endosc. 2005;62:44–7.
4. Yew KC, Chuah SK. Antireflux endoluminal therapies: past and present. Gastroenterol Res Pract. 2013:481417.
5. Kaehler GF, Langner C, Suchan KL, Freudenberg S, Post S. Endoscopic full-thickness resection of the stomach: an experimental approach. Surg Endosc. 2006;20:519–21.
6. Kaehler G, Grobholz R, Langner C, Suchan K, Post S. A new technique of endoscopic full-thickness resection using a flexible stapler. Endoscopy. 2006;38:86–9.
7. Meireles OR, Kantsevoy SV, Assumpcao LR, et al. Reliable gastric closure after natural orifice translumenal endoscopic surgery (NOTES) using a novel automated flexible stapling device. Surg Endosc. 2008;22:1609–13.
8. Magno P, Giday SA, Dray X, et al. A new stapler-based full-thickness transgastric access closure: results from an animal pilot trial. Endoscopy. 2007;39:876–80.
9. Raju GS, Shibukawa G, Ahmed I, et al. Endoluminal suturing may overcome the limitations of clip closure of a gaping wide colon perforation (with videos). Gastrointest Endosc. 2007;65:906–11.
10. Ikeda K, Fritscher-Ravens A, Mosse CA, Mills T, Tajiri H, Swain CP. Endoscopic full-thickness resection with sutured closure in a porcine model. Gastrointest Endosc. 2005;62:122–9.
11. Dray X, Krishnamurty DM, Donatelli G, et al. Gastric wall healing after NOTES procedures: closure with endoscopic clips provides superior histological outcome compared with threaded tags closure. Gastrointest Endosc. 2010;72:343–50.
12. Kantsevoy SV. Endoscopic full-thickness resection: new minimally invasive therapeutic alternative for GI-tract lesions. Gastrointest Endosc. 2006;64:90–1.
13. Hu B, Chung SC, Sun LC, et al. Endoscopic suturing without extracorporeal knots: a laboratory study. Gastrointest Endosc. 2005;62:230–3.
14. Hu B, Chung SC, Sun LC, et al. Eagle claw II: a novel endosuture device that uses a curved needle for major arterial bleeding: a bench study. Gastrointest Endosc. 2005;62:266–70.
15. Kantsevoy SV, Hu B, Jagannath SB, et al. Technical feasibility of endoscopic gastric reduction: a pilot study in a porcine model. Gastrointest Endosc. 2007;65:510–3.
16. Kantsevoy SV. Endoscopic suturing for closure of transmural defects. Tech Gastrointest Endosc. 2015;17:136–40.
17. Conway NE, Swanstrom LL. Endoluminal flexible endoscopic suturing for minimally invasive therapies. Gastrointest Endosc. 2014;81:262–9, e19.
18. Swanstrom LL. Current technology development for natural orifice transluminal endoscopic surgery. Cir Esp. 2006;80:283–8.
19. Mullady DK, Lautz DB, Thompson CC. Treatment of weight regain after gastric bypass surgery when using a new endoscopic platform: initial experience and early outcomes (with video). Gastrointest Endosc. 2009;70:440–4.
20. Ryou M, Mullady DK, Lautz DB, Thompson CC. Pilot study evaluating technical feasibility and early outcomes of second-generation endosurgical platform for treatment of weight regain after gastric bypass surgery. Surg Obes Relat Dis. 2009;5:450–4.
21. Kantsevoy SV, Thuluvath PJ. Successful closure of a chronic refractory gastrocutaneous fistula with a new endoscopic suturing device (with video). Gastrointest Endosc. 2012;75:688–90.
22. Armengol-Miro JR, Dot J, Abu-Suboh Abadia M et al. New endoscopic suturing device for closure of chronic gastrocutaneous fistula in an immunocompromised patient. Endoscopy. 2012;43 Suppl 2 UCTN:E403–404.

23. Kantsevoy SV, Bitner M. Esophageal stent fixation with endoscopic suturing device (with video). Gastrointest Endosc. 2012;76:1251–5.
24. Fujii LL, Bonin EA, Baron TH, Gostout CJ, Wong Kee Song LM. Utility of an endoscopic suturing system for prevention of covered luminal stent migration in the upper GI tract. Gastrointest Endosc. 2013;78:787–93.
25. Rieder E, Dunst CM, Martinec DV, Cassera MA, Swanstrom LL. Endoscopic suture fixation of gastrointestinal stents: proof of biomechanical principles and early clinical experience. Endoscopy. 2012;44:1121–6.
26. Rieder E, Makris KI, Martinec DV, Swanstrom LL. The suture-pulley method for endolumenal triangulation in endoscopic submucosal dissection. Endoscopy. 2011;43 Suppl 2 UCTN:E319–20.
27. Aihara H, Kumar N, Ryou M, Abidi W, Ryan MB, Thompson CC. Facilitating endoscopic submucosal dissection: the suture-pulley method significantly improves procedure time and minimizes technical difficulty compared with conventional technique: an ex vivo study (with video). Gastrointest Endosc. 2014;80:495–502.
28. Kantsevoy SV, Bitner M, Davis JM, Hajiyeva G, Thuluvath PJ, Gushchin V. Endoscopic suturing closure of large iatrogenic colonic perforation. Gastrointest Endosc. 2015;82:754–5.
29. Henderson JB, Sorser SA, Atia AN, Catalano MF. Repair of esophageal perforations using a novel endoscopic suturing system. Gastrointest Endosc. 2014;80:535–7.
30. Kantsevoy SV, Bitner M, Hajiyeva G et al. Endoscopic management of colonic perforations: clips versus suturing closure (with videos). Gastrointest Endosc
31. Kumar N, Thompson CC. A novel method for endoscopic perforation management by using abdominal exploration and full-thickness sutured closure. Gastrointest Endosc. 2014;80:156–61.
32. Armengol-Miro JR, Dot J, Abu-Suboh Abadia M, et al. Endoscopic closure of iatrogenic colonic perforations: randomized controlled trial on animal model and initial clinical experience. Gastrointest Endosc. 2013;77:AB461.
33. Kantsevoy SV, Bitner M, Mitrakov AA, Thuluvath PJ. Endoscopic suturing closure of large mucosal defects after endoscopic submucosal dissection is technically feasible, fast, and eliminates the need for hospitalization (with videos). Gastrointest Endosc. 2013;79:503–7.
34. Armengol-Miro JR, Dot J, Abu-Suboh Abadia M, et al. Full-thickness purely endoscopic resection of colon cancer. Gastrointest Endosc. 2012;75:AB114–5.
35. Armengol-Miro JR, Abu-Suboh Abadia M, Dot J, et al. Full-thickness endoscopic resection of gastrointestinal cancer: from animal experiments to humans. Gastrointest Endosc. 2013;77:AB458.
36. Stavropoulos SN, Modayil R, Friedel D, Brathwaite CE. Endoscopic full-thickness resection for GI stromal tumors. Gastrointest Endosc. 2014;80:334–5.
37. Stavropoulos SN, Modayil R, Friedel D. Current applications of endoscopic suturing. World J Gastrointest Endosc. 2015;7:777–89.
38. Armengol-Miro JR, Dot Bach J, Suboh Abadia MA, et al. Natural orifice translumenal endoscopic surgery (NOTES) for G.I. tract neoplasia. In: Testoni PA, Arcidiacono PG, Mariani A, editors. Endoscopic management of gastrointestinal cancer and precancerous conditions. Turin: Edizoni Minerva Medica; 2015. p. 277–83.

7 Endoluminal Therapy for Treatment of Gastroesophageal Reflux Disease

Pier Alberto Testoni, Sabrina Testoni, and Giorgia Mazzoleni

7.1 Introduction

Gastroesophageal reflux disease (GERD) is a very common disorder that can be currently treated by medical therapy and surgical or endoscopic transoral interventions.

Medical therapy represents the most common approach: proton pump inhibitors (PPIs) relieve symptoms and improve the patient's quality of life in the majority of cases. However, concerns related to potential side effects of continuous long-term medication, drug intolerance, or unresponsiveness and the need of high dosages for long periods to treat symptoms or prevent recurrences have increased in the recent years. Moreover, medical therapy may be inadequate to treat symptoms occurring in the presence of weakly acidic reflux and has high cost in the long term for either patients or healthcare system, if started at a young age and maintained for many years.

On the other hand, patients suffering from a mild GERD are in general reluctant to undergo surgical repair of the valve, considering its invasiveness. Surgery may also have in some cases consequences characterized by long-lasting dysphagia, flatulence, inability to belch or vomit, diarrhea, or functional dyspepsia related to delayed gastric emptying [1–4]. Even for interventions performed in centers of excellence, incisional hernias in the site of trocar insertion have been reported in up to 3 % of cases [5].

P.A. Testoni (✉) • S. Testoni • G. Mazzoleni
Division of Gastroenterology and Gastrointestinal Endoscopy, Vita-Salute San Raffaele University – Scientific Institute San Raffaele, Via Olgettina 60, 20134 Milan, Italy
e-mail: pieralberto.testoni@unisr.it; testoni.pieralberto@hsr.it

R. Conigliaro, M. Frazzoni (eds.), *Diagnosis and Endoscopic Management of Digestive Diseases*, DOI 10.1007/978-3-319-42358-6_7

For these reasons, in the last 15 years, technological innovations have led to the development of a variety of transoral endoscopic techniques as alternatives to antisecretory therapy or antireflux surgery [6]. All these techniques would aim at reinforcing the barrier function of the lower esophageal sphincter (LES), similarly to surgery, and thus controlling reflux but with a lower invasiveness and costs compared to surgery.

Endoluminal therapies gained popularity and showed significant symptom control in the short-term period in the majority of published studies. However, most of them showed disappointing long-term results and have been abandoned [7–9]. Although an American Gastroenterological Association Institute Medical Position Statement established in 2008 that "the current data suggest that at present there are no definitive indications for the use of endoluminal therapy in gastroesophageal reflux disease" [10], transoral procedures have been offered to a selected group of patients with documented symptomatic chronic GERD (pathological reflux at pH and impedance recording and positive correlation between reflux and symptoms), responsiveness to PPI therapy and dependence on antisecretory drugs, hiatal hernias less than 2–3 cm, absence of Barrett's esophagus, and mild esophagitis. Patients with Barrett's esophagus, large hiatal hernias, obesity, severe medical comorbidities, esophageal primary motility disorders, or proximal reflux symptoms have been in general excluded from these transoral approaches.

Endoluminal techniques include three major categories: implantation or injection of foreign materials, application of radiofrequency ablation, and endoscopic tissue apposition techniques.

7.2 Endoluminal Techniques

7.2.1 Implantations and Injections

The theory on the basis of this technique is to instill a bulking agent at the level of LES, in order to increase its natural mechanical barrier to gastroesophageal reflux. Over the years, several attempts with various bulk-forming agents were made, but none remained on the market due to the occurrence of serious adverse events and/or lack of clinical efficacy. The first trials involved injection of polytetrafluoroethylene paste (Teflon, DuPont™, Wilmington, Delaware, USA, and Polytef, Mentor O&O Inc., Santa Barbara, California, USA) and bovine collagen that showed increased gastric yield pressures and decreased esophagitis, but a lack of durability (<6 months) [11].

Subsequent technologies involved the submucosal injection of polymethylmethacrylate (Plexiglass, Artes Medical Inc., San Diego, California, USA) into the LES, but it wasn't effective beyond 6 months [12]. Therefore, all these products were withdrawn from the market.

The most promising of the injectables was Enteryx (Boston Scientific Corporation, Marlborough, Massachusetts, USA), an implantable and biocompatible polymer, consisting of ethylene vinyl alcohol 8% mixed with powder of tantalum, a radiopaque agent, in an organic liquid solution of dimethyl sulfoxide. It was injected as liquid form around the gastroesophageal junction in a circumferential manner. Once injected into the tissue, the agent forms a spongy, more solid material at the target site of injection at the esophagogastric junction (EGJ). It was a reproducible procedure in the event of inadequate control of the symptoms, but not reversible. In an international multicenter study involving 85 patients, Enteryx was effective concerning pH normalization (38.8 % at 12 months) and cessation of PPI therapy (74 % at 6 months). The scores of symptomatic questionnaires were comparable with those obtained with the antisecretory therapy. However, the device was withdrawn from the market because of procedure-related complications, such as chest pain (92 %), dysphagia (20 %), re-intervention (up to 25 % within 2 years), and a case of death due to the injection into the aortic wall [13–15].

Another injectable has recently been developed, Durasphere (Carbon Medical Technologies, St. Paul, Minnesota, USA), that is, a sterile non-pyrogenic bulking agent composed of pyrolytic carbon containing zirconium oxide beads, suspended in a water-based carrier gel containing beta-glucan. Durasphere is injected into the submucosa in order to create increased tissue bulk and subsequent coaptation of the LES. Over time, collagen is deposited around the pyrolytic carbon-coated beads, with the final bulking result due to the combination of the pyrolytic-coated beads and the body's own collagen. A pilot study on ten patients showed that 70 % of patients with mild to moderate GERD was able to discontinue medical treatment at 12-month follow-up, while 90 % of patients had reduced PPI use by 50 %, and 40 % had normalized pH [16]. However, further studies are needed to confirm its safety and effectiveness.

Among implantation techniques, a hydrogel prosthesis has been proposed (Gatekeeper Reflux Repair System, Medtronic Europe Inc., Tolochenaz, Switzerland). The aim of this technique was to narrow the diameter of the distal esophagus through endoscopic implantation of an expandable, removable, and radiopaque prosthesis in polyacrylonitrile hydrogel in the submucosal layer of the gastroesophageal junction. It was a repeatable and reversible procedure and has shown improvement in the control of reflux symptoms at 6-month follow-up. In 68 patients treated by this procedure, distal esophageal acid exposure (measured by pH monitoring), LES pressure, and symptom scores improved. Normalization of pH was observed in 40 % of patients. However, the device was withdrawn from the market due to related complications, such as pharyngeal perforation and severe postprandial nausea [17, 18].

7.2.2 Radiofrequency Ablation

The Stretta System (Mederi Therapeutics, Norwalk, Connecticut, previously Curon Medical, Sunnyvale, California, USA) was first introduced in 2000 and then refined over the years. This technique provides the ablation of the muscular layer by straddling the gastroesophageal junction with radiofrequency energy, performed with low power and controlled temperature. The device consists of a special flexible catheter with a balloon-basket assembly and curved needles, distributed radially, which is inserted orally up to the cardia. Each needle is equipped with titanium electrodes to deliver the radiofrequency energy into the esophageal wall and LES, heating the water molecules of the muscle tissue and leading to collagen contraction and tissue constriction while irrigating the overlying mucosa to prevent thermal injury [19]. The ablation is repeated by rotating the device and varying its linear position between 2 cm above and 2 cm below the Z line. The procedure induces irreversible changes, resulting in tissue healing and thus tightening of the LES.

A randomized controlled trial has shown improvement in both symptom control and quality of life at 6-month follow-up, but the technique did not significantly reduce the need to take PPIs, the LES pressure, and the time of distal esophageal acid exposure [20]. The Stretta System was also able to reduce the frequency of the transient LES relaxation, because of the tissue fibrosis and retraction at the level of gastric cardia [21, 22]. The Stretta procedure reported few adverse events. The most common complications reported in studies of case series included transient epigastric pain (66 %), chest pain (15 %), fever (7 %), tears of the mucosal surface (4 %), esophageal ulceration (4 %), and dysphagia (3 %). Major adverse events were reported in less than 0.1 % of patients [23, 24].

No difference was observed between the Stretta procedure and the laparoscopic fundoplication regarding the quality of life in GERD, but 97 % of patients no longer required therapy with PPIs after laparoscopic surgery compared with 58 % of patients who underwent the Stretta procedure [25].

In a systematic review and meta-analysis (20 studies), involving 1441 patients, the authors found that the Stretta procedure improved GERD symptoms (decreased heartburn symptom in 525 patients (36.4 %) over 24.1 months, decreased quality of life scores in 433 patients (30.0 %) over 19.8 months, and improved DeMeester scores in 267 patients (18.5 %), but did not normalize esophageal acid exposure and did not significantly increase the LES pressure [26]. In an 8-year follow-up on 26 patients, Dughera et al. found a significant decrease in heartburn and GERD-HRQL scores, and 77 % of patients completely stopped PPIs. The only complication reported was a case of severe gastroparesis requiring long-term hospitalization [27].

In summary, Stretta provided safe, effective, and durable suppression of GERD; thus it is strongly recommended by the SAGES (Society of American Gastrointestinal and Endoscopic Surgeons) for "patients who have had symptoms of heartburn, regurgitation or both for 6 months or more, who have been partially or completely responsive to antisecretory pharmacological therapy, and who have declined laparoscopic fundoplication" [28].

7.2.3 Endoscopic Tissue Apposition Techniques

Several endoscopic suturing and apposition devices have been developed, in order to mechanically sustain the LES or improve the antireflux barrier creating tissue plication around the gastroesophageal junction.

The EndoCinch (Bard Endoscopic Technologies, Murray Hill, NJ, USA) was initially approved in the USA in 2000. It consists of a suture system that is attached at the end of a standard flexible endoscope and has a cavity that permits the suction of a tissue fold. The device is inserted until reaching 1 cm downstream the Z line. A T-tag secures the submucosal tissue, and the physician lowers the suturing system to the gastroesophageal junction, where other series of sutures are placed below the LES, in order to create two to three gastric plications, forming a valve that works as a barrier against GER [13]. Several studies have evaluated EndoCinch as compared to sham or laparoscopic fundoplication. A noncontrolled trial, carried out in a single center on 70 patients, demonstrated the long-term failure of the treatment, mainly because of the loss of the sutures. Eighteen months after treatment, 56 patients (80 %) did not get improvement in the severity of reflux symptoms or use of PPIs. Endoscopic examination showed all the sutures in place in 12 patients (17 %) and no suture in 18 patients (26 %). In 54 and 50 patients tested, respectively, any significant change was not observed in the 24-h pH monitoring or pressure in the LES, while the length of the LES was only slightly increased [29]. A double-blinded, randomized study of EndoCinch versus sham demonstrated a significant improvement in the use of PPIs, the GERD symptoms, and the time of acid exposure up to 12-month follow-up, compared with the observation group, but did not show any significant improvement over the sham group. Of the EndoCinch group, 29 % of patients required re-treatment during the 12-month follow-up [30]. Moreover, in a study comparing EndoCinch to laparoscopic fundoplication, the authors found EndoCinch less effective than surgical fundoplication [31]. Thus, although a good safety profile, the device was no longer manufactured due to the lack of long-term efficacy.

Another device no longer available in the market for clinical use was the endoscopic suturing device (ESD, Wilson-Cook Medical, Bloomington, Indiana, USA) that consisted of an external accessory channel, attached to a flexible endoscope, which allowed the passage of the other two components of the device, the flexible systems Sew-Right and Ti-Knot. Sew-Right was a dual system of needles that used a single suture loop to create the tissue plication. The target tissue was sucked into a suction chamber; a suture was then passed through the tissue collected within the chamber. It was used as a continuous and single suture loop to sew two adjacent areas in the proximal stomach in order to form the plication, and it was possible to create two to three plications during a single treatment. Studies revealed the early loss of the sutures; at 6 months, only 5 % of the sutures were found still in place. There were no significant changes in the healing of esophagitis, time of esophageal acid exposure at 24-h pH monitoring, LES pressure, and PPI use [32]. In case series, this procedure has been associated with transient chest pain, abdominal pain, nausea, and self-limited bleeding, with rates similar to those observed with EndoCinch.

The endoscopic full-thickness plication system NDO Plicator (NDO Surgical Inc., Mansfield, MA, USA) was approved by the FDA in 2004. It was designed to create a transmural, full-thickness, serosa-to-serosa plication below the gastroesophageal junction at the angle of His, under endoscopic direct retroflexed view by means of a flexible pediatric endoscope (5.9 mm) inserted through a dedicated channel of the device. A pretied suture-based pledget is delivered to create the plication, performed between the anterior gastric wall and the fundus [33]. A randomized controlled trial on 78 patients who underwent the procedure reported a significant reduction in the time of distal esophageal acid exposure, measured with pH monitoring, PPI use, and improvement of esophagitis at 6 and 12 months [34, 35]. Another randomized trial by Rothstein et al. reported an extended improvement in quality of life and PPI usage at 5 years compared to the sham group [36].

This device was withdrawn from the market, too, because of several complications: persistent abdominal pain (20 %), sore throat (41 %), chest pain (17 %), dysphagia (11 %), burping (14 %), nausea (6 %), pneumothorax (1.6 %), pneumoperitoneum (1.6 %), and gastric perforation (1.6 %) [37].

The treatment of GERD with endoscopic procedures continues to evolve, as two FDA-approved endoluminal platforms now exist, that allow endoscopists to bring the surgical principles of an anterior partial fundoplication to patients without the worry or risk of the post-fundoplication complications seen with traditional laparoscopic surgery. In the last years, transoral incisionless fundoplication (TIF) has been shown to be an effective and promising therapeutic option in alternative to medical and surgical therapy; the procedure achieves long-lasting improvement of GERD symptoms (up to 6 years), cessation or reduction of proton pump inhibitor (PPI) medication in about 75 % of patients, and improvement of functional findings, measured by either pH or impedance monitoring. TIF reconfigures the tissue to obtain a full-thickness gastroesophageal valve from inside the stomach, by serosa-to-serosa plications which include the muscle layers: the new valve is capable to boost the barrier function of the LES with patient's less discomfort and possibly fewer technique-related complications and side effects, compared to surgery.

The endoluminal platform for TIF with the greatest global experience so far is that performed by using the EsophyX® device (EndoGastric Solutions Ltd., Redmond, WA, USA), with over 10,000 procedures performed to date. TIF with this device has been proven to be good, durable, long-term follow-up data in most of the series, mainly using the TIF 2 technique. The newest endoluminal fundoplication device to gain FDA approval was the MUSE™ (Medigus Ultrasonic Surgical Endostapler – Medigus Ltd., Omer, Israel).

EsophyX® constructs an omega-shaped valve 3–5-cm long, in a 250–300° circumferential pattern around the gastroesophageal junction, by deploying multiple nonabsorbable polypropylene fasteners through the two layers (the esophagus and stomach) under endoscopic vision of the operator. MUSE™ staples the fundus of the stomach to the esophagus below the diaphragm using multiple sets of metal stitches placed under an ultrasound-guided technique and creates an anterior fundoplication functionally similar to standard surgical Dor-Thal operation. In the case of sliding hiatal hernia, the procedure can be performed only if the hernia can be reduced below the diaphragm.

7.3 Techniques for Transoral Incisionless Fundoplication

7.3.1 Pre-procedure Evaluation

Preoperative upper GI endoscopy is mandatory to determine the distance between the incisor teeth and both the esophagogastric junction (EGJ) and the diaphragmatic hiatus and the greatest transverse dimension of the hiatus under full gastric distension. In fact, with the current TIF technique, only a hiatal hernia not exceeding 3.0 cm in length can be fully reduced below the diaphragm, while a plication performed in a hiatus with a transverse dimension >3.0 cm can end up in the thorax, situation that reduces the efficacy of the newly created valve. Prior to the procedure, patients should always undergo esophageal manometry, to exclude primary motility disorders, and 24-h pH-impedance monitoring to avoid the inclusion of patients with functional heartburn. If the MUSE device is used, barium swallow should be performed to assess the reducibility of the hernia, being its irreducibility a contraindication to the procedure.

7.3.2 Transoral Fundoplication by EsophyX® Device

The EsophyX® device is composed of:

(a) A handle, wherein controls are located
(b) An 18-mm diameter chassis, through which control channels run and a standard front view 9-mm diameter endoscope can be inserted
(c) The tissue invaginator, constituted of side holes located on the distal part of the chassis, to which external suction can be applied
(d) The tissue mold, which can be brought into retroflection and pushes the tissue against the shaft of the device
(e) A helical screw, which is advanced into the tissue and permits to retract the tissue between the tissue mold and the shaft
(f) Two stylets, which penetrate through the plicated tissue and the tissue mold, and over them polypropylene H-shaped fasteners can be deployed
(g) A cartridge containing 20 fasteners

The device has been recently updated and improved in a new generation instrument: the EsophyX® 2. The fastener deployment is similar to a surgical stapler firing mechanism with a reduction of control complexity and dual fastener deployment and is improved by managing trailing leg; the crossing profile has been reduced with the elimination of tissue mold elbow and increase of tissue mold lateral stiffness; the tissue mold tip covers stylets during deployment.

Details of the first- and second-generation devices are illustrated in Fig. 7.1.

The procedure is performed by two operators: one controls the device and the other one operates the endoscope.

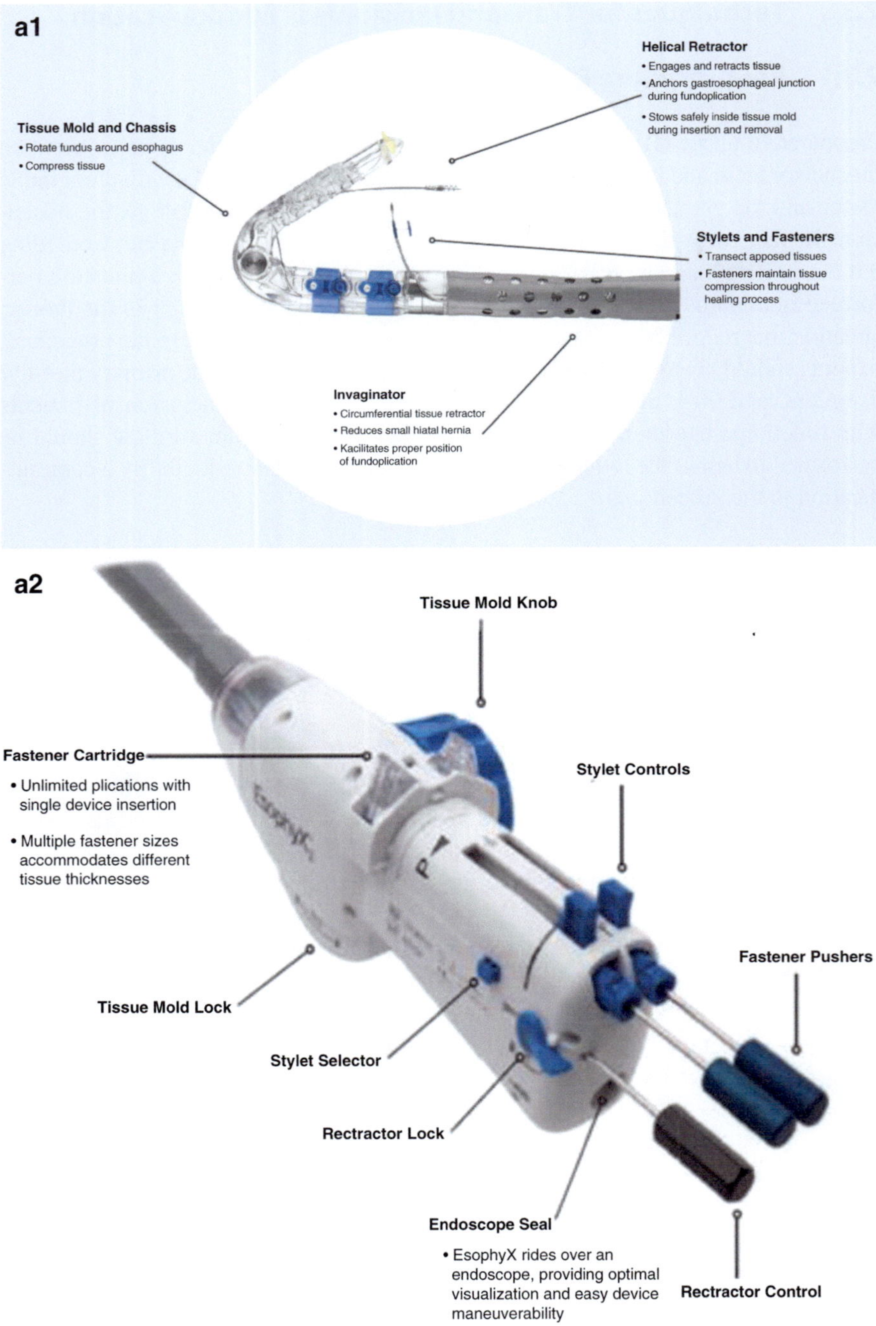

Fig. 7.1 The EsophyX® device: first- and second-generation devices (courtesy of EndoGastric Solutions, Inc. Redmond, WA, USA). (**a1**, **a2**) The device currently used (©*2014 EndoGastric Solutions*, Inc.). (**b1**, **b2**) The new generation device (©*2014 EndoGastric Solutions*, *Inc*.)

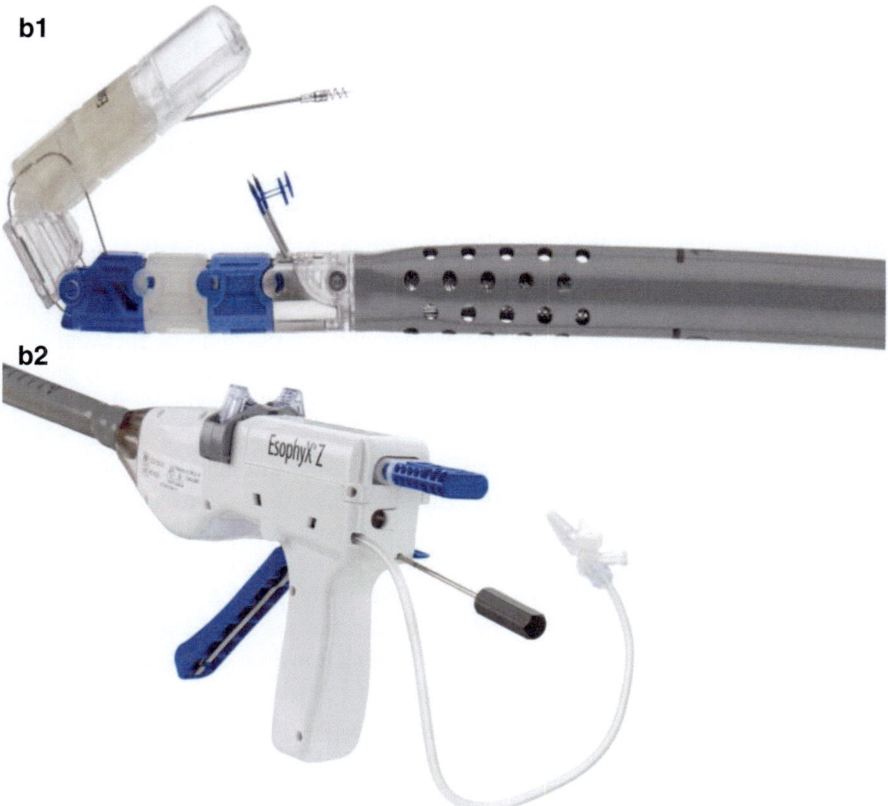

Fig. 7.1 (continued)

The device is inserted transorally with the patient in the left lateral or supine position, under general anesthesia. Hypopharyngeal perforation has been reported in this phase of the procedure if the device is introduced without an adequate caution; in difficult cases, the device can be gently rotated to pass the upper esophageal sphincter.

Once into the stomach, air or CO_2 is insufflated to distend the gastric cavity and permit an adequate vision of the gastric fundus and EGJ; CO_2 is preferable, because it leads to a faster and more sustained gastric insufflation and induces less discomfort to patients. With the endoscope placed in retroflexion position, the lesser curve is located at the 12 o'clock position and the greater curve at the 6 o'clock in the patient placed in left decubitus. Once the tissue mold is retroflexed, it is closed against the EsophyX® device, rotated to 11 or 1 o'clock position (lesser curve), and pulled back to place its tip just inside the esophageal lumen. At this point, the helical screw is advanced to engage the tissue under direct vision just below the Z line, the shaft of the device is advanced caudally, the tissue mold is opened, and the helical screw cable freed from the tissue mold. Then, a tension is applied to helical retractor, while a slight opening and closing of the tissue mold allow the fundus to slide through the tissue mold; in this phase the stomach is being desufflated. Failure to desufflate the stomach during this phase of the procedure limits the size of the fundoplication.

After completing this maneuver, both helical retractor and tissue mold are locked in place; suction is applied to the tissue invaginator for approximately half a minute, and the device is then advanced caudally into the stomach, which has been re-insufflated. The latter maneuver ensures that esophagogastric plication is performed in an intra-abdominal position and reduces hiatal hernia, when present.

Plication is carried out by deploying multiple polypropylenes, H-shaped fasteners advanced over two stylets, one anterior and the other posterior. The fastener deployment process initiates on the far posterior and anterior sides of the esophagogastric valve adjacent to the lesser curvature and then is extended to the greater curvature by rotating the tissue mold axially to slide the stomach over the esophagus, resulting in circumferential tightening and a new valve circumference of >240°. The stylet is advanced under direct endoscopical vision through the tissue molded until its tip is seen by the operator. The fastener is then advanced over the stylet and deployed to create a serosa-to-serosa plication. Once the tip of the fastener becomes visible at the tissue mold, the stylet is pulled back while the fastener is maintained in place; by this way, the leading leg of the fastener is derailed and the fastener is deployed. Fourteen fasteners allowing seven plications are needed to construct a satisfactory circumferential gastroesophageal valve; however, the higher is the number of fasteners deployed, the more continent is the newly created valve. Details of the EsophyX® device's technique are shown in Fig. 7.2.

Endoscopic pre- and post-procedural findings are reported in Fig. 7.3.

Besides the standard procedure, two modified techniques have been reported over time to create the fundoplication. The technique we used in the last years engages the tissue by advancing the helical screw just below the Z line on the far posterior and anterior sides of the esophagogastric valve adjacent to the lesser curvature (11 and 1 o'clock position). Before inserting the stylet, a torque is applied by rotation (clockwise and counterclockwise at 11 and 1 o'clock, respectively) of the tissue mold locked; such a maneuver allows part of the fundus to rotate around the esophageal wall and more tissue to be engaged by the stylet. Four fasteners for each site are deployed at 1 and 11 o'clock and two fasteners for each site in the middle part of the valve, at 4, 6, and 8 o'clock position, to reinforce and prolong caudally the plication. This technique increased by 30 % the success rate of the procedure. With the standard TIF technique, 11/27 patients (40.7 %) didn't take PPI therapy at 12 months; with the application of the rotational TIF technique, 14/22 patients (63.6 %) were full responders.

Bell R. et al. have developed a rotational fundoplication, the so-called Bell Roll maneuver [38]. The helical retractor is engaged at 12 o'clock, and the tissue mold is placed at 6 o'clock; then the tissue mold locked is rotated toward the lesser curve by a radial motion of the handle of the device to the 12 o'clock position. This maneuver rolls the fundus over and around the distal esophagus to the 1 o'clock position.

At the end of the plication, an immediate endoscopy is performed to evaluate the pharynx, the esophageal lumen, the gastric fundus, and the fundoplication.

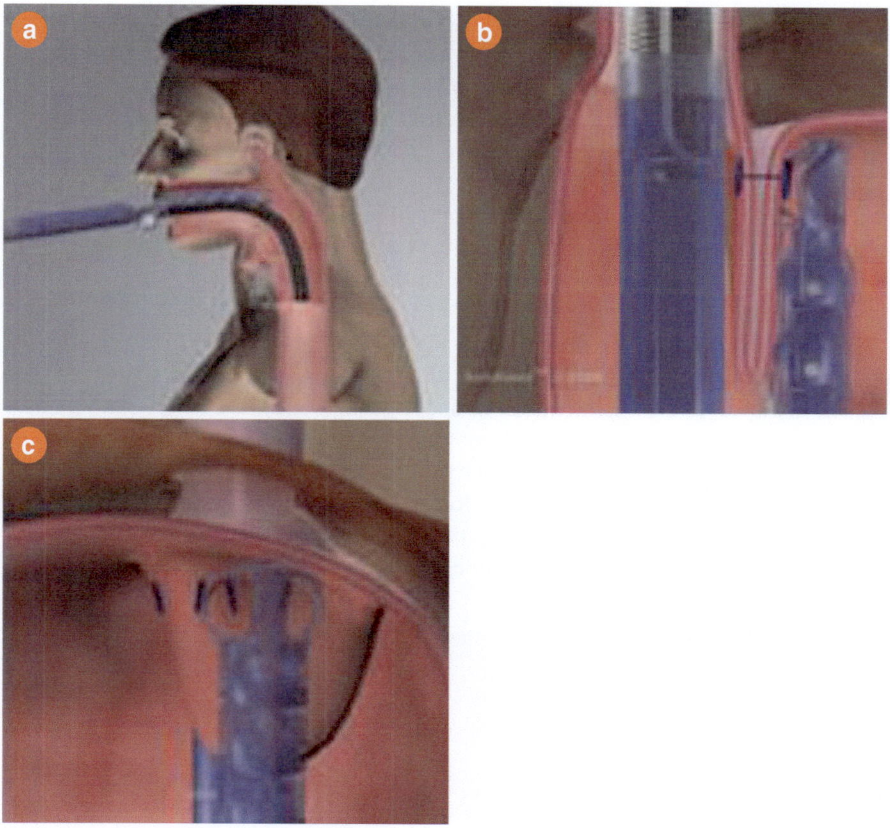

Fig. 7.2 Schematic representation of the procedure with EsophyX® device (Courtesy of EndoGastric Solutions Inc. Redmond, WA, USA). (**a**) The EsophyX® device enters the esophagus through the mouth and is positioned at the gastroesophageal junction; (**b**) the device wraps the fundus around the distal esophagus and fastens a tissue fold; this step is then repeated multiple times to reconstruct a robust, tight valve (**c**) (*©2014 EndoGastric Solutions, Inc.*)

7.3.3 Transoral Fundoplication by MUSE™ System

The MUSE™ system includes the endostapler and a console connected with the endostapler, containing a controller for the camera, ultrasonic range finder and various sensors, a pump for insufflation and irrigation, a suction system, and power and controls for the LED.

The endostapler has:

(a) A handle, wherein controls are located
(b) An insertion tube 15.5 mm in diameter, 66 cm long, containing the suction, insufflation/irrigation channels, and electrical and mechanical cables which operate the device

(c) A rigid section 66 mm in length that contains the cartridge. Each cartridge contains five standard 4.8-mm titanium staples, the ultrasound mirror, one alignment pin funnel, and two anvil screw funnels
(d) The distal tip, similar to that of an endoscope, with suction, irrigation, illumination (via LED), and visualization (via miniature camera) capabilities

The anvil, alignment pin, anvil screw, and ultrasound are all designed to ensure proper alignment and positioning of the device during stapling. The distal tip may be articulated in one direction to align with the rigid section and cartridge, with a bending radius of 26 and 40 mm.

Details of the device are illustrated in Fig. 7.4.

The procedure can be performed by one operator in experienced hands. The patient is placed in the supine position, under general anesthesia with endotracheal intubation. Positive end-expiratory pressure (PEEP) of at least 5 mmHg (7.5-cm H_2O) is administered. After a preliminary endoscopic assessment of the esophagus and stomach and once no contraindications are found, an overtube is placed. Then, the endostapler is inserted transorally through the overtube and gently advanced into the stomach under direct vision; passing the rigid section across the

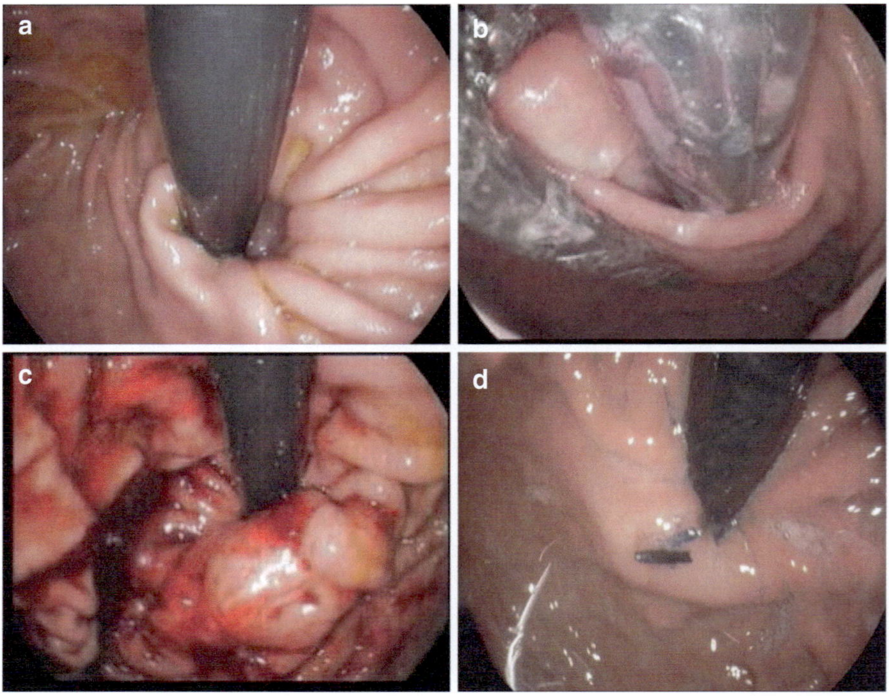

Fig. 7.3 Endoscopic views of the gastroesophageal valve before and immediately after the TIF procedure by EsophyX® device (authors' case). (**a**) The gastroesophageal valve: before the procedure with the EsophyX® device; (**b**) the "Bell Roll" maneuver to create the new gastroesophageal valve; (**c**) the gastroesophageal valve: immediately after the procedure with the EsophyX® device; (**d**) the gastroesophageal valve: 6 months after the procedure

pharyngoesophageal junction may encounter some resistance. In order to avoid applying excessive force and risk to injure the esophagus, the overtube may be withdrawn approximately 5 cm and then advanced with the endostapler as a unit. This maneuver can be repeated until the system reaches the esophageal midbody. Flexing the neck may make passage easier.

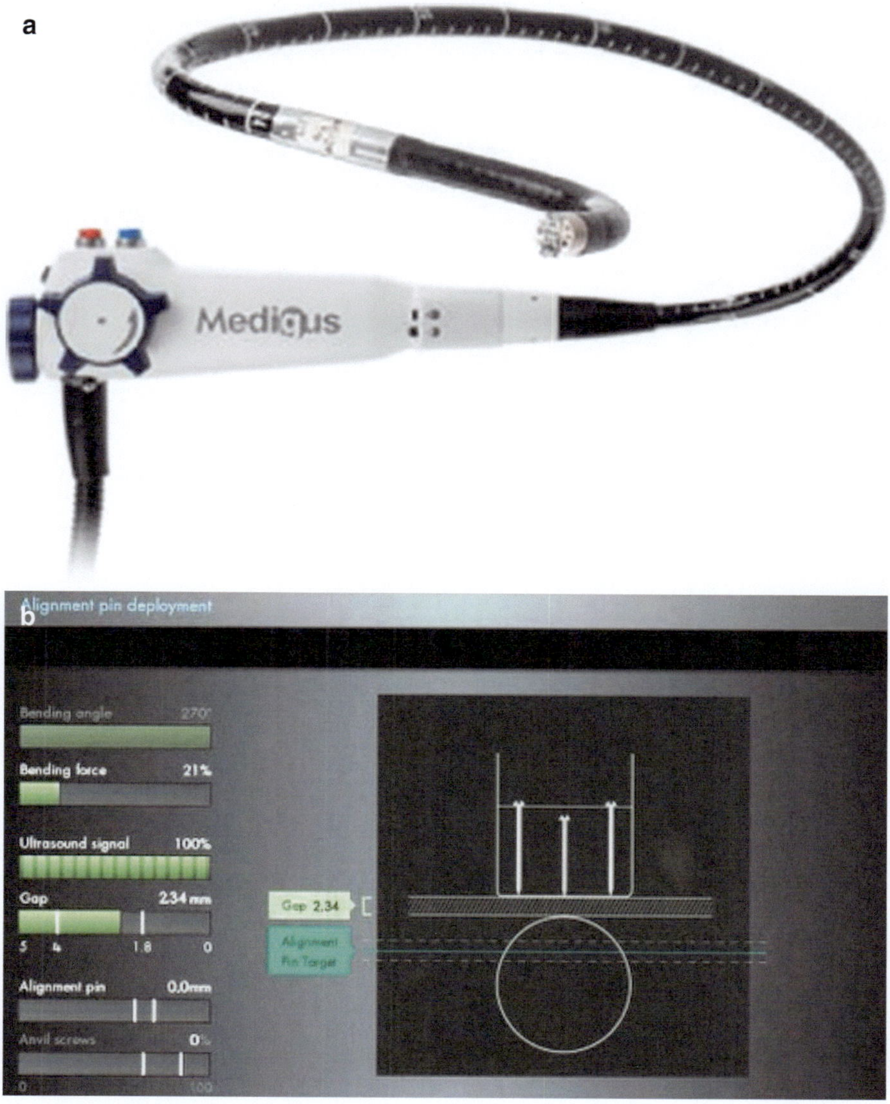

Fig. 7.4 The Medigus Surgical Ultrasonic Endostapler system, MUSE™ (Courtesy of Medigus Ltd., Omer, Israel). (**a**) The MUSE™ system (© *All rights reserved to Medigus Ltd. 2008–2015*); (**b**) the console connected with the endostapler, containing a controller for the camera, ultrasonic range finder, and various sensors (bending angle, bending force, alignment pin, anvil screws, gap) (© *All rights reserved to Medigus Ltd. 2008–2015*)

Once into the stomach, distended by insufflation of air or CO2, the stapler is advanced until the tip is approximately 5 cm past the EGJ and then retroflex by 180° to obtain an adequate vision of the gastric fundus and EGJ to select stapling location.

The most important stapling location is the leftmost location, which is typically performed first. This is the anchoring point for the fundus and should be placed as far to the left of the esophagus as possible. At times, depending on anatomy, it may be easier to perform the first stapling in a more central location. The additional stapling locations should be within 60–180° as long as the rightmost stapling should not be done on the lesser curve, because stapling in the lesser curve may attach the antrum to the esophagus and open the esophagogastric junction rather than close it. Additional staplings may be placed between the leftmost and rightmost. Once the correct location for stapling has been identified, all the procedures are performed under ultrasound guidance. Subsequent phases of the procedure include clamping tissue, deploying alignment pin, advancing anvil screw, stapling, and retrieving anvil screws [29]. Details of the MUSE™ device's technique are shown in Fig. 7.5.

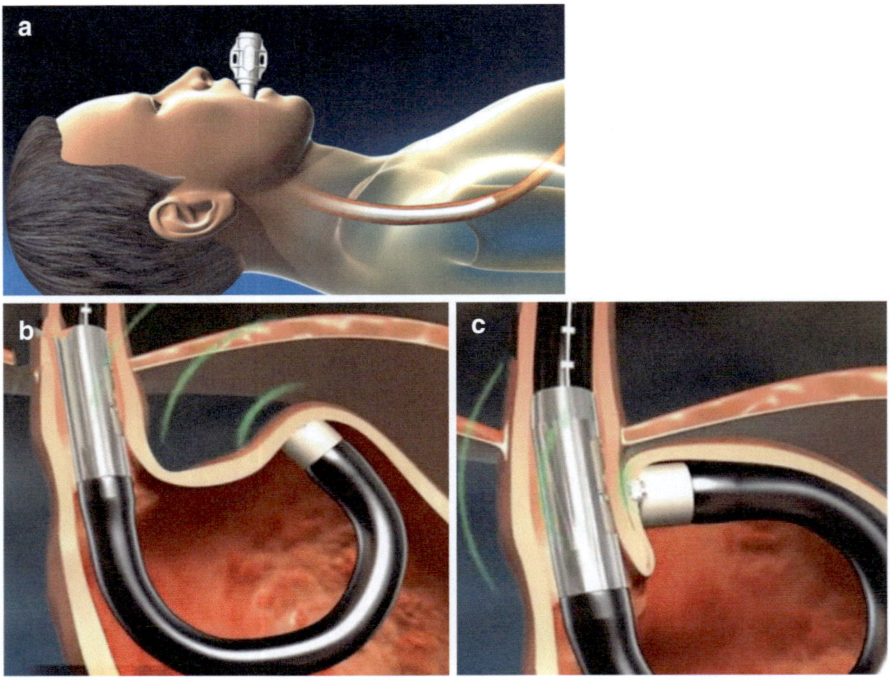

Fig. 7.5 Schematic representation of the Medigus Ultrasonic Surgical Endostapler (MUSE™) procedure (Courtesy of Medigus Ltd., Omer, Israel). (**a**) The endostapler is inserted transorally through the overtube and gently advanced into the stomach under direct vision; (**b**) once in the stomach, distended by insufflation of air or CO2, the stapler is advanced until the tip is approximately 5 cm past the EGJ and then retroflexed 180° to give adequate vision of the gastric fundus and EGJ to select the stapling location. The tissue is clamped and stapled under ultrasonic guidance; (**c**) this step is then repeated at least twice to reconstruct a robust, tight valve. Additional stapling locations should be within 60–180° of the valve circumference. EGJ, esophagogastric junction (*© All rights reserved to Medigus Ltd. 2008–2015*)

Endoscopic pre- and post-procedural findings after TIF with MUSE™ system are reported in Fig. 7.6.

7.3.4 Postoperative Care

Antiemetic prophylaxis with at least two drugs (according to the ASA recommendations for interventions with high risk of post-procedure nausea and vomiting) and full muscle relaxation throughout the procedure are mandatory for TIF. Antiemetic prophylaxis is maintained i.v. for 24 h, while broad-spectrum antibiotic therapy is maintained i.v. for 48 h and then by oral route over a 5-day period.

Almost all patients complain of transient pharyngeal irritation, as a result of insertion and manipulation of the device, and some have mild to moderate epigastric pain in 6 h after the procedure. Pain persisting for 2–4 days may require analgesics and should be considered for esophageal or gastric leak; CT scan and hydrosoluble contrast X-ray investigation should be carried out in these cases. Dysphagia and gas bloating are generally not reported by patients. White blood cell count may be slightly increased after the procedure. At discharge, patients are instructed to follow a liquid diet for the first 2 weeks and a soft diet for the next 4 weeks. PPIs are

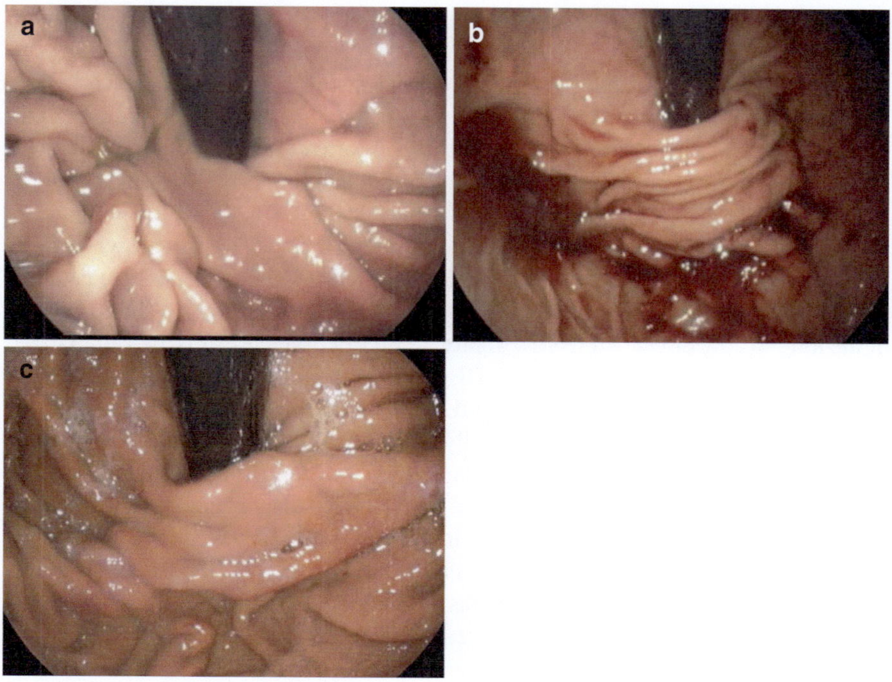

Fig. 7.6 Endoscopic views of the gastroesophageal valve before and after the TIF procedure with the Medigus Ultrasonic Surgical Endostapler (MUSE™) (authors' case). (**a**) The gastroesophageal valve: before the TIF procedure with the MUSE™ system; (**b**) the gastroesophageal valve: immediately after the TIF procedure by MUSE™ system; (**c**) the gastroesophageal valve: 6 months after the TIF procedure by MUSE™ system

discontinued 7 days after the procedure. Patients are also asked to refrain from vigorous exercise for 4 weeks.

7.4 Outcomes

To date, 20 prospective studies and one retrospective study, most of them observational and carried out in a limited number of patients, have been published on short- and medium-term follow-up (1–3 years) after TIF using EsophyX® device [38–58]. One study evaluated patients' outcomes up to 6 years after the procedure [56]. Sixteen studies assessed symptoms by means of the GERD health-related quality of life (HRQL); 11 evaluated pre- and post-procedure pH ± impedance recordings. A multicenter prospective study compared the efficacy of TIF versus omeprazole in a randomized controlled trial [59].

Overall, in 17 studies TIF was proven to discontinue antireflux medications or markedly decrease their dose; three studies arose concerns about the effectiveness of the procedure [45, 46, 49].

In the observational, nonrandomized studies, 6- and 12-month outcomes after TIF showed that 75–84 % and 53–85 % of patients had either discontinued PPI use or halved the dose of PPI therapy. Normalization of esophageal acid exposure, in terms of total acidic refluxes, number of refluxes, and DeMeester score, was reported in 37–89 % of patients.

Twenty-four months after TIF, daily high-dosage PPI dependence was eliminated in 75–93 % of patients. Endoscopic findings comparing fundoplication immediately after the procedure and 2 years later are reported in Fig. 7.7. In the two series reporting a 3-year follow-up, persistent discontinuation of daily PPI ranged from 74 to 84 % of cases [54, 56].

Only one study evaluated outcomes 6 years after TIF in 14/50 patients who underwent the procedure. High-dosage PPI dependence was eliminated in 86 % of patients, and approximately half of them completely stopped PPI use [56], providing evidence of the long-lasting effect of TIF on symptoms and PPI usage. Results are summarized in Fig. 7.8. Unsuccessful outcomes of TIF occurred mainly between 6 and 12 months after the procedure, while between 12 and 36 months, the results did not substantially differ. Six-year results were substantially similar to those reported at 36 months. These findings show that an appropriate patient selection plays a pivotal role in achieving clinical success after TIF and confirm that factors negatively affecting postoperative outcomes play a role early in the postoperative period in most patients. Operator's experience plays an important role in TIF outcomes, too. All TIF failures observed in our series occurred in patients who underwent the procedure early in the operator's learning curve. A retrospective study in 124 unselected patients carried out in two community hospitals and reporting, respectively, 75 and 80 % of patients free of typical and atypical GERD symptoms over a mean follow-up of 7 months confirmed that the operator's experience plays a major role in successful outcomes [52].

Only three prospective, randomized controlled trials have been so far published. Two assessed the 6-month efficacy of TIF versus omeprazole therapy: one showed

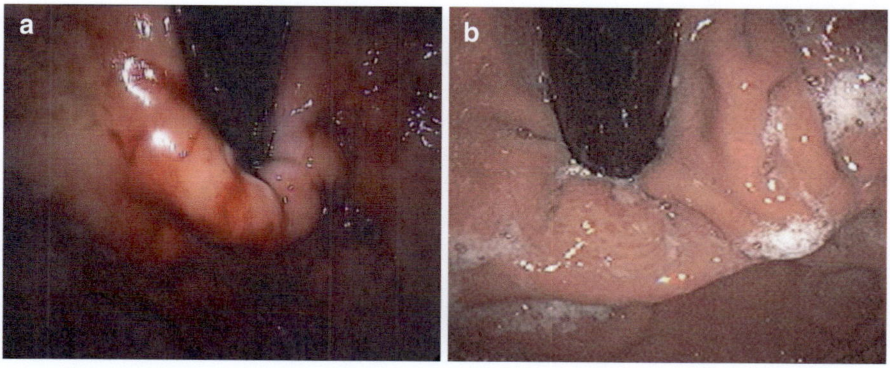

Fig. 7.7 Endoscopic views of the gastroesophageal valve immediately after and 24 months after the TIF procedure with EsophyX® device (authors' case). (**a**) The gastroesophageal valve: immediately after the TIF procedure with EsophyX® device; (**b**) the gastroesophageal valve: 24 months after the TIF procedure with EsophyX® device

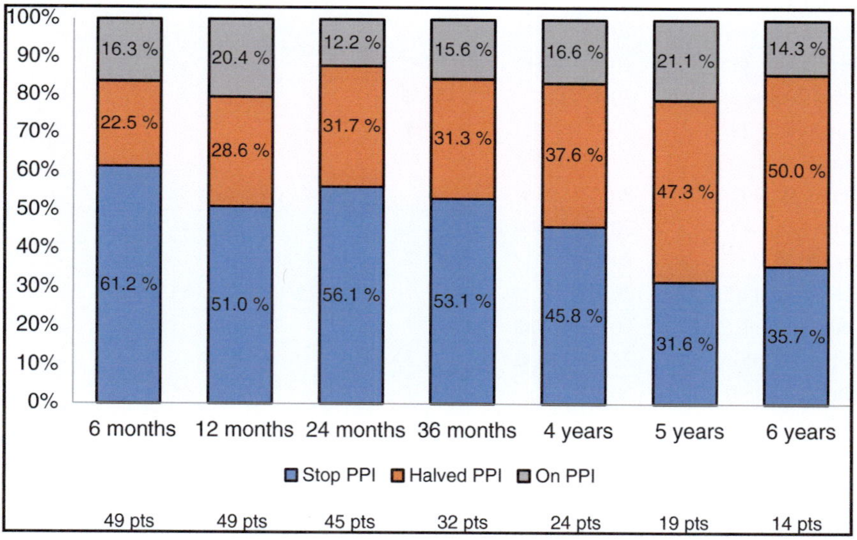

Fig. 7.8 Symptomatic responses 6 months and 1–6 years after TIF with EsophyX® device, classified according to proton pump inhibitor (PPI) use. Patients were grouped as complete responders (who completely stopped using PPI) or partial responders (who halved the previous PPI dose) and nonresponders (who still used the pre-TIF PPI dose): 12 months versus 6 months after TIF $P=0.8$; 24 versus 12 months $P=0.4$; 36 versus 24 months $P=0.7$; 4 years versus 36 months $P=1.0$; 5 versus 4 years $P=1.0$; 6 versus 5 years $P=1.0$

TIF more effective than PPI therapy in treating regurgitation and extraesophageal symptoms (97 % vs 50 % of patients, respectively; $P=0.006$) [58]; the second one proved at intention-to-treat analysis TIF more effective than PPI in eliminating GERD symptoms (67 % vs 45 %, respectively; $P=0.023$) [59]. These data show different outcomes and require additional randomized studies to clarify the efficacy of TIF in treating GERD. The third study compared 3- and 12-month results of TIF and Nissen fundoplication, showing TIF as effective and safe as Nissen fundoplication but with significantly lower hospital stay (2.9±0.8 days vs 6.4±0.7 days, respectively; $P<0.0001$) [60].

Outcomes of TIF, with regard to the effects on PPI usage, are reported in Tables 7.1 and 7.2.

Table 7.1 Symptomatic responses after transoral incisionless fundoplication with the EsophyX® device

Follow-up		6 months	12 months	24 months	36 months	6 years
Cadière et al. [39]	2008	–	85 %	–	–	–
Cadière et al. [41]	2009	–	–	93 %	–	–
Testoni et al. [42]	2010	82 %	76 %	–	–	–
Velanovich et al. [44]	2010	79 %	–	–	–	–
Repici et al. [45]	2010	55 %	47 %	–	–	–
Demyttenaere et al. [43]	2010	–	53 %	–	–	–
Hoppo et al. [46]	2010	–	42 %	–	–	–
Barnes et al. [52]	2011	93 %	–	–	–	–
Bell et al. [47]	2011	75 %	–	–	–	–
Ihde et al. [48]	2011	76 %	–	–	–	–
Trad et al. [51]	2012	–	82 %	–	–	–
Testoni et al. [53]	2012	–	–	75 %	75 %	–
Petersen et al. [50]	2012	58 %	–	–	–	–
Bell et al. [55]	2012	86 %	–	–	–	–
Muls et al. [54]	2013	–	77 %	–	65 %	–
Bell et al. [61]	2013	–	82 %	–	–	–
Bell et al. [57]	2014	–	–	77–80 %	–	–
Trad et al. [58]	2015	93 %	–	–	–	–
Hunter et al. [59]	2015	–	72 %	–	–	–
Testoni et al. [56]	2015	84 %	80 %	88 %	84 %	86 %

Table 7.2 Symptomatic responses after transoral incisionless fundoplication with the MUSE™ system

Follow-up		6 months	12 months	24 months	36 months	6 years
Zacheri et al. [62]	2015	83 %	–	–	–	–
Roy-Shapira et al. [63]	2015	–	82%	73 %	73 %	–

Unsuccessful outcomes after TIF were reported in three studies. Two series found worsening of distal esophageal acid exposure in 66.7 % of cases and persisting of GERD symptoms in 68 % of cases, respectively, in small series with a short follow-up (12 months). An open-label study comparing TIF with robot-assisted Nissen fundoplication in PPI-refractory GERD patients reported complete symptom remission and normalization of esophageal acid exposure time in 30 and 100 % of patients after TIF and 50 and 100 % after Nissen fundoplication [49]. These data suggest that in a challenging clinical setting such as PPI refractoriness, Nissen fundoplication seems more effective than TIF by EsophyX® device.

In case of failure of TIF, surgical fundoplication has been shown feasible, without technical difficulties or increased morbidity. Surgical revision after TIF failure was reported in from 8.1 to 18.0 % of cases [53, 54, 60, 64]. In two studies Nissen fundoplication induced complete disappearance of symptoms in all cases of TIF failure (respectively, 9 and 11 patients) [64, 65]. In our series, however, only one out of the four patients who underwent Nissen fundoplication for persisting GERD symptoms after TIF stopped acid-suppressive therapy: this finding may depend upon the particular subset of patients who underwent TIF in our series, who had only a mild impairment of the gastroesophageal junction and suffered from GERD-related symptoms that could have been generated by a number of complex mechanisms, including increased esophageal sensitivity to refluxate.

On the other hand, re-intervention after laparoscopic fundoplication has been reported in up to 14 % of cases, and TIF has been found effective after failed surgery [61].

Only two studies assessed so far the outcomes after TIF performed by MUSE™ technique (anterior fundoplication): a pilot study with a 5-year follow-up and a multicenter prospective study [62, 63]. The pilot study assessed GERD-related symptoms and PPI use up to 5 years after the procedure in 13 subjects: GERD-related symptom score at 6 months was normalized in 92 % of cases; PPI use was completely stopped or reduced by half in 77 % of cases (54 % off PPI completely) [63]. PPI therapy was abolished or reduced by half in 82 % of patients at 12 months and in 73 % at 36 months; this rate persisted unchanged up to 5 years. Another study assessed outcomes after TIF performed by MUSE™ technique (anterior fundoplication) in a multicenter, prospective international study enrolling 66 patients with a 6-month follow-up [62]. GERD-related symptom scores improved by more than 50 % in 73 % of patients and 64.6 % of them were no longer using daily PPI medication. Among patients who continued to take PPI, 56.5 % reduced by more than 50 % the dose. At 24-h pH recording, the total time with esophageal pH < 4.0 decreased significantly from baseline. There were no post-procedure side effects commonly seen after laparoscopic fundoplication as gas bloating, inability to belch or vomit, dysphagia, or diarrhea.

An important issue regarding all new interventional procedures introduced in clinical practice is the recognition of technique- or patient-related factors that could affect the outcomes.

In our series, from the technical point of view, the number of fasteners deployed and the rotational technique applied were associated with a good outcome; a larger number of fasteners raised the probability of being a responder about fourfold.

Another study reported the number of satisfactory fasteners as critical point for the success of the procedure, too. The rotational technique raised the probability of being a responder by one half, confirming other recent reports. Among patient-related factors affecting postoperative outcomes in our series, preoperative Hill grades III and IV, hiatal hernia larger than 2 cm, and ineffective esophageal motility were associated with a higher rate of unsuccessful results. The defective clearance of refluxate could induce an epithelial sensitization that might produce symptoms, even in the presence of low-volume gastroesophageal reflux. A univariate and multivariate analysis of preoperative factors influencing symptomatic outcomes of TIF by EsophyX was performed on data from 158 consecutive patients identified [57]. Predictors of successful outcomes for patients with typical symptoms have been found in the age ≥50 years, a GERD health-related quality of life score (GERD-HRQL) on PPIs ≥15, a reflux symptom index >13 on PPIs, and the gastroesophageal reflux symptom score ≥18 on PPIs. Age and GERD-HRQL remained significant predictors also at the multivariate analysis. For patients with atypical GERD symptoms only, a GERD-HRQL score ≥15 on PPIs was associated with successful outcomes.

7.5 Complications

The overall complication rate reported in studies so far available for TIF by EsophyX® ranges from 3 to 10 %. Major complications occurred rarely and were bleeding, mucosal tears or perforation requiring endoscopic intervention or surgery, pneumothorax, and mediastinal abscesses. The finding of free air in the abdomen immediately after the procedure is not always a sign of clinically relevant complications. Bleeding requiring transfusions has been reported in about 3–5 % of cases and can occur at the site of the helical retractor insertion. Mediastinal abscesses have been reported in less than 2 % of cases. No procedure-related deaths occurred. In the only study so far published on TIF by Medigus, minor side effects such as chest pain, sore throat, transient atelectasia, shoulder pain, and belching were reported in 5.5–22 % of patients; major complications were reported in 6.2 % of cases (4 out of 64 patients) and were pneumothorax (one case), pneumothorax and esophageal leak (one case), and bleeding (one case). Patients with pneumothorax and esophageal leak and with bleeding required intervention. All major complications occurred in the first 24 patients.

No late complications or long-lasting side effects occurred for both TIF techniques.

Conclusions

In the last years, TIF has been performed only in clinical trials including patients with typical gastroesophageal reflux symptoms responsive or partially responsive to PPI therapy, without hiatal hernia or with small hiatal hernia (<3 cm), who refused lifelong medical therapy, or were intolerant to PPIs or required high dosage of antisecretory maintenance therapy. Patients with grade C and D esophagitis, according to Los Angeles classification and Barrett's esophagus, were excluded from these studies. In the majority of studies, TIF was done by EsophyX® device and was proven effective in the short term in approximately 75 % of patients, eliminating the daily dependence from PPIs in half PPI-responsive GERD patients and markedly reducing the overall PPI dose in the other cases. Similar results were obtained more recently for TIF done with Medigus endostapler, but in few studies.

Such results were confirmed in studies with a follow-up up to 3 years, although few, and in the only follow-up up to 6 years. Troublesome procedure-related persisting side effects were not reported in all the published studies.

Overall outcomes showed that TIF procedure can be an effective and safe alternative therapeutic option to surgery in a selected subset of patients, as were those recruited in the published studies. In available series with 3- to 6-year follow-up, post-TIF results were slightly inferior to those reported in patients operated by Nissen fundoplication, but similar to those with surgical posterior partial (Toupet) or anterior partial (Dor-Thal) fundoplication, without any of the surgery-related side effects such as dysphagia and gas bloat.

Currently, based on clinical results, TIF may be offered as an alternative to surgery in patients suffering from gastroesophageal reflux disease and grade A-B esophagitis, if present, with the sole limitation of the length and reducibility of an eventual hiatal hernia, which is at present the only limiting factor affecting the choice of the intervention. TIF may also be offered to patients who have some risk of developing persistent postsurgical side effects. To date, data supporting the efficacy of TIF in the treatment of severe grades of esophagitis or symptoms associated with oropharyngeal reflux are lacking.

However, as for all new procedures introduced in clinical practice, despite favorable short- and medium-term outcomes, questions still arise about the long-term efficacy of the techniques, mainly for the MUSE, in controlling symptoms and persistence over time of the newly created valve. Therefore, randomized controlled trials are warranted in order to establish the role of TIF in the management of GERD patients, which, among the two techniques, could be more effective and safe.

In addition, preoperative patient-related anatomo-functional findings and procedure-related technical aspects that can help select patients and predict a successful outcome need to be clarified.

References

1. Lundell L, Miettinen P. Continued (5 years) follow up of a randomized clinical study comparing antireflux surgery and omeprazole in GERD. J Am Coll Surg. 2001;192(2):171–9. PMID: 11220717.
2. Draaisma WE, Rijnhart-de Jong HG, Broeders IA, Smout AJ, Furnee EJ, Gooszen HG. Five-year subjective and objective results of laparoscopic and conventional Nissen fundoplication. Ann Surg. 2006;244(1):34–41. PMID: 16794387.
3. Smith CD. Surgical therapy for gastroesophageal reflux disease: indications, evaluation and procedures. Gastrointest Endosc Clin N Am. 2009;19(1):35–48. PMID: 19232279.

4. Broeders JA, Draaisma WA, Bredenoord AJ, Smout AJ, Broeders IA, Gooszen HG. Long-term outcome of Nissen fundoplication in non-erosive and erosive gastro-esophageal reflux disease. Br J Surg. 2010;97(6):845–52. PMID: 20473997.
5. Bowrey DJ, Blom D, Crookes PF, Bremner CG, Johansson JL, Lord RV, Hagen JA, DeMeester SR, DeMeester TR, Peters JH. Risk factors and the prevalence of trocar site herniation after laparoscopic fundoplication. Surg Endosc. 2001;15(7):663–6. PMID: 11591964.
6. Fornari F, Sifrim D. Diagnostic options for patients with refractory GERD. Curr Gastroenterol Rep. 2008;10(3):283–8. PMID: 18625140.
7. Triadafilopoulos G. Endotherapy and surgery for GERD. J Clin Gastroenterol. 2007;41 Suppl 2:S87–96. PMID: 17575537.
8. Portale G, Filipi CJ, Peters JH. A current assessment of endoluminal approaches to the treatment of gastroesophageal reflux disease. Surg Innov. 2004;11(4):225–34. PMID: 15756391.
9. Fry LC, Monkenmuller K, Malfertheiner P. Endoluminal therapy for gastroesophageal reflux disease: evidence from clinical trials. Eur J Gastroenterol Hepatol. 2007;19(12):1125–39. PMID: 17998840.
10. Institute AGA. American gastroenterological medical position statement on the management of gastroesophageal reflux disease. Gastroenterology. 2008;135(4):1383–91. PMID: 18789939.
11. Lehman GA. The history and future of implantation therapy for gastroesophageal reflux disease. Gastrointest Endosc Clin N Am. 2003;13(1):157–65. PMID: 12797435.
12. Feretis C, Benakis P, Dimopoulos C, Dailianas A, Filalithis P, Stamou KM, Manouras A, Apostolidis N. Endoscopic implantation of Plexiglas (PMMA) microsphere for the treatment of GERD. Gastrointest Endosc. 2001;53(4):423–6. PMID: 11275880.
13. Vassiliou MC, von Renteln D, Rothstein RI. Recent advances in endoscopic antireflux techniques. Gastrointest Endosc Clin N Am. 2010;20(1):89–101. PMID: 19951796.
14. Johnson DA, Ganz R, Aisenberg J, Cohen LB, Devière J, Foley TR, Haber GB, Peters JH, Lehman GA. Endoscopic implantation of Enteryx for treatment of GERD: 12-month results of a prospective, multicenter trial. Am J Gastroenterol. 2003;98(9):1921–30. PMID: 14499767.
15. Johnson DA, Ganz R, Aisenberg J, Cohen LB, Deviere J, Foley TR, Haber GB, Peters JH, Lehman GA. Endoscopic, deep mural implantation of Enteryx for the treatment of GERD: 6-month follow-up of a multicenter trial. Am J Gastroenterol. 2003;98(2):250–8. PMID:12591037.
16. Ganz RA. The future of endoscopic esophageal therapy – what comes next. Gastrointest Endosc Clin N Am. 2010;20:147–59. PMID: 19951800.
17. Fockens P. Gatekeeper Reflux Repair System: technique, pre-clinical and clinical experience. Gastrointest Endosc Clin N Am. 2003;13(1):179–89. PMID: 12797437.
18. Fockens P, Bruno MJ, Gabbrielli A, Odegaard S, Hatlebakk J, Allescher HD, Rösch T, Rhodes M, Bastid C, Rey J, Boyer J, Muehldorffer S, van den Hombergh U, Costamagna G. Endoscopic augmentation of the lower esophageal sphincter for the treatment of gastroesophageal reflux disease: multicenter study of the Gatekeeper Reflux Repair System. Endoscopy. 2004;36(8):682–9. PMID: 15280972.
19. Triadafilopoulos G, Utley DS. Temperature-controlled radiofrequency energy delivery for gastro-esophageal reflux disease: the Stretta procedure. J Laparoendosc Adv Surg Tech A. 2001;11(6):333–9. PMID: 11814123.
20. Corley DA, Katz P, Wo JM, Stefan A, Patti M, Rothstein R, Edmundowicz S, Kline M, Mason R, Wolfe MM. Improvement of gastro-esophageal reflux symptoms after radiofrequency energy: a randomized, sham-controlled trial. Gastroenterology. 2003;125(3):668–76. PMID: 12949712.
21. Yeh RW, Triadafilopoulos G. Endoscopic antireflux therapy: the Stretta procedure. Thorac Surg Clin. 2005;15(3):395–403. PMID: 16104130.
22. Di Baise JK, Brand RE, Quigley EM. Endoluminal delivery of radiofrequency energy to gastro-esophageal junction in uncomplicated GERD: efficacy and potential mechanisms of action. Am J Gastroenterol. 2002;97(4):833–42. PMID: 12003416.
23. Galmiche JP, Bruley des Varannes S. Endoluminal therapies for gastroesophageal reflux disease. Lancet. 2003;361(9363):1119–21. PMID: 12672327.
24. Franciosa M, Triadafilopoulos G, Mashimo H. Stretta radiofrequency treatment for GERD: a safe and effective modality. Gastroenterol Res Pract. 2013;2013:783815. PMID: 24078808.

25. Chen D, Barber C, McLoughlin P, Thavaneswaran P, Jamieson GG, Maddern GJ. Systematic review of endoscopic treatments for gastro-esophageal reflux disease. Br J Surg. 2009;96(2):128–36. PMID: 19160349.
26. Perry KA, Banerjee A, Melvin WS. Radiofrequency energy delivery to the lower esophageal sphincter reduces esophageal acid exposure and improves GERD symptoms: a systematic review and meta-analysis. Surg Laparosc Endosc Percutan Tech. 2012;22(4):283–8. PMID: 22874675.
27. Dughera L, Rotondano G, De Cento M, Cassolino P, Cisarò F. Durability of stretta radiofrequency treatment for GERD: results of an 8-year follow-Up. Gastroenterol Res Pract. 2014;2014:531907. PMID: 24959175.
28. Auyag ED, Carter P, Rauth T, Fanelli RD, SAGES Guidelines Committee. SAGES clinical spotlight review: endoluminal treatments for gastroesophageal reflux disease (GERD). Surg Endosc. 2013;27(8):2658–72. PMID: 23801538.
29. Schiefke I, Zabel-Langhennig A, Neumann S, Feisthammel J, Moessner J, Caca K. Long term failure of endoscopic gastroplication (EndoCinch). Gut. 2005;54(6):752–8. PMID: 15888777.
30. Schwartz MP, Wellink H, Gooszen HG, Conchillo JM, Samsom M, Smout AJ. Endoscopic gastroplication for the treatment of gastroesophageal reflux disease: a randomized, sham-controlled trial. Gut. 2007;56(1):20–8. PMID: 16763053.
31. Mahmood Z, Byrne PJ, McMahon BP, Murphy EM, Arfin Q, Ravi N, Weir DG, Reynolds JV. Comparison of transesophageal endoscopic placation (TEP) with laparoscopic Nissen fundoplication (LNF) in the treatment of uncomplicated reflux disease. Am J Gastroenterol. 2006;101(3):431–6. PMID: 16542276.
32. Schiefke I, Neumann S, Zabel-Langhennig A, Moessner J, Caca K. Use of an endoscopic suturing device (the "ESD") to treat patients with gastroesophageal reflux disease, after unsuccessful EndoCinch endoluminal gastroplication: another failure. Endoscopy. 2005;37(8):700–5. PMID: 16032486.
33. Chuttani R. Endoscopic full-thickness plication: the device, technique, pre-clinical and early clinical experience. Gastrointest Endosc Clin N Am. 2003;13(1):109–16. PMID: 12797431.
34. von Renteln D, Schiefke I, Fuchs KH, Raczynski S, Philipper M, Breithaupt W, Caca K, Neuhaus H. Endoscopic full-thickness plication for the treatment of GERD by application of multiple Plicator implants: a multicenter study (with video). Gastrointest Endosc. 2008;68(5):833–44. PMID: 18534586.
35. von Renteln D, Schiefke I, Fuchs KH, Raczynski S, Philipper M, Breithaupt W, Caca K, Neuhaus H. Endoscopic full-thickness plication for the treatment of gastroesophageal reflux disease using multiple Plicator implants: 12-month multicenter study results. Surg Endosc. 2009;23(8):1866–75. PMID: 19440792.
36. Pleskow D, Rothstein R, Kozarek R, Haber G, Gostout C, Lo S, Hawes R, Lembo A. Endoscopic full-thickness placation for the treatment of GERD: five-year long-term multicenter results. Surg Endosc. 2008;22(2):326–32. PMID: 18027032.
37. Ozawa S, Yoshida M, Kumai K, Kitajima M. New endoscopic treatments for gastroesophageal reflux disease. Ann Thorac Cardiovasc Surg. 2005;11(3):146–53. PMID: 16030472.
38. Bell RC, Cadière GB. Transoral rotational esophagogastric fundoplication: technical, anatomical, and safety considerations. Surg Endosc. 2011;25(7):2387–99. PMID: 21184101.
39. Cadière GB, Buset M, Muls V, Rajan A, Rösch T, Eckardt AJ, Weerts J, Bastens B, Costamagna G, Marchese M, Louis H, Mana F, Sermon F, Gawlicka AK, Daniel MA, Devière J. Antireflux transoral incisionless fundoplication using EsophyX: 12-month results of a prospective multicenter study. World J Surg. 2008;32(8):1676–88. PMID: 18443855.
40. Bergman S, Mikami DJ, Hazey JW, Roland JC, Dettorre R, Melvin WS. Endolumenal fundoplication with Esophyx: the initial North American experience. Surg Innov. 2008;15(3):166–70. PMID: 18757375.
41. Cadière GB, Van Sante N, Graves JE, Gawlicka AK, Rajan A. Two-year results of a feasibility study on antireflux transoral incisionless fundoplication using Esophyx. Surg Endosc. 2009;23(5):957–64. PMID: 19288158.
42. Testoni PA, Corsetti M, Di Pietro S, Castellaneta AG, Vailati C, Masci E, Passaretti S. Effect of transoral incisionless fundoplication on symptoms, PPI use, and pH-impedance refluxes of GERD patients. World J Surg. 2010;34(4):750–7. PMID: 20091308.

43. Demyttenaere SV, Bergman S, Pham T, Anderson J, Dettorre R, Melvin WS, Mikami DJ. Transoral incisionless fundoplication for gastro-esophageal reflux disease in an unselected patient population. Surg Endosc. 2010;24(4):854–8. PMID: 19730949.
44. Velanovich V. Endoscopic, endoluminal fundoplication for gastroesophageal reflux disease: initial experience and lesson learned. Surgery. 2010;148(4):646–51. PMID: 20708763.
45. Repici A, Fumagalli U, Malesci A, Barbera R, Gambaro C, Rosati R. Endoluminal fundoplication (ELF) for GERD using Esophyx: a 12-month follow-up in a single-center experience. J Gastrointest Surg. 2010;14(1):1–6. PMID: 19902310.
46. Hoppo T, Immanuel A, Schuchert M, Dubrava Z, Smith A, Nottle P, Watson DI, Jobe BA. Transoral incisionless fundoplication 2.0 procedure using EsophyX™ for gastroesophageal reflux disease. J Gastrointest Surg. 2010;14(12):1895–901. PMID: 20878257.
47. Bell RC, Freeman KD. Clinical and pH-metric outcomes of transoral esophagogastric fundoplication for the treatment of gastroesophageal reflux disease. Surg Endosc. 2011;25(6):1975–84. PMID: 21140170.
48. Ihde GM, Besancon K, Deljkich E. Short-term safety and symptomatic outcomes of transoral incisionless fundoplication with or without hiatal hernia repair in patients with chronic gastroesophageal reflux disease. Am J Surg. 2011;202(6):740–6. PMID: 22014853.
49. Frazzoni M, Conigliaro R, Manta R, Melotti G. Reflux parameters as modified by EsophyX or laparoscopic fundoplication in refractory GERD. Aliment Pharmacol Ther. 2011;34(1):67–75. PMID: 21539587.
50. Petersen R, Filippa L, Wassenaar EB, Martin AV, Tatum R, Oelschlager BK. Comprehensive evaluation of endoscopic fundoplication using the Esophyx device. Surg Endosc. 2012;26(4):1021–7. PMID: 22042587.
51. Trad KS, Turgeon DG, Deljkich E. Long-term outcomes after transoral incisionless fundoplication in patients with GERD and LPR symptoms. Surg Endosc. 2012;26(3):650–60. PMID: 21959689.
52. Barnes WE, Hoddinott KM, Mundy S, Williams M. Transoral incisionless fundoplication offers high patient satisfaction and relief of therapy-resistant typical and atypical symptoms of GERD in community practice. Surg Innov. 2011;18(2):119–29. PMID: 21307014.
53. Testoni PA, Vailati C, Testoni S, Corsetti M. Transoral incisionless fundoplication (TIF 2.0) with Esophyx for gastroesophageal reflux disease: long-term results and findings affecting outcome. Surg Endosc. 2012;26(5):1425–35. PMID: 22170317.
54. Muls V, Eckardt AJ, Marchese M, Bastens B, Buset M, Devière J, Louis H, Rajan A, Daniel MA, Costamagna G. Three-year results of a multicenter prospective study of transoral incisionless fundoplication. Surg Innov. 2013;20(4):321–30. PMID: 22968006.
55. Bell RC, Mavrelis PG, Barnes WE, Dargis D, Carter BJ, Hoddinott KM, Sewell RW, Trad KS, DaCosta GB, Ihde GM. A prospective multicenter registry of patients with chronic gastroesophageal reflux disease receiving transoral incisionless fundoplication. J Am Coll Surg. 2012;215(6):794–809. PMID: 22939637.
56. Testoni PA, Testoni S, Mazzoleni G, Vailati C, Passaretti S. Long-term efficacy of transoral incisionless fundoplication with Esophyx (TIF 2.0) and factors affecting outcomes in GERD patients followed for up to 6 years: a prospective single-center study. Surg Endosc. 2015;29(9):2770–80. PMID: 25480624.
57. Bell RC, Fox MA, Barnes WE, Mavrelis PG, Sewell RW, Carter BJ, Ihde GM, Trad KS, Dargis D, Hoddinott KM, Freeman KD, Gunsberger T, Hausmann MG, Gill BD, Wilson E. Univariate and multivariate analysis of preoperative factors influencing symptomatic outcomes of transoral fundoplication. Surg Endosc. 2014;28(10):2949–58. PMID: 24879134.
58. Trad KS, Barnes WE, Simoni G, Shughoury AB, Mavrelis PG, Raza M, Heise JA, Turgeon DG, Fox MA. Transoral incisionless fundoplication effective in eliminating GERD symptoms in partial responders to proton pump inhibitor therapy at 6 months: the TEMPO randomized clinical trial. Surg Innov. 2015;22(1):26–40. PMID: 24756976.
59. Hunter GJ, Kahrilas PJ, Bell RC, Wilson EB, Trad KS, Dolan JP, Perry KA, Oelschlager BK, Soper NJ, Snyder BE, Burch MA, Melvin WS, Reavis KM, Turgeon DG, Hungness ES, Diggs

BS. Efficacy of transoral fundoplication vs omeprazole for treatment of regurgitation in a randomized controlled trial. Gastroenterology. 2015;148(2):324–33. PMID: 25448925.
60. Svoboda P, Kantorová I, Kozumplík L, Scheer P, Radvan M, Radvanová J, Krass V, Horálek F. Our experience with transoral incisionless plication of gastroesophageal reflux disease: NOTES procedure. Hepatogastroenterology. 2011;58(109):1208–13. PMID: 21937380.
61. Bell RC, Hufford RJ, Fearon J, Freeman KD. Revision of failed traditional fundoplication using Esophyx transoral fundoplication. Surg Endosc. 2013;27(3):761–7. PMID: 23052519.
62. Zacheri J, Roy-Shapira A, Bonavina L, Bapaye A, Kiesslich R, Schoppmann SF, Kessler WR, Selzer DJ, Broderick RC, Lehman GA, Horgan S. Endoscopic anterior fundoplication with the Medigus Ultrasonic Surgical Endostapler (MUSE) for gastroesophageal reflux: 6-month results from a multi-center prospective trial. Surg Endosc. 2015;29(1):220–9. PMID: 25135443.
63. Roy-Shapira A, Bapaye A, Date S, Pujari R, Dorwat S. Trans-oral anterior fundoplication: 5-year follow-up of pilot study. Surg Endosc. 2015;29(12):3717–21. PMID: 25783833.
64. Fumagalli Romario U, Barbera R, Repici A, Porta M, Malesci A, Rosati R. Nissen fundoplication after failure of endoluminal fundoplication: short-term results. J Gastrointest Surg. 2011;15(3):439–43. PMID: 21207179.
65. Furnée EJ, Broeders JA, Draaisma WA, Schwartz MP, Hazebroek EJ, Smout AJ, van Rijn PJ, Broeders IA. Laparoscopic Nissen fundoplication after failed Esophyx fundoplication. Br J Surg. 2010;97(7):1051–5. PMID: 20632271.

The Point on the POEM: Comparison Between Different Techniques and Outcomes

8

Jennifer L. Maranki, Rani Modayil, and Stavros N. Stavropoulos

8.1 Introduction

Peroral endoscopic myotomy (POEM) has emerged as a natural orifice transluminal endoscopic surgery (NOTES) alternative to laparoscopic Heller myotomy (LHM) for the treatment of achalasia. Since the first human POEM, performed in Yokohama, Japan, by Haruhiro Inoue and reported in 2009, POEM has enjoyed explosive growth and became the subject of comprehensive documents by the major US endoscopic societies, the American Society for Gastrointestinal Endoscopy (ASGE) and Society of American Gastrointestinal and Endoscopic Surgeons (SAGES) [1, 2].

8.2 Standard Technique

The standard POEM technique involves four main steps (see Figs. 8.1 and 8.2). First, a submucosal injection with saline and indigo carmine along either the anterior or posterior esophagus is made several centimeters proximal to the

J.L. Maranki, MD, MSc
Division of Gastroenterology and Hepatology, Temple University School of Medicine, Philadelphia, PA, USA

R. Modayil, MD
Division of Gastroenterology and Hepatology, Winthrop University Hospital, Mineola, NY, USA

S.N. Stavropoulos, MD (✉)
Program for Advanced GI Endoscopy (PAGE), Winthrop University Hospital, Mineola, NY, USA

Columbia University College of Physicians and Surgeons, New York, NY, USA

Temple University School of Medicine, Philadelphia, PA, USA
e-mail: sstavropoulos@winthrop.org

R. Conigliaro, M. Frazzoni (eds.), *Diagnosis and Endoscopic Management of Digestive Diseases*, DOI 10.1007/978-3-319-42358-6_8

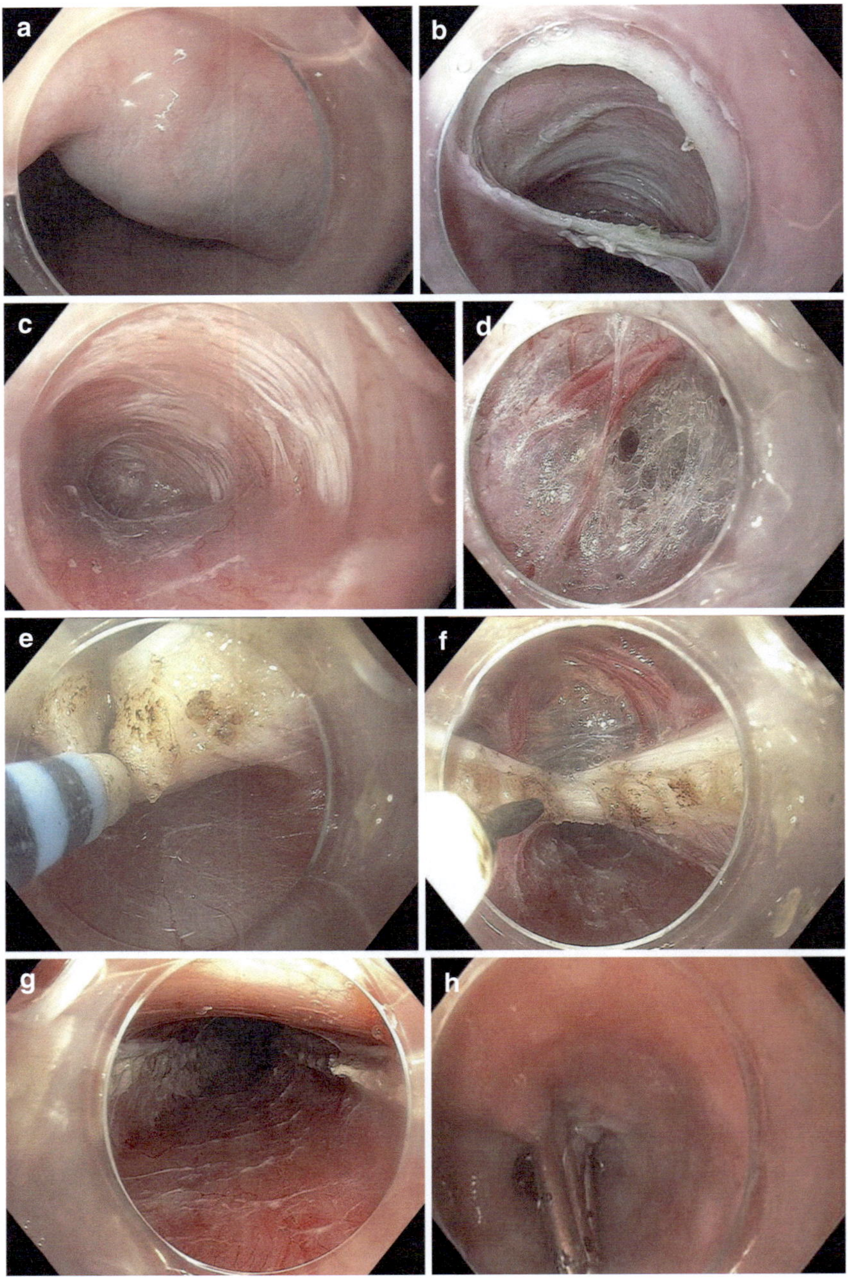

Fig. 8.1 (**a**) Submucosal injection is performed with saline stained with indigo carmine. (**b**) Mucosotomy is performed along the right anterior wall of the esophagus. (**c**) Submucosal dissection is performed with hybrid knife. (**d**) Vessels noted during dissection in the submucosal tunnel are coagulated. (**e**) Myotomy is initiated 2 cm below site of mucosotomy. (**f**) Full-thickness myotomy is extended to gastric cardia. (**g**). Final full-thickness myotomy is seen as endoscope is withdrawn from the submucosal tunnel. (**h**) Mucosotomy is closed with endoscopic clips

gastroesophageal junction (GEJ). Next, using the submucosal tunnel technique initially developed by Sumiyama and Gostout, a mucosotomy is created, and the submucosa is dissected, creating a submucosal tunnel [3]. The submucosal tunnel is extended into the cardia of the stomach. The myotomy is initiated 2 cm distal to the mucosotomy. The lower esophageal sphincter (LES) myotomy is completed. The submucosal tunnel mucosotomy site is then closed with either hemoclips or endoscopic suturing (see Fig. 8.3) [4].

8.2.1 Variations in Technique

Among high-volume centers, there are variations in the technique of POEM, including in the orientation (e.g., "anterior" vs "posterior") and thickness of the myotomy (full-thickness vs circular-layer-only myotomy) (see Figs. 8.4 and 8.5), and devices used for dissection (see Fig. 8.7) and for tunnel closure (see Fig. 8.3) [1].

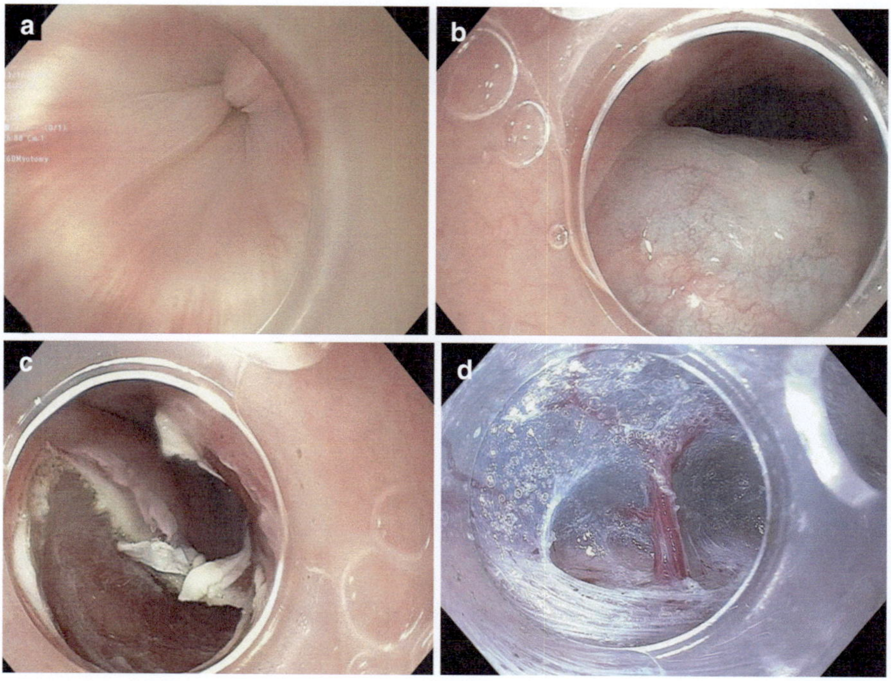

Fig. 8.2 (**a**) Prior to POEM, there is evidence of a tightly puckered LES. (**b**) Submucosal injection is performed with saline stained with indigo carmine. (**c**) Mucosotomy is performed along the right posterior wall of the esophagus. (**d**) Submucosal dissection is performed with hybrid knife and submucosal vessels are coagulated. (**d**) Submucosal tunnel is extended into the gastric cardia. (**e**) Myotomy is initiated 2 cm below site of mucosotomy. (**f**) Final full-thickness myotomy is seen as endoscope is withdrawn from the submucosal tunnel. (**e**) Mucosotomy is closed with an endoscopic suturing device. (**f**) After POEM, the LES appears patulous

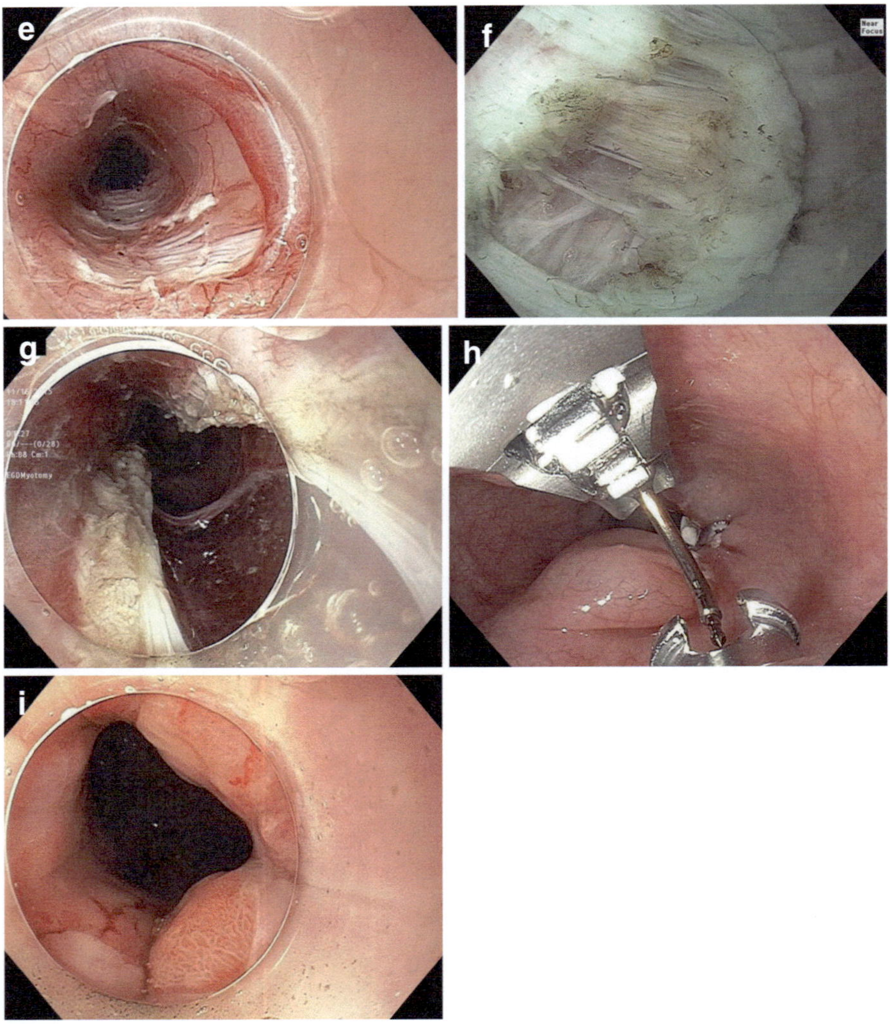

Fig. 8.2 (continued)

Fig. 8.3 A Closure of POEM tunnel orifice in a posterior POEM with the tunnel opening at the 5 o'clock position. (**a**) We use a single running suture for closure starting at the distal, left margin of the defect as shown here. (**b**) We attempt to penetrate mucosa and submucosa but not muscularis propria to avoid ischemia and pain or even possible injury to mediastinal structures. (**c**) We proceed with suture placement through the right margin of the defect. (**d**) The single running suture has been completed and has approximated the edges of the defect, and the needle has been dropped in order to serve as a T-tag securing the suture at the proximal end of the defect. (**e–f**) The cinch catheter is inserted over the long suture leading to the start of the running suture in the distal end of the defect; the suture is tightened and the cinch is deployed securing the suture at the start of the suture line in the distal end of the defect. (**g**) Completed closure of mucosotomy with endoscopic suturing. (**h**) For comparison purposes, we show here closure of the tunnel with endoscopic clips

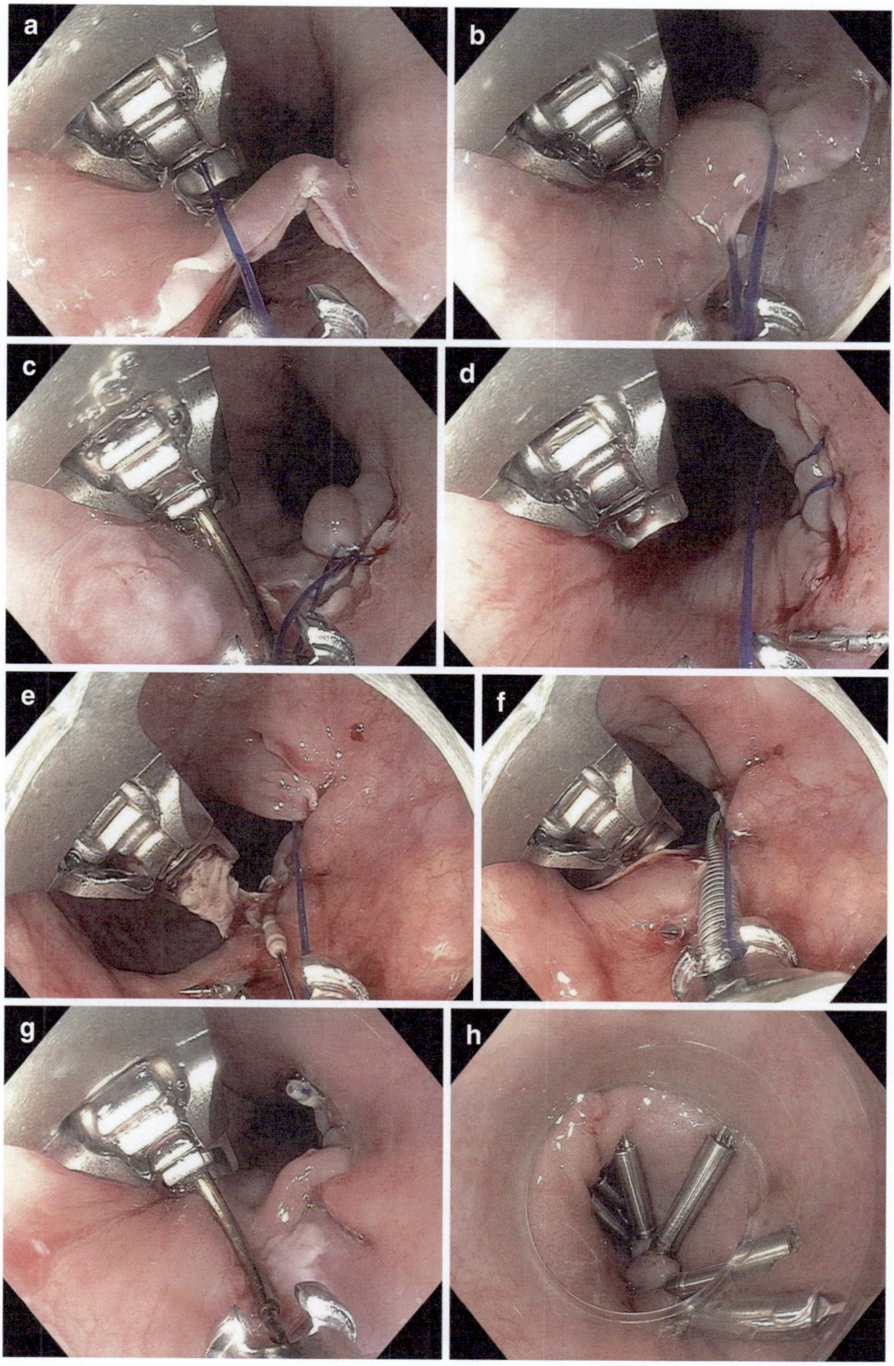
a
b
c
d
e
f
g
h

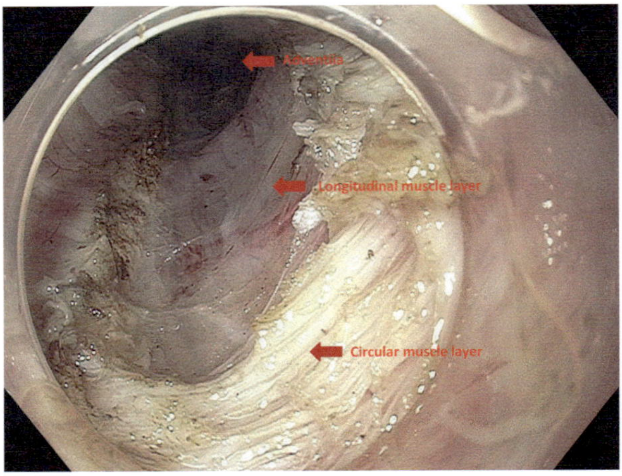

Fig. 8.4 Demonstrates for illustration purposes full-thickness myotomy and circular-layer-only myotomy in the same patient. In the initial portion of the myotomy, the circular muscle is dissected and the longitudinal muscle layer is preserved, whereas more distally full-thickness myotomy has been performed with visualization of the adventitia

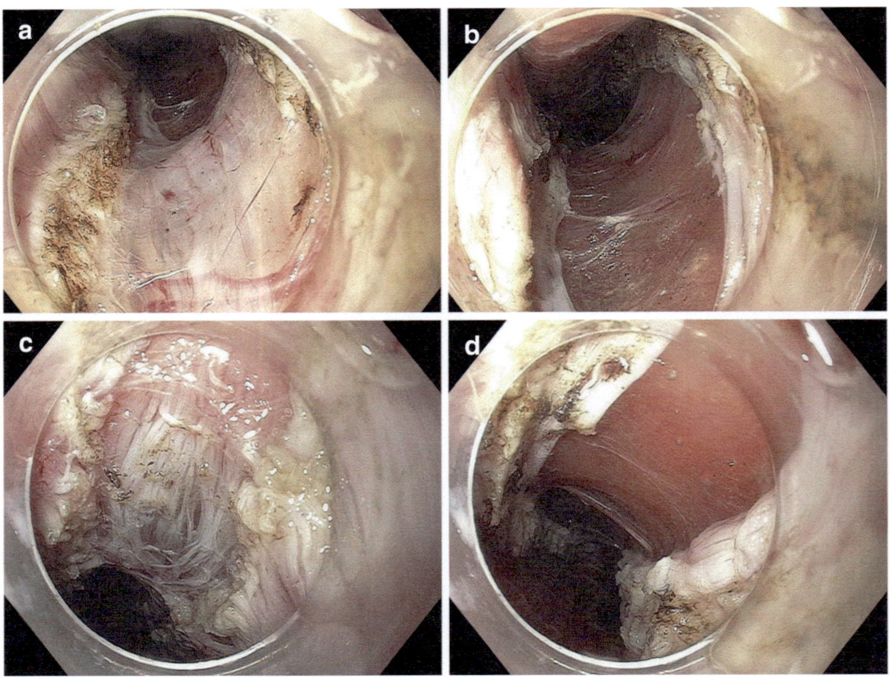

Fig. 8.5 Partial versus full-thickness myotomy. (**a**) Posterior myotomy. The cut edges of the circular muscle are seen between 5 and 8 o'clock, and the longitudinal muscle layer is preserved. (**b**) Posterior myotomy. Full-thickness myotomy is performed exposing the adventitia/mediastinal pleura which appears as a transparent thin membrane through which the right lung can be visualized. (**c**) Anterior myotomy. The cut edges of the circular muscle are seen between 2 and 4 o'clock, and the longitudinal muscle layer is preserved. (**d**) Anterior myotomy. Full-thickness myotomy is performed exposing the adventitia and pericardium that appear as a thin transparent membrane

8.3 Orientation

The orientation of POEM can vary depending on the practice of various centers but also depending on esophageal lesions such as diverticula or ulcerations, sigmoidization, or scarring from a prior myotomy that can force a certain orientation independent of the individual preference of the operator. In general a typical anterior myotomy is performed at 2 o'clock using the usual convention (the orientation that results in a myotomy that is centered along the clasp fibers at the lesser curvature of the EGJ and cardia) (see Fig. 8.1). A posterior myotomy is typically performed at 5–6 o'clock (just to the right of the spine) (see Fig. 8.2). A greater curvature myotomy at the 8 o'clock position has also been reported [5]. The anterior, or lesser curvature (LC), approach was initially adopted during the development of POEM as it reflects the surgical Heller myotomy approach, with access to the gastroesophageal junction from the ventral surface. The POEM procedure with this anterior, lesser curvature myotomy (at the 2 o'clock position) has shown excellent results [6–9]. However, excellent results have also been reported by centers that favor a posterior approach [10, 11]. It has been proposed that one of the benefits of the anterior approach is that the sling fibers, a natural reflux barrier supporting the angle of His, are not disrupted, thereby helping to minimize post-procedural gastroesophageal reflux disease (GERD) [5, 12]. However, data supporting the validity of this hypothesis are still lacking. Our group is currently near completion of enrollment of patients in a single-center randomized study comparing anterior and posterior orientation. Furthermore, we recently presented preliminary data from a comparison of anterior and posterior POEMs in our large single-operator series using data from a prospectively maintained database (Stavropoulos SN, et al. *Gastrointestinal Endoscopy*. 81(5):Supp AB 188–119). In this study we analyzed all POEMs performed at our center, 248 consecutive POEMs (120 anterior, 128 posterior), all successfully completed, with no aborted POEMs or surgical conversions, between 10/2009 and 10/2015. No learning curve bias expected as we performed a similar percentage of anterior POEMs in the first 3 years of our series (48/91, 53 %), as in the last 2 years (72/157 46 %). There were no differences in the Eckardt score, including failures (post-POEM Eckardt score >3, 5/110 A vs 4/117 P, NS), accidental mucosal injuries including nontransmural minor blanching (29 % vs 23 %), with prolonged stay of >5 days (one patient in each group). There was no difference in significant AEs, but it should be noted that there was paucity of such events in our series with no leaks, no tunnel bleeds, and no surgical/IR interventions. Posterior POEM was significantly faster overall (97 min A, 79 min P, $P=0.0007$) including a faster closure (suturing 177, clips 71) (9.6 min A, 7.9 min P, $P=0.02$). More patients had pain requiring narcotics in posterior POEM (17 % A vs 27 % P, $P=0.007$). There was a trend for less acid exposure in anterior POEM: +BRAVO studies 21/58 (36 %) A vs 29/58 (50 %) P, $P=0.13$, reflux esophagitis 22/57 (38 %) A vs 33/60 (55 %) P, $P=0.076$. Based on these results, we calculated a sample size of 120 (including 20 % dropout) for an anterior vs posterior randomized trial to demonstrate that posterior POEM is faster. However, a larger number may be required to demonstrate a difference in incidence of reflux at 95 % confidence. We have currently enrolled 94 pts in this RCT. Therefore, high-quality data comparing these two approaches should be forthcoming in the near future.

Nevertheless, currently there is no consensus regarding the optimal orientation. The international POEM survey (IPOEMS) [13] revealed that as early as 2013, several pioneering centers performed myotomy in orientations other than the anterior 2 o'clock orientation (see Fig. 8.6). Notably the center with the highest POEM volume and fastest procedure times (Zhongshan Hospital, Shanghai) favored a posterior 5–6 o'clock orientation. The operators at this center favor the posterior approach due to their belief that performing the myotomy posteriorly is technically easier and thus potentially faster and safer. Our data presented above certainly support this contention. In the posterior approach, the muscle incision occurs directly along the long axis of the endoscope since the endoscope lies posteriorly in the esophagus due to gravity and has its therapeutic channel (from which the dissection knife exits) posteriorly (at the 7 o'clock position on the tip of the endoscope). By contrast during an anterior myotomy, the myotomy plane is located across from the endoscope, which, in the usual technique, causes the myotomy to proceed by hooking and cutting sequentially bundles of muscle fibers which results in slower completion of the myotomy [14]. Haruhiro Inoue, one of the operators who has strongly

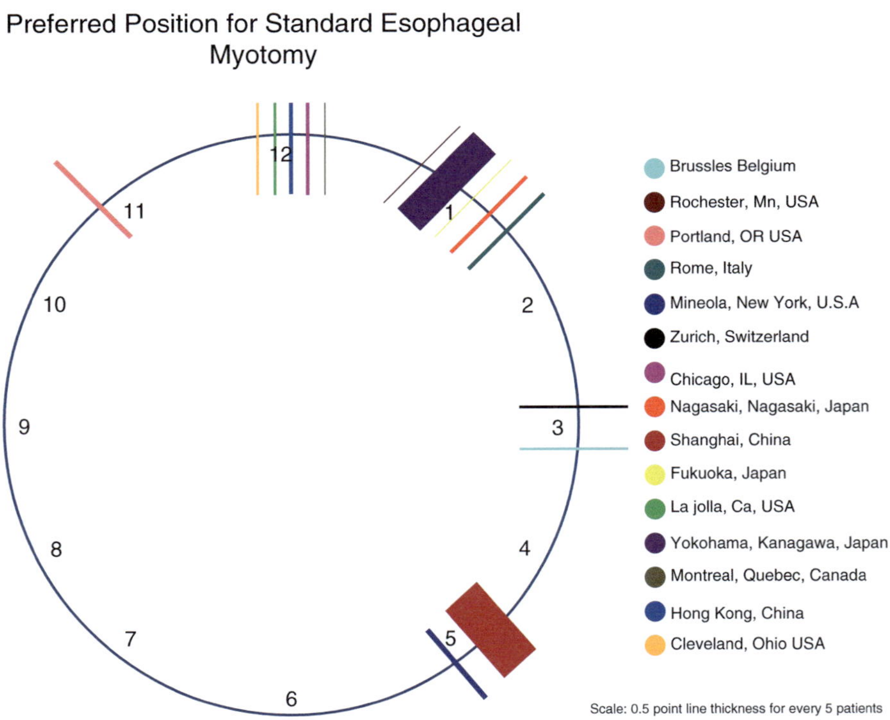

Fig. 8.6 Preferred orientation for POEM by pioneering centers participating in the International POEM Survey conducted in 2012 and published in Surgical Endoscopy in 2013. Bar thickness corresponds to center volume at the time of the survey (From Stavropoulos et al. 2013 [13])

favored an anterior POEM orientation, has noted recently, anecdotally, that he believes that there may be a higher preponderance of large paraesophageal and paragastric vessels in the EGJ and cardia anteriorly, a concern that in at least certain situations may favor a posterior approach.

As noted above in patients with lesions such as large diverticula, these lesions force an orientation located away from the lesion. Similarly, in patients that have previously undergone failed myotomy laparoscopically or perorally, there may be significant scar tissue in the orientation of the prior myotomy making re-do myotomy via POEM more technically difficult. In these cases, a posterior orientation [15] or even a greater curvature (GC) orientation in the 8 o'clock position [5] provides a path that avoids the prior scar tissue. It has also been suggested that a GC orientation allows clear identification of the LES because of the angle of His which is located along the greater curve [5]. In 2015 Onimaru and colleagues reported their experience with 21 achalasia patients who underwent POEM with GC myotomy. They were successful in identifying the angle of His in all patients, and they achieved significant reductions in LES pressures and Eckardt scores after the procedure. They deemed GC POEM to be safe as no adverse events were observed. However, reflux esophagitis was documented in 52 %, with clinical GERD symptoms occurring in 9.5 %, in all of whom they were controlled with proton pump inhibitor (PPI) therapy [5]. It should be noted, however, that a GC myotomy is substantially more challenging than an anterior or posterior myotomy and is also potentially riskier in that it involves dissection of the esophagus in close proximity to the aorta. Therefore, this technique should be employed by expert POEM operators only when an anterior or posterior orientation is not possible due to lesions or scar tissue from prior manipulations.

8.4 Depth of Myotomy

Another modification in the technique of POEM is to perform a full-thickness myotomy rather than a myotomy limited to the circular muscle as advocated by Haruhiro Inoue (see Figs. 8.4 and 8.5). Preservation of the longitudinal muscle has been recommended to avoid entering the pleural space, but in practice, limiting the myotomy to the circular muscle is challenging, as the longitudinal muscle layer is often very thin and easily breached by air insufflation, mechanical trauma from the endoscope, or electrocautery damage [14]. Further, for long-term reduction in LES pressure, full-thickness myotomy, as is performed with a Heller myotomy, may be beneficial. In the largest series comparing the two techniques, Li et al. in 2013 reported their retrospective study with 103 patients undergoing full-thickness myotomy and 131 patients receiving circular myotomy. Full-thickness procedure times were faster, but short-term symptom relief and manometry outcomes were comparable between the two groups, and there was no difference in complication rates [10]. Similarly, Duan et al. reported faster procedure times, comparable treatment success rates, and no increase in adverse events with full-thickness myotomy [16].

8.5 Tools

The conventional technique of POEM uses standard injection needle for creation of the submucosal space and a cutting knife, such as the triangle-tip (TT) knife (Olympus Corp, Tokyo, Japan) (see Fig. 8.7a) for submucosal dissection and myotomy. The injection needle and knife are repeatedly exchanged through the working channel of the scope to allow for adequate submucosal cushioning and subsequent dissection [6]. Another technical modification that has been made to the original POEM procedure is the water-jet-assisted POEM, using a combined injection/cutting knife (HybridKnife (HK), ERBE, Tubingen, Germany) (see Fig. 8.7b). This device allows injection and dissection in a single instrument [17]. In their randomized controlled trial of 100 patients comparing POEM performed with the TT knife versus the HK, Zhou's group reported that the hybrid knife produced significant decreases in POEM procedure time (22.9 vs 35.9 min ($p<0.0001$) and fewer minor bleeding episodes, with no differences in complications of treatment success [17]. This improvement in procedure times was mostly attributed to less replacement of accessories. Even though our group has consistently used the hybrid knife to perform tunnel dissection and full-thickness myotomy for all but the first 18 cases of our series (currently numbering 290 POEMs), in our initial POEMs in 2009, when no specialized ESD knives were available in the USA, we employed a balloon inflation technique for submucosal tunnel creation. This technique was described in detail at our 2010 GIE case report with video demonstration of our first POEM (and also the first POEM to be performed anywhere outside of Japan) [18]. In brief, after initial submucosal saline injection and mucosal incision to allow entry into the submucosal space, we performed blunt insertion of a 5.5 cm long, 12 mm diameter

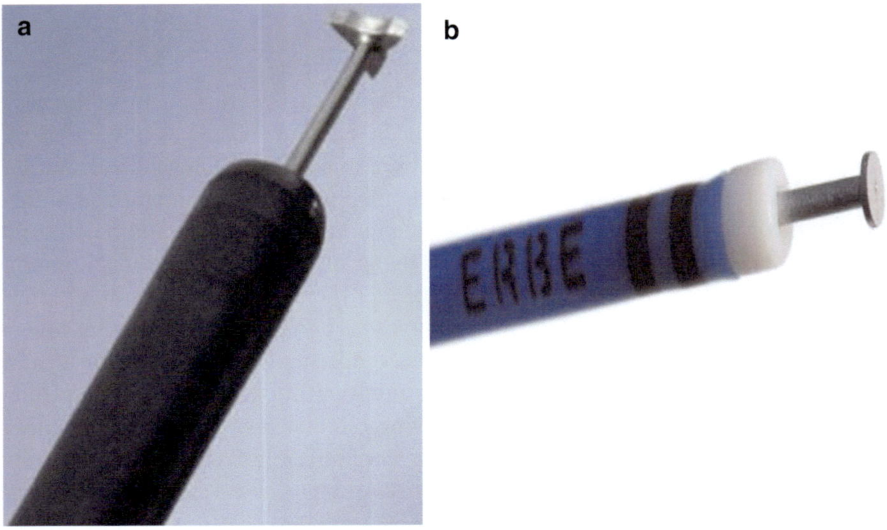

Fig. 8.7 (**a**) Triangle-tip knife Olympus Corp., Tokyo, Japan. (**b**) HybridKnife, ERBE, Tubingen, Germany

dilation balloon (CRE wire-guided dilator; Boston Scientific, Marlborough, MA, USA) followed by dilation of the submucosa to 12 mm. The endoscope was then inserted to the distal terminus of the tunnel created by the dilation, and the process was repeated two or three additional times extending the tunnel to the gastric cardia. This technique results in rapid creation of the tunnel within 5–10 min (much faster than what can be achieved by the standard electrosurgical dissection using an ESD knife). However, this technique carries the risk of inadvertent insertion of the balloon through the mucosa or muscularis propria during the blunt insertion stage, which would result in perforation. Because of this risk, we rapidly transitioned to electrosurgical dissection after the first few POEMs. The technique however does carry promise as it results in rapid and relatively bloodless submucosal tunneling and could provide a superior alternative with properly designed balloons that lack the stiffness of CRE balloons and allow more precise and safe dissection through submucosal tissue and do so even in settings with significant submucosal fibrosis (e.g., POEM after extensive prior Botox injections). Christopher Gostout has been a stalwart advocate of this technique even for ESD [19]. Anecdotally the Oregon Clinic group has used this technique for the initial portion of the tunnel to facilitate endoscope insertion into the submucosal space, and some other groups reportedly use biliary balloons or even biopsy forceps (repeatedly inserting the forceps and opening its jaws) to create the submucosal tunnel without any electrosurgical energy, but peer-reviewed publications are lacking.

8.6 Techniques for Mucosal Closure

Closure of the submucosal flap is another area of modification from the original POEM procedure. Reliable closure of the mucosal site is critical in preventing leakage of esophageal contents into the peritoneal space. Most groups use hemostatic clips to approximate the edges of the tunnel entry site [6, 7, 20, 21]. Saxena et al. describe their experience using an over-the-scope clipping device (OTSC, Ovesco Endoscopy AG, Tubingen, Germany) in two patients. In both patients, initial attempt at closure using hemostatic clips was unsuccessful but OTSC closure was successful [22]. Swanstrom's group at the Oregon Clinic reported a retrospective case-controlled study evaluating closure with hemostatic clips versus endoscopic suturing using the Apollo OverStitch device [23]. Of the 124 POEM cases assessed, endoscopic suturing was employed in 10 (8 %). Five cases were included in the study and were matched to five cases using conventional clip methods. No complications were noted in either group, and postoperative contrast esophagrams were negative in all patients. Closure time was shorter for the endoscopic clip group (16 +/− 12 min) as compared to the OverStitch device group (33 +/− 11 min), $p=0.044$. The very long median closure time with endoscopic suturing is not explained and was the main reason for a cost advantage with endoscopic clips (the device costs were not too dissimilar with the OR time difference accounting for most of the cost difference according to the authors). The authors concluded that endoscopic suturing seems best suited for cases of difficult mucosotomy closure [23]. A larger, retrospective study by our group at Winthrop, to avoid learning curve bias from early cases, compared the most recent 25 consecutive closures of the mucosotomy with clips to the most recent 25 consecutive closures with OverStitch. There were no significant differences in closure time (8.8 min for endoclips and 10.1 min for OverStitch), cost ($916 versus $818), and hospital stay (1.9 days versus 1.7 days) [24].

8.7 Technique of Simultaneous Tunnel and Muscle Dissection

In 2015 Liu reported on a new technique for accomplishing the POEM procedure that combines the steps of submucosal tunneling and myotomy. The procedure was performed in two patients, with an average procedure time of 24 min with less bleeding. The authors hypothesized based on these very preliminary findings that the simultaneous cutting of the submucosa and muscularis propria may result in a more efficient procedure [25].

8.8 Distal to Proximal ("Retrograde") Myotomy

The conventional POEM is performed in antegrade fashion: the submucosal tunnel is created several centimeters proximal to the GEJ and extended beyond the GEJ into the cardia. The subsequent myotomy is similarly initiated proximally and extended distally into the cardia. Ponsky and colleagues reported on their experience with "retrograde myotomy" in five patients, initiating the myotomy at the distal end of the submucosal tunnel, in the cardia, and proceeding in "retrograde" fashion to perform the myotomy across the GEJ extending it to approximately 3 cm distal to the mucosotomy forming the entry to the tunnel [26]. The authors felt that this approach resulted in an easier, faster procedure. We have occasionally utilized this technique in patients with extremely tight LES in whom the sphincter could "shut the endoscope out of the cardia" during proximal to distal myotomy, requiring forceful forward pressure which may not be as effective in the presence of a partially completed proximal myotomy that may allow "buckling" of the endoscope into the mediastinum. We do not recommend this "retrograde" myotomy technique for routine use due to its increased risk as the knife is cutting away from the esophageal lumen (toward the mediastinum/peritoneum) and there is limited visualization of the tissue to be cut since the leading edge of the incision is hidden by the muscle tissue yet to be cut.

8.9 Techniques for Confirming Adequate Cardiomyotomy

One of the key issues in the POEM procedure is ensuring that the submucosal tunnel has been extended 2–3 cm beyond the GEJ into the cardia to ensure complete ablation of the LES high-pressure zone. A variety of indicators that suggest that the GEJ or cardia has been reached include:

1. Endoscopic measurements (using the markers on the endoscope to measure depth of insertion from the incisors)
2. Narrowing of the submucosal space at the GEJ with resistance to endoscope insertion caused by the LES followed by prompt expansion of the submucosal space in the cardia with increased overall vascularity of the submucosa
3. Slender palisading vessels along the mucosal flap, indicating the distal-most aspect of the esophagus
4. Spindle-like veins on the surface of the muscularis propria near the GEJ
5. Large-caliber arborizing, perforating vessels in the cardia, usually branches of the left gastric artery
6. Aberrant inner longitudinal muscle bundles at the GEJ originating from circular muscle fibers and inserting into circular muscle fibers after a short course of 2–3 cm
7. Visualization of a blue hue on intraluminal inspection of the mucosa of the cardia (due to the blue color of the injectate) [1]

A transillumination auxiliary technique, initially described by Baldaque-Silva and colleagues, allows confirmation that the tunnel was extended into the cardia by inserting transnasally an ultrathin endoscope, in parallel with the orally inserted gastroscope used to perform the POEM procedure. The ultrathin scope is advanced to the level of the stomach and placed in the retroflexed position with visualization of the cardia, while the gastroscope is kept within the tunnel with its tip at the tunnel terminus. The light intensity of the thin endoscope is diminished, and the light from the gastroscope within the submucosal tunnel is identified, thereby confirming its position in the cardia [27]. Inoue's group compared this technique to conventional identification of the cardia by the indicators listed above in a prospective randomized controlled trial with 100 consecutive achalasia patients undergoing POEM. POEM was completed with high rates of technical and clinical success in both groups, with low adverse events, but the double-scope transillumination group had myotomy extension in 34 % of cases, which led to an increase in the length of the cardiomyotomy from 2.6 to 3.2 cm ($p=0.01$) [28]. Despite the extension of the myotomy in a third of the patients in the transillumination group (suggesting that the final length of the cardiomyotomy of the control group may have not been of adequate length in a third of patients), there were no differences in clinical success rates, and no differences in post-procedure GERD, thus raising doubts about the clinical significance of these findings. Some drawbacks of this technique are that it may require two operators, is cumbersome, requiring a second endoscopy tower and endoscope, and adds significant time to the procedure (17 min in this study). However, this technique may be beneficial for difficult cases such as those on patients with sigmoid end-stage achalasia or for operators early on the POEM learning curve.

Another technique for reliably identifying an adequate myotomy extension into the cardia involves the use of fluoroscopy. Kumbhari reported using either a hemoclip attached to the GEJ or the fluoroscopically guided placement of a 19-gauge needle on the skin at the level of the GEJ to help accurately assess the length of the myotomy in 24 consecutive patients undergoing the POEM procedure. Based on the fluoroscopic information, the submucosal tunnel was extended in 21 % of patients, with minor increases in procedure time (4 min for the hemoclip group and 2 min for the 19-gauge needle group) [29]. Others have used fluoroscopy for reorienting the submucosal tunnel in a downward direction, particularly in cases of sigmoid achalasia esophagus [30]. It should be noted, however, that these techniques require performing POEMs in a fluoroscopy room tying up this room for at least 2 h. Given the small benefit of this technique, which would be expected to be even smaller after the early portion of the POEM learning curve, it is unclear whether this would represent appropriate resource utilization in busy endoscopy suites with one or two fluoroscopy rooms.

8.10 Functional Assessment to Ensure Adequacy of the Myotomy

Real-time measurement of the GEJ distensibility with a balloon-based imaging probe that uses impedance planimetry has been used intraprocedurally to assess the adequacy of the myotomy [31]. The device EndoFLIP (Crospon Ltd, Galway, Ireland) provides measurements that include cross-sectional area (CSA), minimal diameter, compliance, and distensibility indices. The device had previously been used to assess the GEJ pre-procedurally and on follow-up evaluation 3 months after the POEM [32]. Rieder used the EndoFLIP device on four patients undergoing POEM and compared values to healthy volunteers. Pre- and post-myotomy data were obtained. In the group undergoing POEM, pre-procedure diameter, CSA, and distensibility were lower than in healthy volunteers. These parameters improved significantly during the intraprocedural (immediate post-myotomy) assessment, becoming more like those of the healthy volunteers [31]. The device was used intraprocedurally during POEM and laparoscopic Heller procedures demonstrating similar improvements in GEJ distensibility intraoperatively [33]. Unlike other objective measurements of the adequacy of the myotomy, the EndoFLIP device has the ability to give a real-time assessment of the myotomy, potentially allowing for optimization of the myotomy at the time of the POEM. Recently, EndoFLIP was used to assess the degree that each of the POEM stages (submucosal tunnel dissection, esophageal body myotomy, short cardiomyotomy, long cardiomyotomy) contributed to improved GEJ physiology [34]. Interestingly, this study found that submucosal tunnel dissection prior to any myotomy resulted in a marked improvement in EGJ physiology. Myotomy extension across the LES to 2 cm distal to the EGJ onto the gastric wall resulted in normalization of EGJ distensibility, whereas subsequent extension and additional centimeter to 3 cm distal to the EGJ did not increase compliance further. These data suggest no further improvement in GEJ; patency would be expected from extending the myotomy more than 2 cm into the cardia [34]. The same group has examined the use of proprietary software to analyze real-time pre-POEM EndoFLIP data to obtain insights in achalasia pathophysiology. They found that esophageal contractility not observed with manometry can be detected in patients with achalasia using FLIP topography, and they speculated that the presence and patterns of contractility detected with FLIP topography may represent variations in pathophysiology, such as mechanisms of panesophageal pressurization in patients with type II achalasia. These findings could have implications for additional subclassification to supplement prediction of the achalasia disease course [35].

8.11 POEM for Non-achalasia Motility Disorders

The POEM procedure has been successfully expanded to non-achalasia motility disorders of the esophagus, namely, spastic disorders such as diffuse esophageal spasm (DES), nutcracker esophagus, and jackhammer esophagus [36–38]. In these disorders, the length of the myotomy is substantially longer, up to 20 cm or so, owing to the pathophysiology of these motility disorders which involves spasticity or hypercontractility of as much as 2/3 s of the esophagus. Sharata and colleagues reported on 25 non-achalasia patients within a larger cohort of 100 patients undergoing POEM [39]. Twelve had nutcracker esophagus, five had DES, and there were eight cases of hypertensive non-relaxing LES. When compared to their counterparts with achalasia, this non-achalasia group had somewhat less dysphagia relief (70 % versus 97 % in the achalasia group), less chest pain relief (75 % versus 100 %), and higher rates of heartburn and regurgitation [39]. A multicenter retrospective analysis of outcomes in 73 patients with DES, Jackhammer, and type 3 achalasia that had POEM at 12 different centers revealed mildly lower efficacy in pain relief than dysphagia relief (not statistically significant however) and significantly lower efficacy in Jackhammer compared to DES and spastic achalasia [40].

In a small single-center series with 25 achalasia and eight spastic non-achalasia patients, dysphagia improved in 92 % of patients with achalasia vs 75 % of those with non-achalasia disorders, and chest pain resolved in 100 % of patients with achalasia (8/8) vs 80 % of patients with non-achalasia (4/5) [41].

8.11.1 POEM Outcomes

POEM efficacy is determined by several metrics including a decrease of the Eckardt score to ≤3, LES pressure decrease (>50 % decrease), and improvement of esophageal emptying as assessed by a timed barium esophagram [1]. There are currently no published randomized controlled trials comparing POEM to Heller myotomy or pneumatic dilation. There are many series reported in the literature, with therapeutic success rates ranging from 82 to 100 %, the majority achieving efficacy in greater than 95 % [1, 6–9, 20, 32, 42–48]. Table 8.1 summarizes POEM efficacy data from series with significant number of cases and/or follow-up (defined in our review as ≥150 patient-years of follow-up, e.g., 50 cases with mean follow-up ≥3 months, 30 cases with ≥6 month mean follow-up, etc.) [8, 11, 30, 39, 46, 47, 49–56]. Werner and colleagues reported long-term results by combining the patients from three

Table 8.1 POEM series with efficacy data

Location	Year	# of patients	Mean age (years)	Mean follow-up (months)	Eckardt score (pre/post)	LES pressure (pre/post) (mmHg)	Post-POEM timed barium esophagram	Efficacy
Europe MCT [8]	2013	70	45	12	6.9/1	27.6/8.9		82.4 %
Portland, Oregon [39]	2014	100	58 (18–83)	21.5	6/1	44.3/19.6	In 55 pts, median emptying at 1 min 93 %: 100 % emptying 100 %: 80–100 % emptying	96 %
Chicago, Illinois [49]	2014	41	45	15	7/1	28/11	In 16 pts, median height 1 min 6 ± 4 cm 2 min 6 ± 4 cm 5 min 5 ± 3 cm ($p < 0.001$)	92 %
Rome, Italy [50]	2014	100	48 (18–75)	11	8.1/1.1	41.4/19		94.5 %
Nagasaki, Japan [46]	2014	28	52 (19–48)	16	6.7/0.7	71.2/21		100 %
Mineola, New York [11]	2015	93	52 (18–93)	22	78/0.44	43/18		96 %
Europe MCT [47]	2015	80	44.9 (9–88)	29	7.7/1.5	31.9/10.1	In 32 pts, 93.75 %: >70 % emptying at 5 min	78.5 %
Hyderabad, India [30]	2015	212	39.3 (9–74)	12	7.2/1.2	37.5/15.2	In 82 pts, mean 5 min emptying 71.5 %	92 %

Yokohama, Japan [51]	2015	500	43 (3–89)	12–24	6/1.7	28.7/14		88.5 %
Shanghai, China [52]	2015	32	43.6 (18–72)	30	7.8/1.4	37.9/12.9		96.8 %
Liuzhou, China [53]	2015	35	40.2 (15–63)	6	6.83/0.46	29.5/10.3		100 %
Columbus, Ohio [54]	2015	45	52.2	10	4/0	–		100 %
Fukuoka, Japan [55]	2016	100	48 (9–91)	3	5.9/0.8	43.6/20.9		99 %
Baltimore, Maryland [56]	2015	60	48	3.9	8/1.19	29/11		94 %

centers (Rome, Hamburg, Portland) that had completed a minimum of 2 years of follow-up totaling 79 patients in a multicenter retrospective analysis [47]. They observed an initial clinical response in 96 %, but clinical recurrences occurred in 17.7 % at maximum follow-up ≥2 years (mean 29 months). Older age and the presence of post-procedure endoscopic reflux signs were independent predictors of treatment success. Interestingly, almost 50 % of recurrences were among the first ten cases at each one of the three participating centers, suggesting that the more modest 2-year outcomes may have been due to a learning curve effect. Reflux esophagitis, while mild, was seen on endoscopy at 2 years in 37.5 % of patients [47].

In our data from Winthrop, Patel and colleagues reported outcomes and the learning curve on the first 93 consecutive POEMs in achalasia patients [11]. At mean follow-up of 22 months, clinical success was achieved in 96 % with a 2 % adverse event rate with no severe adverse events. Efficiency was attained at 40 POEMs and mastery after 60 POEMs. This learning curve is somewhat longer than previously reported by Kurian and colleagues, who defined mastery at 20 cases, as evidenced by an overall decrease in procedure time [48]. However, that study had methodological limitations as no plateau phase was documented, and the data analyzed were based on only 40 cases with multiple operators involved.

In the largest POEM series to date, Inoue reported outcomes in 500 patients, with 105 patients at more than 3 years post POEM [51]. The procedure was technically successful in all patients. The median total length of the myotomy was 14.0 cm, with a median of 11.0 cm in the esophagus and 3.0 cm in the stomach. Typically, an anterior myotomy was performed, with a greater curvature myotomy performed in cases of previous Heller myotomy, suspected severe submucosal fibrosis, and adhesions on the lesser curve. Adverse events occurred in 3.2 % and included pneumothorax, bleeding, mucosal injuries, postoperative hematomas, pleural effusion, and inflammation of the lesser omentum. Most were managed conservatively. Two-month outcomes showed significant reductions in Eckardt scores and LES pressures. Clinical success (as defined by a post-POEM Eckardt score of less than two or a decrease from the pre-POEM score by at least four points) was achieved in 91.7 %. On endoscopy, 65 % had signs of reflux esophagitis, but only 17 % of patients complained of GERD symptoms. In terms of long-term outcomes, overall success (as defined above) persisted at 91 %, and 19 % complained of GERD symptoms. At 3 years, with interview data available in 61/105 patients (58.1 %) and manometry and endoscopy data in 16/105 patients (15 %), overall success remained high at 88.5 %, with symptomatic GERD in 21 % and signs of reflux esophagitis in 56 %. All reflux symptoms were effectively managed with proton pump inhibitors [51]. A number of limitations should be noted:

1. Significant differences in this Asian series compared to Western series (we offer a comparison with the most recent update of the POEM data from our center, the largest single-operator series in the USA ([57] (see Table 8.2)). The following important differences should be noted:
    1. There are several differences in the patient populations:

Table 8.2 POEM series with GERD data including pH studies

Location	GERD symptoms	Erosive esophagitis	+pH study
Chicago, Illinois [49]	15/41 (15 %)	13/22 (59 %)	4/13 (31 %)
Portland, Oregon [39]	12/100 (15 %)	20/73 (27 %)	26/68 (38 %)
Rome, Italy [50]	19/103 (18 %)	21/103 (20 %)	52/103 (50 %)
Mineola, New York [57]	40/174 (23 %)	29/86 (34 %)	29/84 (36 %)
Fukuoka, Japan [55]	9/100 (9 %)	66/100 (66 %)	22/86 (25.6 %)

   (a) Significantly younger patient population by more than a decade in the Inoue series compared to our US series (mean age of 43 vs 54)
   (b) Much lower numbers of patients previously treated with Botox (6 pts, 1 %) and Heller (10 pts, 2 %) in the Inoue series compared to our series (21 % prior Botox and 16 % prior Heller)
   (c) Significantly lower proportion of advanced achalasia patients with esophageal dilation to >6 cm, 21 patients (4 %) in the Inoue series versus 68 patients (27 %) in our series
2. An unusual efficacy definition was used (post-POEM Eckardt <2 or decrease of the Eckardt score by ≥4 points) that differs from the definition used by all the other published POEM series and most LHM series (i.e., decrease of the Eckardt score to ≤3). This makes comparison with efficacy in other series less straightforward.
3. There is a significant amount of missing follow-up data, e.g., even though 105 pts were at >3 years from their POEM, Eckardt score data were only available in 61 (58 %) and follow-up endoscopy in only 16 (15 %).

8.12 Incidence of GERD After POEM

Early POEM series noted a GERD prevalence of <10 % [6, 20, 58]. This finding was likely due to GERD being assessed for via unstructured interviews and symptoms scores. Once objective GERD investigations including pH studies and endoscopy were employed, it became evident that GERD was more prevalent than previously stated. Tables 8.2 and 8.3 summarizes GERD data from series with comprehensive GERD assessment (defined in our review as series that included all three main GERD assessment components, i.e., presence of GERD symptoms, presence of reflux esophagitis, and acid exposure as assessed by pH studies, or at least two of these, provided one was pH studied). Only four series so far have presented data on significant numbers of post-POEM patients (≥25) for all three parameters used to assess GERD: symptom score, endoscopy, and pH testing [39, 49, 55, 59]. Based on these data, 9–23 % of patients had GERD symptoms, 20–66 % had endoscopic manifestations of GERD (erosive esophagitis which was mostly mild LA Grade A or B esophagitis), and 26–50 % had positive pH testing. The three-center Rome-Hamburg-Portland series with 2-year follow-up noted that 37 % of patients were on PPIs at ≥2 year

Table 8.3 Comparing US and Asian large series

	Stavropoulos et al. [57]	Inoue et al. [51]
No. of patients	248	500
Age	54 (10–93)	43 (3–89)
Prior treatment	120 pts previously treated 33 pneumatic dilation 57 suboptimal balloon dilation 53 Botox injection 39 Heller myotomy 3 POEM	195 previously treated 179 pneumatic dilation 6 Botox injection 10 Heller myotomy
Sigmoid esophagus	45 sigmoid	77 sigmoid
Advanced achalasia stage (esophageal dilation to >6 cm)	68	21
Mean procedure time	89 min (30–240)	90 min (70.8–119)
Mean myotomy length	13.7 cm (3–26)	14 cm (12–16)
Pre- and post Eckardt	7.8/0.8	6/1
Pre- and post LES pressure	43.3 mmHg/18.5 mmHg	25.4 mmHg/13.4 mmHg
Clinical success	3 month 224/236–95 % 6 month 199/211–94 % 12 month 174/183–95 %	2 month 386/423–91.3 % 12–24 month 260/286–91 % 36 month 54/61–88.5 %

follow-up and the same proportion had esophagitis on endoscopy, but no pH testing was reported [47]. In this study, as noted above, the presence of GERD was the strongest predictor of POEM success with an odds ratio of almost 7. This is understandable since POEM by effectively disrupting the LES and achieving dysphagia relief simultaneously predisposes to GERD. It is recommended that POEM operators do not compromise the efficacy of their myotomies in order to minimize GERD, as repeat procedures for recurrent dysphagia is a thornier problem than dealing with the usually mild or moderate, PPI-responsive GERD. Vigilance is necessary to avoid long-term complications from untreated silent GERD such as Barrett's esophagus and adenocarcinoma and peptic stricture formation. All post-POEM patients should have endoscopy and pH study within a year post POEM. After this initial period, we would recommend patient interview and endoscopy at 1–2-year intervals to screen for squamous dysplasia and carcinoma, assess for evidence of GERD, and also, in conjunction with timed Barium study performed at 1–2 year intervals, monitor for signs and symptoms of disease progression leading to relapse that may require further salvage therapy. GERD-related complications were the most prevalent reason for late failure after LHM with Dor fundoplication [60]. PPIs are usually effective for post-POEM GERD. For the minority of patients with true GERD that does not respond to PPI therapy, Dor or Toupet fundoplication would also be very feasible after POEM since no periesophageal scarring or adhesions were noted on laparoscopy after POEM at a center that performed LHM in two patients in whom the response after POEM was inadequate. High-quality studies of patients that have had LHM with fundoplication have demonstrated abnormal acid exposure in 18–42 % of subjects which is not too dissimilar to the rates observed after POEM [61–63]. It appears that the "loose" Dor or Toupet fundoplication performed in achalasia patients is only partially effective in preventing GERD. POEM's seeming equivalence to LHM with fundoplication in terms of GERD incidence likely relates to preservation of extraesophageal hiatal structures including the phrenoesophageal membrane which are thought to maintain the angle of His and serve as a barrier to reflux. This concept is supported by the lower rates of GERD in studies of LHM performed with minimal dissection of the hiatus and particularly the phrenoesophageal membrane [64, 65].

8.13 POEM Versus LHM

Three US studies have compared retrospectively the first consecutive POEMs performed by a surgical operator to that operator's most recent consecutive laparoscopic Heller myotomies [44, 66, 67]. POEM was found to be equivalent or superior to LHM in all outcomes assessed. Significantly better dysphagia relief for POEM was noted in the largest of the three studies with the other two smaller studies showing equal dysphagia relief. The larger study was the only one that assessed acid exposure by pH studies and showed equivalence between POEM and LHM (39 % vs 32 % abnormal pH studies, NS). POEM was also shown to be significantly faster than the LHM in all three studies with some studies showing additionally less post-procedure pain, quicker return to normal activities, and shorter hospitalization for POEM. There was no difference in the low rate of adverse events in any of the three studies. Results are expected in 2017 from two European multicenter studies randomizing patients between balloon dilation and POEM or LHM and POEM.

Conclusion

POEM is a NOTES approach to Heller myotomy that has proven to be as efficacious as LHM but less invasive. We have seen rapid adoption of POEM as a viable treatment for achalasia, with consistently excellent treatment results and a favorable adverse event profile that rival the previous gold standard of therapy, the LHM. The basic technique is now established, but evolution of the technique with minor adjustments and variations continues. The incidence of post-POEM GERD may be higher than the very low rate reported in early publications but may not be significantly higher than the rate of GERD after LHM with Dor fundoplication as reported in high-quality surgical studies. GERD is manageable by medical therapy, but vigilance is required for its early detection and treatment to avoid any long-term adverse events such as development of Barrett's esophagus or peptic strictures.

References

1. Stavropoulos SN, Desilets DJ, Fuchs KH, et al. Per-oral endoscopic myotomy white paper summary. Surg Endosc. 2014;28:2005–19.
2. Committee AP, Chandrasekhara V, Desilets D, et al. The American Society for Gastrointestinal Endoscopy PIVI (preservation and incorporation of valuable endoscopic innovations) on per-oral endoscopic myotomy. Gastrointest Endosc. 2015;81:1087–100.e1.
3. Sumiyama K, Gostout CJ, Rajan E, Bakken TA, Knipschield MA, Marler RJ. Submucosal endoscopy with mucosal flap safety valve. Gastrointest Endosc. 2007;65:688–94.

4. Stavropoulos SN, Modayil R, Friedel D. Per oral endoscopic myotomy for the treatment of achalasia. Curr Opin Gastroenterol. 2015;31:430–40.
5. Onimaru M, Inoue H, Ikeda H, et al. Greater curvature myotomy is a safe and effective modified technique in per-oral endoscopic myotomy (with videos). Gastrointest Endosc. 2015;81:1370–7.
6. Inoue H, Minami H, Kobayashi Y, et al. Peroral endoscopic myotomy (POEM) for esophageal achalasia. Endoscopy. 2010;42:265–71.
7. Swanstrom LL, Kurian A, Dunst CM, Sharata A, Bhayani N, Rieder E. Long-term outcomes of an endoscopic myotomy for achalasia: the POEM procedure. Ann Surg. 2012;256:659–67.
8. Von Renteln D, Fuchs KH, Fockens P, et al. Peroral endoscopic myotomy for the treatment of achalasia: an international prospective multicenter study. Gastroenterology. 2013;145:309–11. e1–3.
9. Chiu PW, Wu JC, Teoh AY, et al. Peroral endoscopic myotomy for treatment of achalasia: from bench to bedside (with video). Gastrointest Endosc. 2013;77:29–38.
10. Li QL, Chen WF, Zhou PH, et al. Peroral endoscopic myotomy for the treatment of achalasia: a clinical comparative study of endoscopic full-thickness and circular muscle myotomy. J Am Coll Surg. 2013;217:442–51.
11. Patel KS, Calixte R, Modayil RJ, Friedel D, Brathwaite CE, Stavropoulos SN. The light at the end of the tunnel: a single-operator learning curve analysis for per oral endoscopic myotomy. Gastrointest Endosc. 2015;81:1181–7.
12. Kahrilas PJ. Anatomy and physiology of the gastroesophageal junction. Gastroenterol Clin North Am. 1997;26:467–86.
13. Stavropoulos SN, Modayil RJ, Friedel D, Savides T. The International Per Oral Endoscopic Myotomy Survey (IPOEMS): a snapshot of the global POEM experience. Surg Endosc. 2013;27:3322–38.
14. Li QL, Zhou PH. Perspective on peroral endoscopic myotomy for achalasia: Zhongshan experience. Gut Liver. 2015;9:152–8.
15. Onimaru M, Inoue H, Ikeda H, et al. Peroral endoscopic myotomy is a viable option for failed surgical esophagocardiomyotomy instead of redo surgical Heller myotomy: a single center prospective study. J Am Coll Surg. 2013;217:598–605.
16. Duan T, Zhou J, Yan Y, et al. Per Oral endoscopic myotomy for severe achalasia: the comparison of full thickness myotomy and circular myotomy. Gastrointest Endoscopy. 2015;81(5S):AB 118.
17. Cai MY, Zhou PH, Yao LQ, et al. Peroral endoscopic myotomy for idiopathic achalasia: randomized comparison of water-jet assisted versus conventional dissection technique. Surg Endosc. 2014;28:1158–65.
18. Stavropoulos SN, Harris MD, Hida S, Brathwaite C, Demetriou C, Grendell J. Endoscopic submucosal myotomy for the treatment of achalasia (with video). Gastrointest Endosc. 2010;72:1309–11.
19. Takizawa K, Knipschield MA, Gostout CJ. Submucosal endoscopy with mucosal resection (SEMR): a new hybrid technique of endoscopic submucosal balloon dissection in the porcine rectosigmoid colon. Surg Endosc. 2013;27:4457–62.
20. Costamagna G, Marchese M, Familiari P, Tringali A, Inoue H, Perri V. Peroral endoscopic myotomy (POEM) for oesophageal achalasia: preliminary results in humans. Dig Liver Dis Off J Ital Soc Gastroenterol Ital Assoc Stud Liver. 2012;44:827–32.
21. Ponsky JL, Marks JM, Pauli EM. How i do it: per-oral endoscopic myotomy (POEM). J Gastrointest Surg Off J Soc Surg Aliment Tract. 2012;16:1251–5.
22. Saxena P, Chavez YH, Kord Valeshabad A, Kalloo AN, Khashab MA. An alternative method for mucosal flap closure during peroral endoscopic myotomy using an over-the-scope clipping device. Endoscopy. 2013;45:579–81.
23. Pescarus R, Shlomovitz E, Sharata AM, et al. Endoscopic suturing versus endoscopic clip closure of the mucosotomy during a per-oral endoscopic myotomy (POEM): a case–control study. Surg Endosc. 2015;30:2132–5.

24. Stavropoulos SN, Modayil R, Friedel D. Current applications of endoscopic suturing. World J Gastrointest Endoscopy. 2015;7:777–89.
25. Liu BR, Song JT, Omar Jan M. Video of the month. Modified peroral endoscopic myotomy. Am J Gastroenterol. 2015;110:499.
26. Ponsky JL, Marks JM, Orenstein SB. Retrograde myotomy: a variation in per oral endoscopic myotomy (POEM) technique. Surg Endosc. 2014;28:3257–9.
27. Baldaque-Silva F, Marques M, Vilas-Boas F, Maia JD, Sa F, Macedo G. New transillumination auxiliary technique for peroral endoscopic myotomy. Gastrointest Endosc. 2014;79:544–5.
28. Grimes KL, Inoue H, Onimaru M, et al. Double-scope per oral endoscopic myotomy (POEM): a prospective randomized controlled trial. Surg Endosc. 2015;30:1344–51.
29. Kumbhari V, Besharati S, Abdelgelil A, et al. Intraprocedural fluoroscopy to determine the extent of the cardiomyotomy during per-oral endoscopic myotomy (with video). Gastrointest Endosc. 2015;81:1451–6.
30. Ramchandani M, Reddy DN, Darisetty S, et al. Peroral endoscopic myotomy for achalasia cardia: treatment analysis and follow up of over 200 consecutive patients at a single center. Dig Endoscopy Off J Japan Gastroenterol Endoscopy Soc. 2015;28:19–26.
31. Rieder E, Swanstrom LL, Perretta S, Lenglinger J, Riegler M, Dunst CM. Intraoperative assessment of esophagogastric junction distensibility during per oral endoscopic myotomy (POEM) for esophageal motility disorders. Surg Endosc. 2013;27:400–5.
32. Verlaan T, Rohof WO, Bredenoord AJ, Eberl S, Rosch T, Fockens P. Effect of peroral endoscopic myotomy on esophagogastric junction physiology in patients with achalasia. Gastrointest Endosc. 2013;78:39–44.
33. Teitelbaum EN, Boris L, Arafat FO, et al. Comparison of esophagogastric junction distensibility changes during POEM and Heller myotomy using intraoperative FLIP. Surg Endosc. 2013;27:4547–55.
34. Teitelbaum EN, Sternbach JM, El Khoury R, et al. The effect of incremental distal gastric myotomy lengths on EGJ distensibility during POEM for achalasia. Surg Endosc. 2016;30:745–50.
35. Carlson DA, Lin Z, Kahrilas PJ, et al. The functional lumen imaging probe detects esophageal contractility Not observed with manometry in patients with achalasia. Gastroenterology. 2015;149:1742–51.
36. Khashab MA, Saxena P, Kumbhari V, et al. Peroral endoscopic myotomy as a platform for the treatment of spastic esophageal disorders refractory to medical therapy (with video). Gastrointest Endosc. 2014;79:136–9.
37. Shiwaku H, Inoue H, Beppu R, et al. Successful treatment of diffuse esophageal spasm by peroral endoscopic myotomy. Gastrointest Endosc. 2013;77:149–50.
38. Sharata A, Kurian AA, Dunst CM, Bhayani NH, Reavis KM, Swanstrom LL. Peroral endoscopic myotomy (POEM) is safe and effective in the setting of prior endoscopic intervention. J Gastrointest Surg Off J Soc Surg Aliment Tract. 2013;17:1188–92.
39. Sharata AM, Dunst CM, Pescarus R, et al. Peroral endoscopic myotomy (POEM) for esophageal primary motility disorders: analysis of 100 consecutive patients. J Gastrointest Surg Off J Soc Surg Aliment Tract. 2015;19:161–70; discussion 70.
40. Khashab MA, Messallam AA, Onimaru M, et al. International multicenter experience with peroral endoscopic myotomy for the treatment of spastic esophageal disorders refractory to medical therapy (with video). Gastrointest Endosc. 2015;81:1170–7.
41. Hoppo T, Thakkar SJ, Schumacher LY, et al. A utility of peroral endoscopic myotomy (POEM) across the spectrum of esophageal motility disorders. Surg Endosc. 2016;30:233–44.
42. Swanstrom LL, Rieder E, Dunst CM. A stepwise approach and early clinical experience in peroral endoscopic myotomy for the treatment of achalasia and esophageal motility disorders. J Am Coll Surg. 2011;213:751–6.
43. Ren Z, Zhong Y, Zhou P, et al. Perioperative management and treatment for complications during and after peroral endoscopic myotomy (POEM) for esophageal achalasia (EA) (data from 119 cases). Surg Endosc. 2012;26:3267–72.

44. Hungness ES, Teitelbaum EN, Santos BF, et al. Comparison of perioperative outcomes between peroral esophageal myotomy (POEM) and laparoscopic Heller myotomy. J Gastrointest Surg Off J Soc Surg Aliment Tract. 2013;17:228–35.
45. Lee BH, Shim KY, Hong SJ, et al. Peroral endoscopic myotomy for treatment of achalasia: initial results of a korean study. Clin Endoscopy. 2013;46:161–7.
46. Minami H, Isomoto H, Yamaguchi N, et al. Peroral endoscopic myotomy for esophageal achalasia: clinical impact of 28 cases. Dig Endoscopy Off J Japan Gastroenterol Endoscopy Soc. 2014;26:43–51.
47. Werner YB, Costamagna G, Swanstrom LL, et al. Clinical response to peroral endoscopic myotomy in patients with idiopathic achalasia at a minimum follow-up of 2 years. Gut. 2015;65:899–906.
48. Kurian AA, Dunst CM, Sharata A, Bhayani NH, Reavis KM, Swanstrom LL. Peroral endoscopic esophageal myotomy: defining the learning curve. Gastrointest Endosc. 2013;77:719–25.
49. Teitelbaum EN, Soper NJ, Santos BF, et al. Symptomatic and physiologic outcomes one year after peroral esophageal myotomy (POEM) for treatment of achalasia. Surg Endosc. 2014;28:3359–65.
50. Familiari P, Gigante G, Marchese M, et al. Peroral endoscopic myotomy for esophageal achalasia: outcomes of the first 100 patients with short-term follow-up. Ann Surg. 2014;263:82–7.
51. Inoue H, Sato H, Ikeda H, et al. Per-oral endoscopic myotomy: a series of 500 patients. J Am Coll Surg. 2015;221:256–64.
52. Hu JW, Li QL, Zhou PH, et al. Peroral endoscopic myotomy for advanced achalasia with sigmoid-shaped esophagus: long-term outcomes from a prospective, single-center study. Surg Endosc. 2015;29:2841–50.
53. Liu XJ, Tan YY, Yang RQ, et al. The outcomes and quality of life of patients with achalasia after peroral endoscopic myotomy in the short-term. Ann Thorac Cardiovasc Surg Off J Assoc Thorac Cardiovasc Surg Asia. 2015;21:507–12.
54. Jones EL, Meara MP, Schwartz JS, Hazey JW, Perry KA. Gastroesophageal reflux symptoms do not correlate with objective pH testing after peroral endoscopic myotomy. Surg Endoscopy. 2016;30:947–52.
55. Shiwaku H, Inoue H, Yamashita K, et al. Peroral endoscopic myotomy for esophageal achalasia: outcomes of the first over 100 patients with short-term follow-up. Surg Endosc. 2016;30(11):4817–26.
56. Khashab MA, El Zein M, Kumbhari V, et al. Comprehensive analysis of efficacy and safety of peroral endoscopic myotomy performed by a gastroenterologist in the endoscopy unit: a single-center experience. Gastrointest Endosc. 2015;83:117–25.
57. Stavropoulos SN, Modayil R, Braithwaite C, et al. Outcomes of a Large Prospective Series on Per Oral Endoscopic Myotomy (POEM) for Achalasia: An Effective and Durable Treatment Modality That Can Safely Be Performed in the Endoscopy Suite. Gastrointest Endoscopy. 2016;83(5S):AB479–80.
58. von Renteln D, Inoue H, Minami H, et al. Peroral endoscopic myotomy for the treatment of achalasia: a prospective single center study. Am J Gastroenterol. 2012;107:411–7.
59. Familiari P, Greco S, Gigante G, et al. Gastroesophageal reflux disease after peroral endoscopic myotomy: analysis of clinical, procedural and functional factors, associated with gastroesophageal reflux disease and esophagitis. Dig Endoscopy Off J Japan Gastroenterol Endoscopy Soc. 2015;28:33–41.
60. Csendes A, Braghetto I, Burdiles P, Korn O, Csendes P, Henriquez A. Very late results of esophagomyotomy for patients with achalasia: clinical, endoscopic, histologic, manometric, and acid reflux studies in 67 patients for a mean follow-up of 190 months. Ann Surg. 2006;243:196–203.
61. Kumagai K, Kjellin A, Tsai JA, et al. Toupet versus Dor as a procedure to prevent reflux after cardiomyotomy for achalasia: results of a randomised clinical trial. Int J Surg. 2014;12:673–80.
62. Khajanchee YS, Kanneganti S, Leatherwood AE, Hansen PD, Swanstrom LL. Laparoscopic Heller myotomy with Toupet fundoplication: outcomes predictors in 121 consecutive patients. Arch Surg. 2005;140:827–33; discussion 33–4.

63. Rawlings A, Soper NJ, Oelschlager B, et al. Laparoscopic Dor versus Toupet fundoplication following Heller myotomy for achalasia: results of a multicenter, prospective, randomized-controlled trial. Surg Endosc. 2012;26:18–26.
64. Simic AP, Radovanovic NS, Skrobic OM, Raznatovic ZJ, Pesko PM. Significance of limited hiatal dissection in surgery for achalasia. J Gastrointest Surg Off J Soc Surg Aliment Tract. 2010;14:587–93.
65. Zurita Macias Valadez LC, Pescarus R, Hsieh T. Laparoscopic limited Heller myotomy without anti-reflux procedure does not induce significant long-term gastroesophageal reflux. Surg Endosc. 2015;29:1462–8.
66. Ujiki MB, Yetasook AK, Zapf M, Linn JG, Carbray JM, Denham W. Peroral endoscopic myotomy: a short-term comparison with the standard laparoscopic approach. Surgery. 2013;154:893–7; discussion 7–900.
67. Bhayani NH, Kurian AA, Dunst CM, Sharata AM, Rieder E, Swanstrom LL. A comparative study on comprehensive, objective outcomes of laparoscopic Heller myotomy with per-oral endoscopic myotomy (POEM) for achalasia. Ann Surg. 2014;259:1098–103.

News in ESD

9

Kazuya Inoki, Takahisa Matsuda, and Yutaka Saito

9.1 Introduction

The development of endoscopic submucosal dissection (ESD) was critical in the history of endoscopy because it enhanced the value of therapeutic endoscopy and provided a less invasive therapy for many patients [1–7]. Although ESD is an attractive procedure for many endoscopists, mastery of ESD is difficult because it requires sophisticated endoscopic techniques. To improve the safety and success rate of ESD, we must continue to develop advanced endoscopic techniques, devices, and strategies.

9.2 Devices

The high-frequency knives used for ESD are roughly classified as tip knives or insulation-tipped diathermic knives (IT knife: Olympus Co., Tokyo, Japan). Both devices have advantages and disadvantages. The strong advantage of the IT knife is its fast speed of incision and dissection. The "IT" means "insulation tip." The tip of the knife restricts the flow of current thus reducing the chances of the

K. Inoki (✉) • Y. Saito
Endoscopy Division, National Cancer Center Hospital, Tokyo, Japan
e-mail: kinoki@ncc.go.jp

T. Matsuda
Endoscopy Division, National Cancer Center Hospital, Tokyo, Japan

Cancer Screening Division, Research Center for Cancer Prevention and Screening, National Cancer Center, Tokyo, Japan

R. Conigliaro, M. Frazzoni (eds.), *Diagnosis and Endoscopic Management of Digestive Diseases*, DOI 10.1007/978-3-319-42358-6_9

device inadvertently damaging tissues. However, manipulating the IT knife is difficult and sometimes requires dissection of lesions without direct visualization of the cutting location when moving the IT knife parallel to the muscularis propria. Thanks to their strong electric current, tip knives are useful for lesions with abundant fibrosis. However, it requires very precise scope manipulation and the cutting speed is slow.

The IT knife series consists of IT knife, IT knife 2, and IT knife nano. Typical tip knives include the Dual knife (Olympus Co., Tokyo, Japan), the Jet-B knife (XEMEX Co., Tokyo, Japan), the Flush knife (Fujifilm Medical Co., Tokyo, Japan), and the Hook knife (Olympus Co., Tokyo, Japan). The Jet-B knife and Flush knife have a water-jet function that enables submucosal injection without exchanging devices. In 2015, a new Dual knife and Hook knife were developed. They have the water-jet function, which many tip knives now possess, and are called the Dual knife J and Hook knife J (Olympus Co., Tokyo, Japan). In addition, a thinner Flush knife BT-S has been developed that enables easier fluid suction during use.

During the procedure, hemostasis forceps should be used to control bleeding, because using clips often disrupts continuation of ESD. There are two types of hemostatic forceps: monopolar and bipolar. Coagrasper (Olympus Co., Tokyo, Japan) is a monopolar type and is frequently used, especially with gastric cases. Slightly larger forceps called Coaglasper G (Olympus Co., Tokyo, Japan) have also been developed because some vessels encountered during gastric ESD are too thick to occlude immediately even if using the Coaglasper. Bipolar-type hemostatic forceps are frequently used for procedures of the colon and esophagus to reduce the risk of delayed perforation. A well-known bipolar-type forceps is the Hemostat-Y (Pentax Co., Tokyo, Japan), and recently a rotatable, bipolar-type hemostatic forceps called Tighturn (XEMEX Co., Tokyo, Japan) has been released.

9.3 How to Create Countertraction

The main reason ESD is difficult is that we have no direct countertraction, unlike in surgical procedures. However, the use of gravity and the attached cap are often very effective to create countertraction. Especially in colorectal cases, you can use gravity by changing the position of the patient. Several other relatively easy methods have been developed. They are the "clip and line method" [8] (Fig. 9.1a– c), the "S-O (Sakamoto and Osada) clip method" [9] (Fig. 9.2a, b), the "clip flap

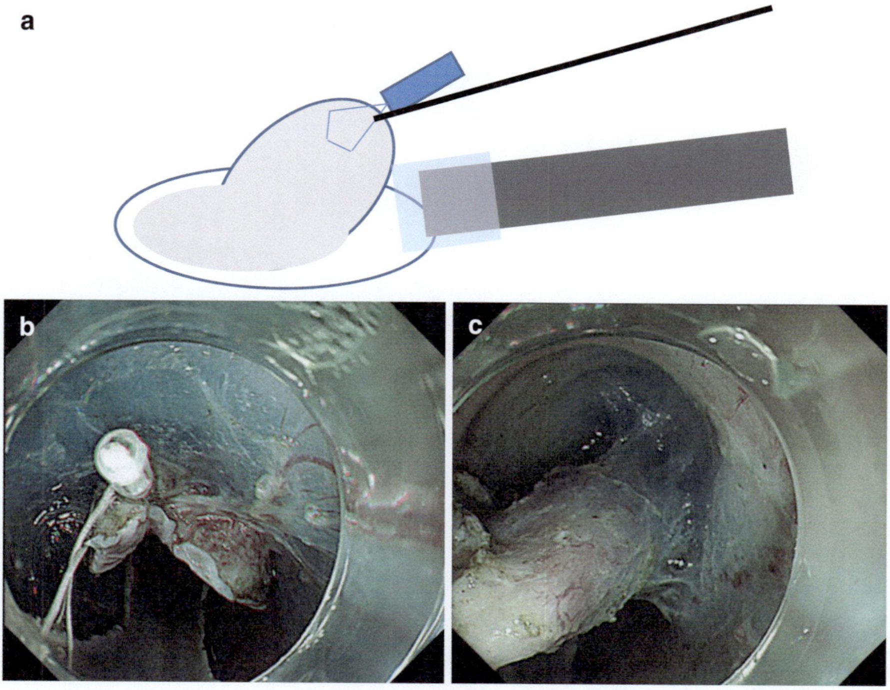

Fig. 9.1 (**a**) Schematic diagram of the clip and line method. (**b**, **c**) Good countertraction was made in esophageal ESD using the clip and line method

method" [10] (Fig. 9.3), and the "pocket creation method" [11]. The former three methods use clips and the last one is a newly developed strategy for ESD. The clip and line method is useful for esophageal, and sometimes gastric, ESD; you can achieve good tension and visibility of the submucosal layer by pulling back the string slightly. The S-O clip method uses a rubber strip or spring and is useful for colorectal lesions. The clip flap method is a relatively easy but helpful approach where an endoclip is substituted for the initial mucosal flap. The dissection may then become easier if traction can be achieved by going under the lesion. In addition, good traction can be achieved using the clip flap method if the submucosa is only slightly dissected. The pocket creation method is a novel strategy for colorectal ESD. It can provide traction and maintain the lifting created from the fluid injection for a longer period.

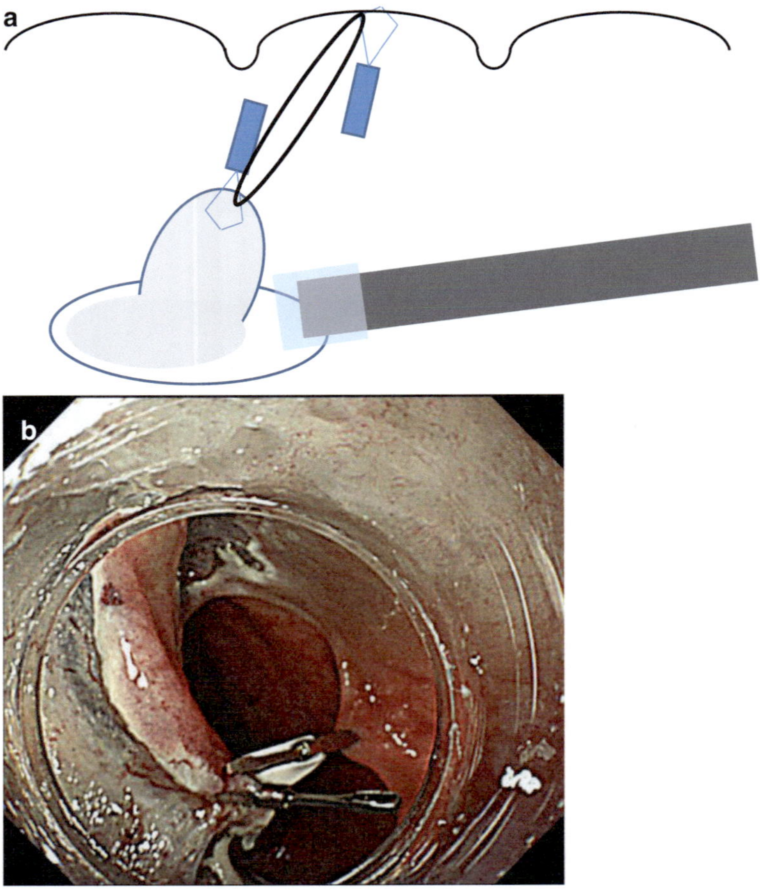

Fig. 9.2 (**a**) Schematic diagram of the S-O clip method. (**b**) Countertraction was made in colonic ESD by using clips and rubber band

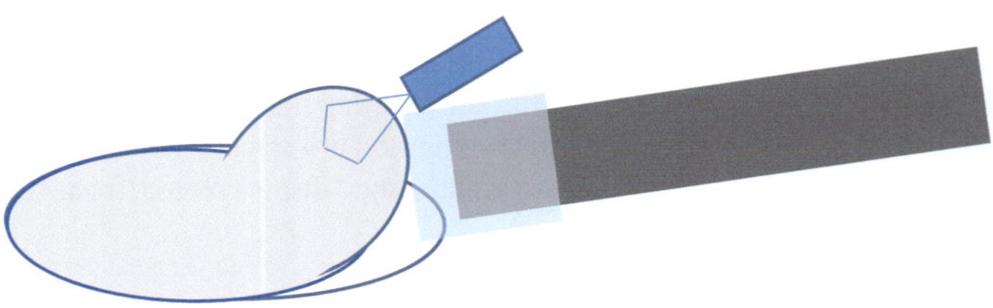

Fig. 9.3 Schematic diagram of the clip flap method. A clip is substituted for the initial mucosal flap

Conclusion

Many new devices and strategies have been developed, and while we have a long way to go before we have mastered ESD, applying these methods will make ESD procedures safer and easier.

References

1. Ono H, Kondo H, Gotoda T, et al. Endoscopic mucosal resection for treatment of early gastric cancer. Gut. 2001;48:225–9.
2. Yamamoto H, Kawata H, Sunada K, et al. Successful en-bloc resection of large superficial tumors in the stomach and colon using sodium hyaluronate and small-caliber-tip transparent hood. Endoscopy. 2003;35:690–4.
3. Fujishiro M, Yahagi N, Kakushima N, et al. Outcomes of endoscopic submucosal dissection for colorectal epithelial neoplasms in 200 consecutive cases. Clin Gastroenterol Hepatol. 2007;5(6):674–7.
4. Saito Y, Uraoka T, Matsuda T, et al. Endoscopic treatment of large superficial colorectal tumors: a cases series of 200 endoscopic submucosal dissections (with video). Gastrointest Endosc. 2007;66(5):966–73. Epub 2007 May 24.
5. Tamegai Y, Saito Y, Masaki N, et al. Endoscopic submucosal dissection: a safe technique for colorectal tumors. Endoscopy. 2007;39(5):418–22.
6. Toyonaga T, Man-i M, Chinzei R, et al. Endoscopic treatment for early stage colorectal tumors: the comparison between EMR with small incision, simplified ESD, and ESD using the standard flush knife and the ball tipped flush knife. Acta Chir Iugosl. 2010;57(3):41–6.
7. Saito Y, Uraoka T, Yamaguchi Y, et al. A prospective, multicenter study of 1111 colorectal endoscopic submucosal dissections (with video). Gastrointest Endosc. 2010;72(6):1217–25. Epub 2010 Oct 27.
8. Oyama T. Counter traction makes endoscopic submucosal dissection easier. Clin Endosc. 2012;45(4):375–8.
9. Sakamoto N, Osada T, Shibuya T, et al. Endoscopic submucosal dissection of large colorectal tumors by using a novel spring-action S-O clip for traction (with video). Gastrointest Endosc. 2009;69(7):1370–4.
10. Yamamoto K, Hayashi S, Nakabori T et al. Endoscopic submucosal dissection using endoclips to assist in mucosal flap formation (novel technique: "clip flap method"). Endoscopy. 2012;44 Suppl 2 UCTN:E334–5.
11. Hayashi Y, Sunada K, Takahashi H et al. Pocket-creation method of endoscopic submucosal dissection to achieve en bloc resection of giant colorectal subpedunculated neoplastic lesions. Endoscopy. 2014;46 Suppl 1 UCTN:E421–2.

ERCP in Altered Anatomy

10

Per-Ola Park and Maria Bergström

ERCP is the standard technique for dealing with pathology of the common bile duct, such as bile duct stones or strictures due to malignant or benign processes. However, ERCP in patients with surgically altered anatomy, such as Roux-en-Y gastric bypass (RYGBP), total gastrectomy, Billroth II procedure or Whipple procedure (Fig. 10.1), is challenging. Several more or less invasive methods have been described for endoscopic biliary interventions in these patients.

10.1 ERCP Using Balloon Enteroscopy

Balloon enteroscopy can be performed to reach through the Roux limb, via the entero-entero anastomosis, and further on through the biliary limb into the duodenum to find the papilla.

Balloon enteroscopy has been available since the beginning of 2000, first described by Yamamoto [1]. There are two current technical solutions: the double-balloon technique from Fujinon and the single-balloon technique from Olympus. Both require specialised equipment and expertise that are not widely available. A long Roux limb can be technically challenging as well as the different anatomic constructions of the entero-entero anastomosis, both varying with type of reconstruction (Fig. 10.2). One major problem with balloon enteroscopy ERCP is the lack of efficient accessories. The enteroscope is long, 2 m, and the working channel is only 2.8 mm, making it impossible to use standard ERCP accessories. There are only a few specialised accessories for these procedures on the market, and some are not possible to use over a guidewire. Another drawback is the lack of elevator at the tip of the endoscope and the fact that the papilla is reached and visualised from below. All these factors make both cannulation and therapy challenging. A cap on

P.-O. Park (✉) • M. Bergström, MD, PhD
Department of Surgery, South Älvsborg Hospital, Borås, Sweden
e-mail: per-ola.park@telia.com

R. Conigliaro, M. Frazzoni (eds.), *Diagnosis and Endoscopic Management of Digestive Diseases*, DOI 10.1007/978-3-319-42358-6_10

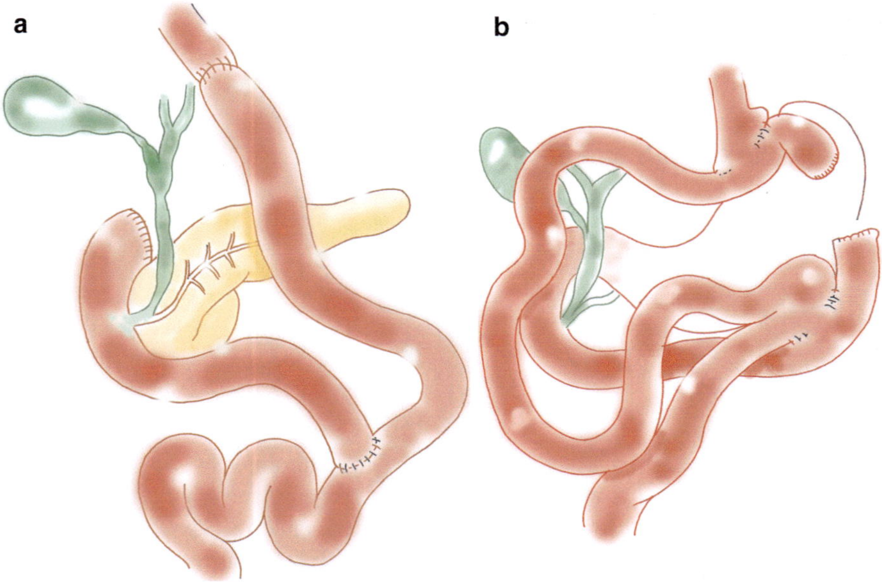

Fig. 10.1 Roux-en-Y reconstructions: (**a**) as performed after gastrectomy, resembling the situation after a BII resection or a Whipple procedure. (**b**) As performed during a gastric bypass procedure

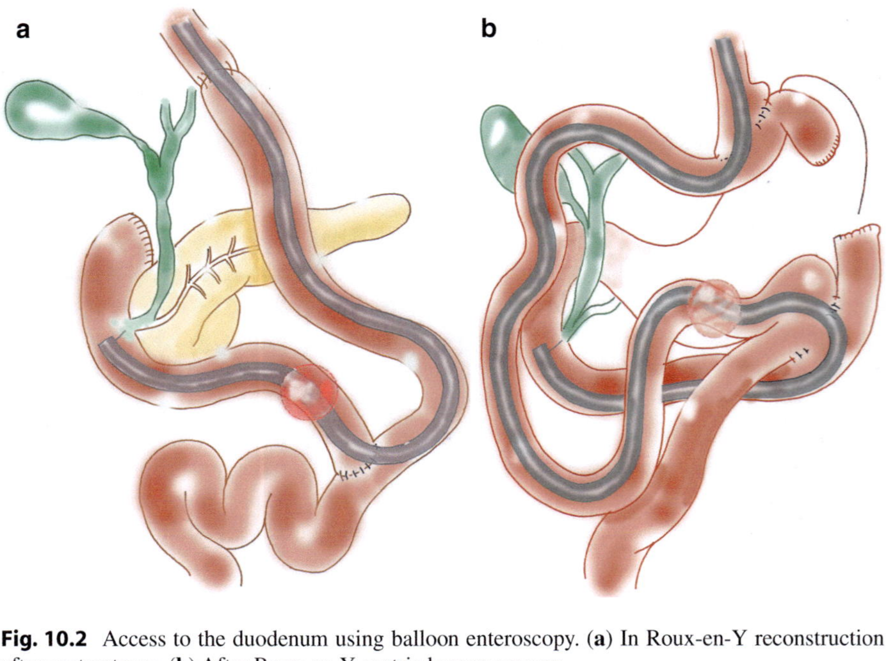

Fig. 10.2 Access to the duodenum using balloon enteroscopy. (**a**) In Roux-en-Y reconstruction after gastrectomy. (**b**) After Roux-en-Y gastric bypass surgery

the tip of the endoscope has been proposed to fixate the papilla during cannulation, making the procedure easier.

In a recent review article by Inamdar, the success rates for reaching the papilla in patients with altered anatomy differed between 55 and 100% [2]. The pooled enteroscopy success rate for all kinds of altered anatomy was 81% (CI 75–86%). The major reason for failure was difficulty to identify the biliary limb at the entero-entero anastomosis or trouble with intubating this limb with its marked angulation. The pooled diagnostic success rate for all attempted enteroscopies was 69% (CI 61–78%), and the pooled success rate for completed interventions was 62% (CI 53–71%). In patients with a successful enteroscopy, reaching the duodenum, the rate for interventional success was 79%. Schreiner et al. suggest that a successful balloon enteroscopy-aided ERCP is less likely in RYGBP patients with an alimentary limb of more than 150 cm [3].

10.2 Percutaneous Transhepatic Techniques

The percutaneous transhepatic cholangiography (PTC) technique has been used for many years for diagnostic and interventional purposes in the biliary tree. Direct transhepatic cholangioscopy, utilising the PTC access for endoscopy, was first described in 1974 by Takada. Today the PTC technique is often used as an alternative to ERCP for internal or external drainage of the biliary tree in situations with difficult cannulation. This access route can be used for interventions similar to those carried out using standard ERCP techniques. In patients with altered anatomy, the PTC technique offers an access route into the biliary system possible to use for primary interventions, for direct cholangioscopy and for aiding in enteral endoscopic interventions with rendezvous technique.

We have used this technique for rendezvous procedures aiming at ERCP in patients with altered anatomy. A guidewire was introduced through the PTC catheter through the papilla and advanced down to the entero-entero anastomosis to meet a balloon enteroscope. The guidewire was grasped by a snare from the endoscope which then could be manipulated up to the papilla (Fig. 10.3). Biliary interventions were then performed over the existing guidewire. Different endoscopes can be used for these rendezvous interventions, depending on the length of the Roux limb (in gastric bypass – enteroscope, after Whipple procedure or total gastrectomy – therapeutic gastroscope).

10.3 Percutaneous Transgastric Access

In gastric bypass patients, a gastrostomy placed in the remnant stomach can be used as an access port for ERCP (Fig. 10.4). The gastrostomy can be achieved using various techniques:

(a) Radiologic ultrasound-guided puncture of the remnant stomach

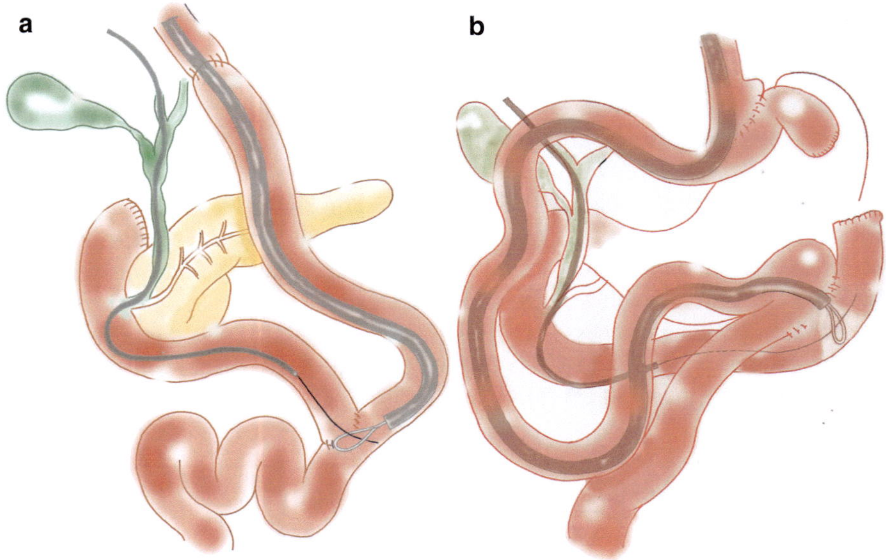

Fig. 10.3 Access to the duodenum and bile ducts using rendezvous techniques with a preplaced PTC access. The endoscope meets the transhepatic guidewire at the entero-entero anastomosis. (**a**) In Roux-en-Y reconstruction after gastrectomy. (**b**) After Roux-en-Y gastric bypass surgery

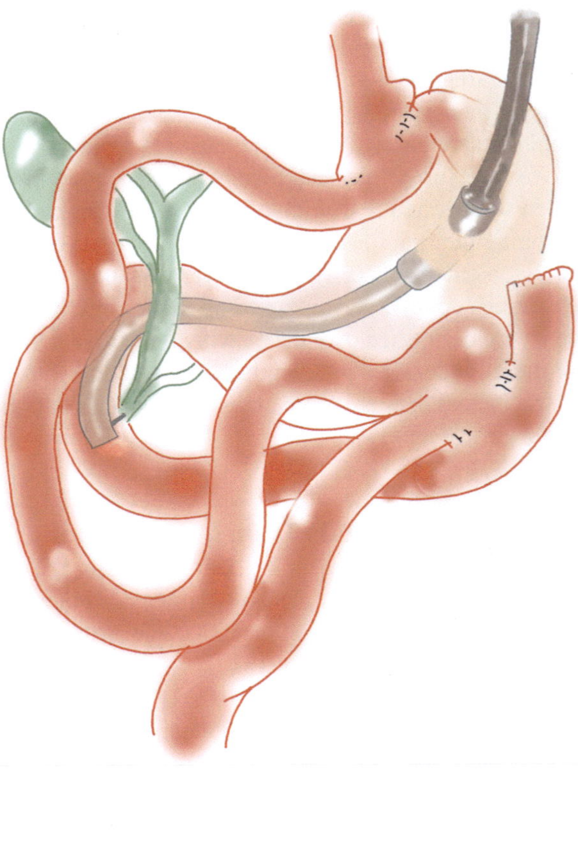

Fig. 10.4 Percutaneous access to the remnant stomach in Roux-en-Y gastric bypass. This access can be achieved using different techniques, as described in the text, but they all result in the possibility to insert the duodenoscope percutaneously

(b) Balloon enteroscopy into the remnant stomach followed by PEG placement
(c) Laparoscopic assisted gastrostomy

ERCP performed through a gastrostomy is technically similar to an ordinary per oral procedure as a standard duodenoscope is used together with standard accessories.

If the gastrostomy has been achieved using traditional endoscopic or radiologic PEG techniques, the stoma has to be established before it can be safely used for access. Achieving a secure gastrostomy takes about 4 weeks making this technique unsuitable in acute situations. To access the stomach with a duodenoscope, the stoma needs to be dilated to at least 15 mm. After the procedure a large diameter gastrostomy tube needs to be placed to secure the stoma. Tod Barron has described a technique, using balloon enteroscopy, creating an endoscopic gastrostomy for immediate access by placing a covered stent in the stoma [4]. The stent diameter allowed for passage of the duodenoscope and kept the stomach attached to the abdominal wall. Postoperatively a 26Fr gastrostomy tube was left in place for 4 weeks.

The technique for laparoscopic assisted access to the remnant stomach was first described by Pimentel in 2004 [5] and has since been repeated and described by several authors [6]. Using this technique, a laparoscopic port (15 mm) is placed through the skin into the stomach under direct laparoscopic vision. The abdominal cavity is then exsufflated and an ERCP can be performed through the port. After completion of the ERCP, the stomach incision can be surgically closed and no gastrostomy tube is needed. The entire procedure can be performed as day care surgery. The laparoscopic approach is well suited for acute situations but needs the assistance of a skilled minimal invasive surgeon.

If further ERCP interventions are required, the stoma can be preserved by leaving a gastrostomy tube in place, regardless of the type of initial stomach access.

10.4 EUS-Assisted Transgastric Techniques

New techniques using EUS for gaining access to the biliary tree are currently being developed. Recent reports describe both direct puncture of bile ducts in the left liver lobe and puncture of the remnant stomach from the pouch or the Roux limb in gastric bypass patients (Fig. 10.5).

The direct puncture technique can be used in all kinds of altered anatomy and is the same technique as in direct puncture of the common bile duct from the duodenal bulb [7]. It can only be used in cases with dilated bile ducts. When the access to the left bile duct has been established, direct drainage can be achieved by placement of a covered metal stent draining the bile into the pouch or Roux limb. Just as in PTC techniques, a guidewire can be introduced through this access into the common bile duct and out through the papilla for rendezvous attempts, brush cytology or stent placement [8].

In gastric bypass anatomy, EUS can be used to puncture the remnant stomach from the pouch or the Roux limb. This technique has recently been described by

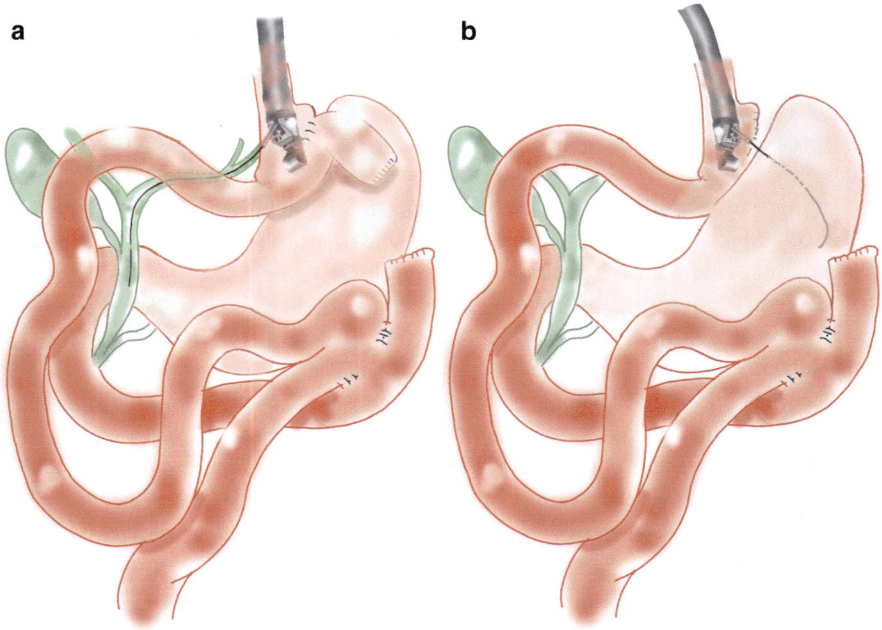

Fig. 10.5 EUS-guided techniques; (**a**) direct puncture of the left liver lobe. (**b**) Puncture of the remnant stomach through from the pouch

Kedia et al. Access was established by placement and dilatation of a lumen-apposing metal stent into the remnant stomach. A conventional ERCP was then performed via the stent. After the procedure the fistula was closed using endoscopic suturing with Overstitch [9]. The technique allows for acute interventions but requires advanced EUS competence.

10.5 Discussion

Performing ERCP in patients with altered anatomy is demanding and challenging and requires specialised equipment and expertise that are not widely available, why these procedures mostly will take place in tertiary or sometimes in secondary centres. The algorithm for solving the ERCP challenge in these patients depends on the available expertise and on which pathologic problem that needs to be solved. Very often a multidisciplinary approach is required. Regardless of which technique that is utilised, the procedure will be time-consuming and will involve advanced anaesthesia.

If the biliary tract pathology is a bile duct stone and the Roux limb is shorter than 150 cm, balloon enteroscopy might be the first choice, if available, despite a fairly low success rate.

However, if the pathology is a stricture or suspected malignancy, the success rate drops significantly and the "PEG" technique or a traditional PTC might be preferred in gastric bypass-operated patients. In other altered anatomy situations, PTC with or without rendezvous will be the most available option. In gastric bypass patients, the combined laparoscopic gastrostomy and ERCP may be the best alternative as it can be performed in day care surgery as well as in acute situations. One drawback is that it has to be performed in the operating theatre with full anaesthesia and that the patient has to be fit for surgery. In patients who previously have undergone laparotomy, intra-abdominal adhesions might cause technical problems. One advantage with the "PEG" technique is that it allows for the ERCP to be performed using standard duodenoscopes and accessories. By leaving a gastrostomy-tube in place after the procedure, the papilla can easily be reached later on, as in a normal ERCP, for re-interventions at the endoscopic unit.

The EUS techniques still have to be developed and evaluated. However, these techniques require a highly skilled interventional EUS endoscopist which is not even available at every tertiary endoscopic centre.

In conclusion the balloon enteroscopy is the least invasive method but at the moment with lower success rate compared with the surgical "PEG" ERCP or PTC. The lack of sufficient accessories for balloon enteroscopy ERCP is presently a drawback that probably will be solved in the near future. For each institution, the primary choice of method for performing ERCP in patients with altered anatomy, will depend on locally available resources and expertise.

References

1. Yamamoto H, et al. Total enteroscopy with a nonsurgical steerable double-balloon method. Gastrointest Endosc. 2001;53(2):216–20.
2. Inamdar S, et al. Systematic review and meta-analysis of single-balloon enteroscopy-assisted ERCP in patients with surgically altered GI anatomy. Gastrointest Endosc. 2015;82(1):9–19.
3. Schreiner MA, et al. Laparoscopy-assisted versus balloon enteroscopy-assisted ERCP in bariatric post-Roux-en-Y gastric bypass patients. Gastrointest Endosc. 2012;75(4):748–56.
4. Baron TH, et al. Novel approach to therapeutic ERCP after long-limb Roux-en-Y gastric bypass surgery using transgastric self-expandable metal stents: experimental outcomes and first human case study (with videos). Gastrointest Endosc. 2012;75(6):1258–63.
5. Pimentel RR, et al. Laparoscopy-assisted transgastrostomy ERCP after bariatric surgery: case report of a novel approach. Gastrointest Endosc. 2004;59(2):325–8.
6. Facchiano E, et al. Laparoscopy-assisted transgastric endoscopic retrograde cholangiopancreatography (ERCP) after Roux-en-Y gastric bypass: technical features. Obes Surg. 2015;25(2):373–6.
7. Artifon EL, Perez-Miranda M. EUS-guided choledochoduodenostomy for malignant distal biliary obstruction palliation: an article review. Endosc Ultrasound. 2012;1(1):2–7.
8. Gomez V, Topazian MD. EUS-guided therapy for obstructive jaundice through a gastric pouch in the setting of prior Roux-en-Y gastric bypass. Gastrointest Endosc. 2016;83(4):828–9.
9. Kedia P, et al. EUS-directed transgastric ERCP for Roux-en-Y gastric bypass anatomy: a minimally invasive approach. Gastrointest Endosc. 2015;82(3):560–5.

Endoscopic and Surgical Management of Zenker's Diverticulum: New Approaches

11

Mauro Manno, Micaela Piccoli, Marzio Frazzoni, and Rita Conigliaro

11.1 Introduction

Zenker's diverticulum (ZD) is a posterior pharyngoesophageal pouch that forms through pulsion forces in an area of relative hypopharyngeal wall weakness between the oblique fibers of the inferior pharyngeal constrictor and the horizontal fibers of the cricopharyngeus (CP) muscles [1]. Poor upper esophageal sphincter (UES) compliance has been regarded as the main pathophysiologic mechanism. This dysfunction creates a high-pressure zone eventuating in increased pulsion forces and subsequent ZD formation. This entity most commonly presents in the elderly and can be associated with a plethora of potential symptoms, of which dysphagia is most common.

11.2 Pathophysiology

Although a complete understanding of the pathogenesis of ZD has not yet been reached, it is generally accepted that ZD is likely to be a multifactorial disorder. The noncompliant cricopharyngeal muscle shows structural changes in terms of histological reduction in muscle component combined with qualitative fiber alterations,

M. Manno
Digestive Endoscopy Unit, Ramazzini Hospital, Carpi, Modena, Italy

M. Piccoli
General Surgery, Baggiovara Hospital, Modena, Italy

M. Frazzoni, MD (✉)
Digestive Pathophysiology Unit, Baggiovara Hospital, Modena, Italy
e-mail: marziofrazzoni@gmail.com

R. Conigliaro
Digestive Endoscopy Unit, Baggiovara Hospital, Modena, Italy

R. Conigliaro, M. Frazzoni (eds.), *Diagnosis and Endoscopic Management of Digestive Diseases*, DOI 10.1007/978-3-319-42358-6_11

increase in fibrotic tissue, and significant increase of the collagen to elastin ratio. The aging process might play a role because of the loss of tissue elasticity and the decrease in muscle tone [1].

The hypothesized mechanisms relate to increased intraluminal pressure leading to an outpouching in the triangle of Killian, an area of relative wall weakness located posteriorly in the hypopharynx between two strong muscles, the CP and the inferior pharyngeal constrictor. This posterior pouch includes only mucosa and submucosa, so that ZD should be considered as a pseudodiverticulum.

The forces that determine this dehiscence are less clear. Accurate manometric measurements are difficult to achieve. The most likely mechanism proposed is decreased compliance of the UES with failure to open completely and a subsequent increase in the hypopharyngeal pressure gradient. It should be noted that this change in compliance is not equivalent to a change in UES pressure, which has been inconsistently shown.

Other contributing factors include an increase in intrabolus pressure due to the stiffness of the CP and hypopharynx. Finally, some investigators have also variably demonstrated incoordination of pharyngeal contraction and UES opening.

11.3 Symptoms and Diagnosis

Zenker's diverticula typically present in middle-aged adults and elderly individuals, especially during the seventh and eighth decades of life. It occurs predominately in men, and the overall prevalence of ZD among the general population is believed to be between 0.01 and 0.11 % [1]. The incidence varies based on region, being more common in Northern than Southern Europe. It has been described more frequently in the United States, Canada, and Australia than in Japan and Indonesia. It is unclear if these differences in prevalence reflect differences in longevity or anatomical differences between geographic areas. However, although Zenker's diverticula are the most common type that cause symptoms, its incidence and prevalence may be underestimated as many diverticula may remain clinically silent and many elderly patients with small pouches and minimal symptoms may not seek medical advice.

The vast majority of patients complain of dysphagia and regurgitation. Cervical borborygmus is almost pathognomonic of ZD. As dysphagia increases, symptoms become more severe with resultant weight loss and malnutrition. Hoarseness, cough, and aspiration pneumonia have also been described. Regurgitation of undigested foods and halitosis may occur because of stasis of food in the pouch.

In most cases, the diagnosis of ZD is suspected based on clinical symptoms and confirmed by contrast esophagography.

11.4 Surgical Treatment

Many experts still consider open surgery as the standard management of symptomatic ZD. However, clinically relevant adverse events are associated with open diverticulectomy, including mediastinitis, recurrent laryngeal nerve injury, esophageal stricture, fistula, esophageal perforation, hematoma, wound infection, pneumonia, and even death, with an 11 % median incidence of major morbidity [1].

In a pilot study, we showed for the first time the feasibility of a robot-assisted left transaxillary approach for the surgical management of ZD [2]. The patient was placed supine under general anesthesia. Similarly to transaxillary robotic thyroidectomy, the neck was slightly extended, and the left arm was raised and fixed to obtain the shortest distance from the axilla to the anterior neck. Under direct vision, a 4–5 cm skin incision was made in the left axilla, and the subplatysmal skin flap from the axilla to the anterior neck area was dissected over the anterior surface of the pectoralis major muscle using the Johann grasper or a monopolar electrical cautery. Next, to maintain adequate working space, an external retractor was inserted through the skin incision in the axilla. A suction tube was connected in order to avoid field fogging. The myocutaneous flap was raised until the sternal and clavicular heads of the sternocleidomastoideus muscle were visualized; then the dissection continued through the two sternocleidomastoideus branches. Next, the external retractor placed beneath the strap muscle was replaced with a larger one to obtain an adequate working space. Robotic docking was then performed. Four robotic arms were used during the operation, all through the axillary incision. The dual-channel endoscope was placed on the central arm, and the Harmonic curved shears together with the Maryland dissector were placed on the right side of the scope. ProGrasp forceps were inserted on the left side of the scope. All vessel dissections were performed using the Harmonic curved shears. Under robotic guidance, the thyroid was drawn medially by the ProGrasp forceps in order to identify and spare the inferior thyroid artery and the inferior laryngeal nerve. It was necessary to cut the middle thyroid vein in all cases and the omohyoid muscle in two cases. The prevertebral fascia was identified and the diverticulum isolated. Under endoscopic control, the loose connective tissue surrounding the pouch was dissected to identify the neck of the diverticulum on the posterior pharyngeal wall (Fig. 11.1). The neck was fully exposed by tractioning the diverticulum to the left with the Maryland dissector (Fig. 11.2). A complete myotomy was then performed with a robotic monopolar hook allowing dissection and resection: the myotomy included the cricopharyngeal muscle and the first 5 cm of the circular layer of the cervical esophagus. Then a surgical linear stapler (Endopath RTS-FLEX Endoscopic Articulating Linear Cutter 35 mm; Ethicon Endo-Surgery, LLC) with a blue cartridge was inserted through the axilla and applied to the neck of the diverticulum (Fig. 11.3). The complete diverticulum removal was endoscopically confirmed. Intravenous

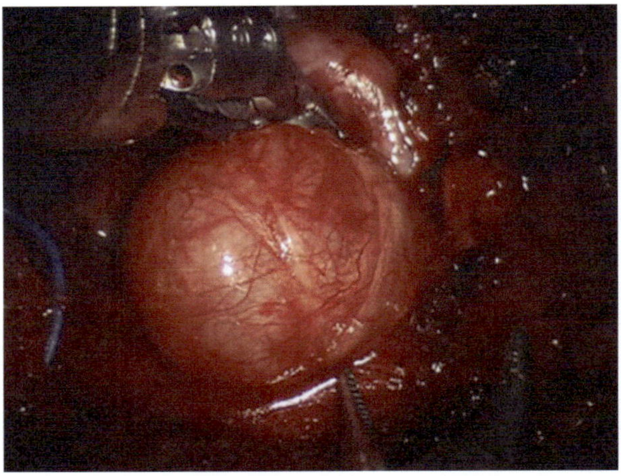

Fig. 11.1 Isolation and exposition of the diverticulum under endoscopic control

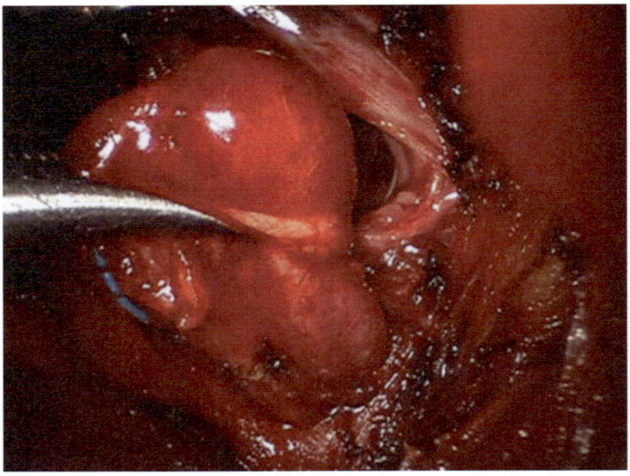

Fig. 11.2 The neck has been isolated and the diverticulum is fully exposed

broad-spectrum antibiotics were administered for 72 h after intervention. The advantages afforded by robotic technology could contribute to prevent both transient and definitive palsy of the recurrent laryngeal nerve and to render the cricopharyngeal myotomy safer with sparing of the esophageal mucosa. In our preliminary series, no relevant complication was registered. These preliminary results are encouraging, but we acknowledge that the robot-assisted transaxillary Zenker's diverticulectomy is a technically demanding procedure. Skill in thyroid and robotic surgery is required, as well as in esophageal surgery. Enthusiasm must be tempered by caution, and our results need to be confirmed in larger patient cohorts.

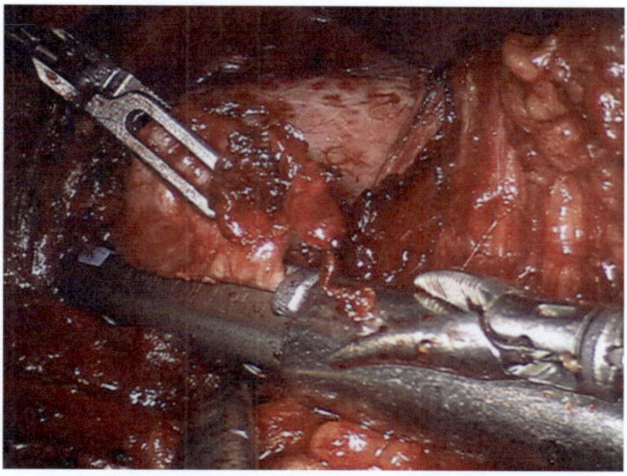

Fig. 11.3 The surgical linear stapler has been applied to the neck of the diverticulum

11.5 Endoscopic Treatment

The open surgical approach is associated with adverse events, including fistulae and infection. A transoral approach lessens these risks by avoiding an incision. In experienced hands, flexible or rigid endoscopic diverticulotomy is currently considered as a first-choice option in the management of ZD because it gives symptom relief comparable to open surgical diverticulectomy with less morbidity, shorter hospital stay, and, in the case of a flexible endoscopic approach, without the need of general anesthesia.

Rigid endoscopic diverticulectomy is carried out by dividing the common wall with a rigid diverticuloscope. The methods adopted to divide the common wall have evolved from electrocautery to carbon dioxide laser therapy to the now more commonly performed stapling [1].

Flexible endoscopy shares the same principles as rigid endoscopy: it consists of dividing the septum thus creating a common cavity. However, the technique still needs to be standardized because a variety of different modalities and endoscopic devices have been used, including freehand cut, guidewire-assisted and diverticuloscope-assisted myotomy, argon plasma coagulation, monopolar forceps, and needle knife for cutting the septum [3–10]. In this line, three different needles have been used: a standard needle knife [5], the hook knife [6] (Fig. 11.4), and most recently the IT knife 2 [7] (Fig. 11.5). Flexible endoscopic treatment of ZD can be performed in deep sedation with propofol or under general anesthesia and endotracheal intubation according to local practice. Antibiotic prophylaxis is recommended in high-risk patients. A soft diverticuloscope (ZD overtube; Cook Endoscopy, Winston – Salem, North Carolina, USA) (Fig. 11.6) permits to expose, stretch, and fix the septum (Fig. 11.7). It has two distal flaps of 40 and 30 mm that protect the anterior esophageal and posterior diverticular wall, respectively. The

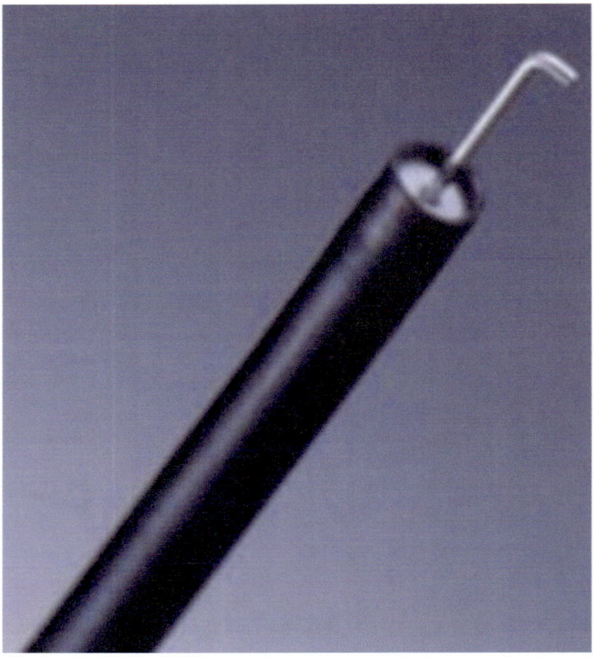

Fig. 11.4 The hook knife (Olympus Co., Ltd)

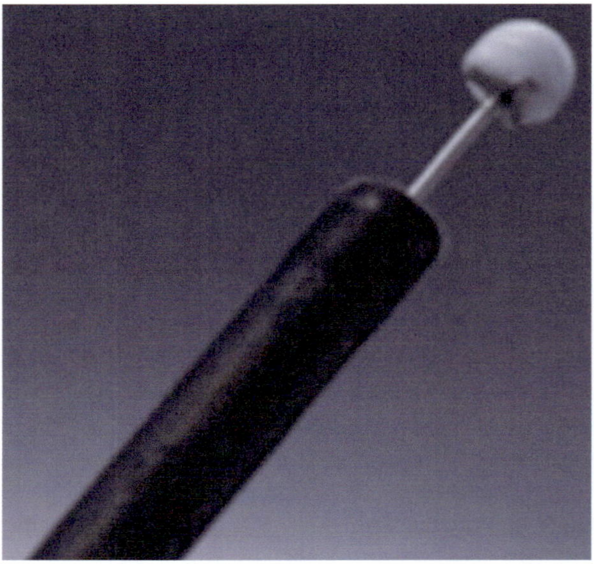

Fig. 11.5 IT knife 2 (Olympus Co., Ltd.)

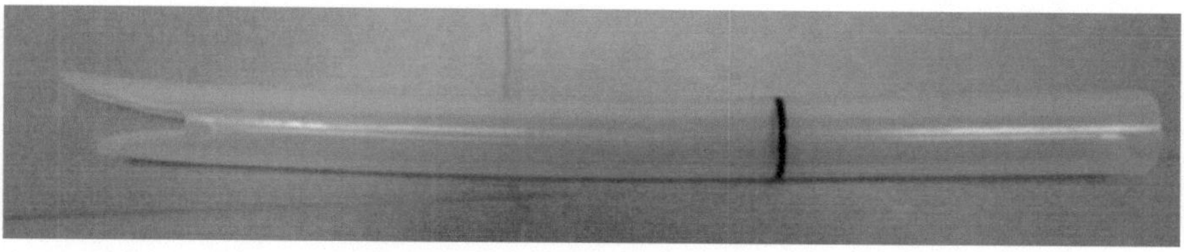

Fig. 11.6 Diverticuloscope (ZD overtube; Cook Endoscopy)

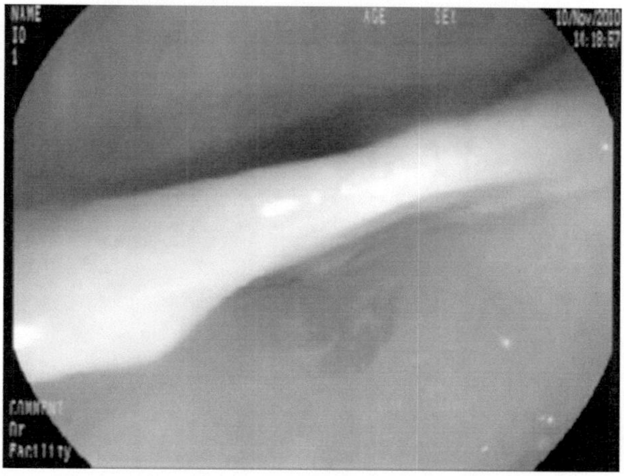

Fig. 11.7 Septum exposure with diverticuloscope

overtube is advanced over the endoscope up to a black marker indicating the average distance between the septum and teeth line. Under endoscopic vision, the septum is displayed [5]. Once the septum is properly exposed, different cutting methods can be applied. Myotomy can be done using standard needle knife, monopolar forceps, argon plasma coagulation, hook knife, or, most recently, IT knife 2 [3–10]. IT knife 2 seems to guarantee a more precise cut compared with other devices, allowing a more stable position by putting the insulated rounded tip on the septum of the diverticulum and cutting it toward a caudal direction (Figs. 11.8 and 11.9). In our study [7], 21 procedures in 19 patients were performed registering two dysphagia recurrences (in the first two cases) and no complications.

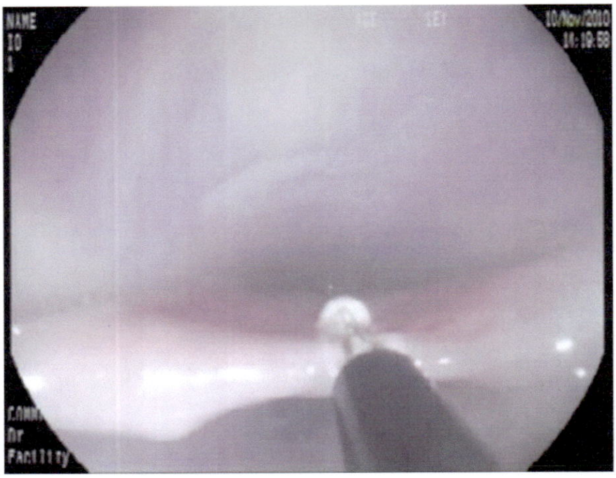

Fig. 11.8 Cut of the septum with IT knife 2

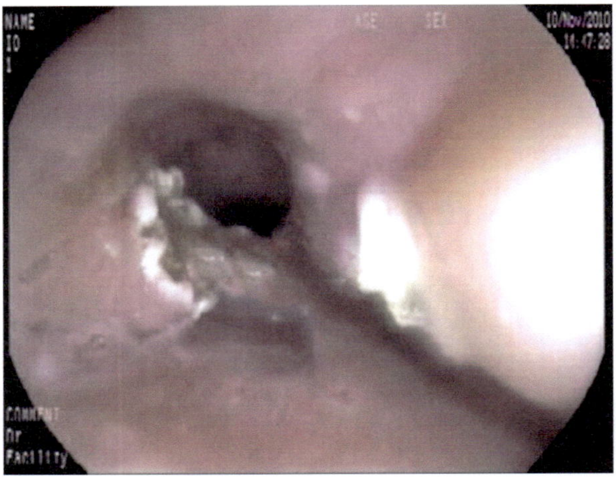

Fig. 11.9 Completion of myotomy

Conclusions

The flexible endoscopic procedure is simpler and less costly than the surgical procedure, particularly when the robotic option is considered, and the median hospital stay is shorter (3 days vs. 7 days at our institution). However, for large-size (>6 cm) diverticula, we still regard the surgical option as more effective and still preferable, unless the patient is unfit for surgery.

In conclusion, flexible endoscopic treatment of ZD seems/appears effective and safe, the choice between different options depending on local expertise and availability of advanced techniques.

References

1. Law R, Katzka DA, Baron TH. Zenker's diverticulum. Clin Gastroenterol Hepatol. 2014;12:1773–82.
2. Melotti G, Piccoli M, Mullineris B, et al. Zenker diverticulectomy: first report of robot-assisted transaxillary approach. J Robot Surg. 2015;9:75–8.
3. Bizzotto A, Iacopini F, Landi R, et al. Zenker's diverticulum: exploring treatment options. Acta Otorhinolaryngol Ital. 2013;33:219–29.
4. Rabenstein T, May A, Michel J, et al. Argon plasma coagulation for flexible endoscopic Zenker's diverticulotomy. Endoscopy. 2007;39:141–5.
5. Costamagna G, Iacopini F, Tringali A. Flexible endoscopic Zenker's diverticulotomy: cap-assisted technique vs diverticuloscope-assisted technique. Endoscopy. 2007;39:146–52.
6. Repici A, Pagano N, Romeo F, et al. Endoscopic flexible treatment of Zenker's diverticulum: a modification of the needle-knife technique. Endoscopy. 2010;42:532–5.
7. Manno M, Manta R, Caruso A, et al. Alternative endoscopic treatment of Zenker's diverticulum: a case series (with video). Gastrointest Endosc. 2014;79(1):168–70.
8. Evrard S, Le Moine O, Hassid S, et al. Zenker's diverticulum: a new endoscopic treatment with a soft diverticuloscope. Gastrointest Endosc. 2003;58:116–20.
9. Vogelsang A, Preiss C, Neuhaus H, et al. Endotherapy of Zenker's diverticulum using the needle-knife technique: long- term follow-up. Endoscopy. 2007;39:131–6.
10. Case DJ, Baron T. Flexible endoscopic management of Zenker diverticulum: the Mayo Clinic experience. Mayo Clin Proc. 2010;85:719–22.

Cholangioscopy Systems: State of the Art

12

Raffaele Manta and Michel Kahaleh

12.1 Introduction

Peroral cholangioscopy (POC) permits direct visualization of the biliary tree for diagnostic procedures and provides endoscopic guidance for therapeutic interventions.

POC is traditionally conducted using a mother-baby scope system. However, POC using this system is cumbersome, labor intensive, and difficult. A small caliber baby scope can be broken easily, is expensive, and is difficult to handle with limited irrigation and suction, and it has a small working channel of 1.2 mm diameter. The mother-baby scope system is also operated by two skilled endoscopists using two endoscopic systems. Therefore, routine clinical application of this system has been given up or limited to few endosocpic centers [1]. A single-operator cholangioscopic system has been developed as a new type of POC system, and nowadays POC can be performed by using a dedicated cholangioscope that is advanced through the accessory channel of a duodenoscope or by direct insertion of a small-diameter endoscope (ultraslim upper endoscope) directly into the bile duct for visualization of the biliary mucosa and lumen.

R. Manta, MD (✉)
U.O.C. Gastroenterologia ed Endoscopia Digestiva, Nuovo Ospedale Civile S.Agostino-Estense, Viale Giardini 1355, Baggiovara-Modena, Italy
e-mail: r.manta@libero.it; r.manta@ausl.mo.it

M. Kahaleh, MD, AGAF, FACG, FASGE
Professor of Medicine Chief, Endoscopy, Medical Director Pancreas Program, Division of Gastroenterology and Hepatology, Department of Medicine, Weill Cornell Medical College, 1305 York Avenue, 4th Floor, New York,10021 NY, Italy

R. Conigliaro, M. Frazzoni (eds.), *Diagnosis and Endoscopic Management of Digestive Diseases*, DOI 10.1007/978-3-319-42358-6_12

12.2 Direct Cholangioscopy

Compared to ductoscopy using a dedicated cholangioscope, the direct approach has several advantages and disadvantages. Three major advantages compared with other POC systems should be underlined: Direct POC provides high-quality endoscopic imaging with the ease of performance of enhanced endoscopy using narrow band imaging (NBI) and enables detection of smaller and more obscure lesions. A large, 2-mm-diameter working channel can be extended for interventional procedures, including for tissue sampling, and permits 5-Fr instruments. The direct POC system uses a conventional endoscope with a standard endoscopic setup by a single operator and avoids problems associated with simultaneous operation of multiple endoscopes such as the need of human resources, coordination of movements, and costs [2].

According to disadvantages ultraslim endoscopes present larger outer diameters, generally 5–6 mm; therefore, they can be used only after a large endoscopic sphincterotomy and/or sphincteroplasty and in patients with dilated bile ducts (>8 mm). The most profound disadvantage of direct peroral cholangioscopy is the difficulty associated with traversing the biliary sphincter to gain access to the bile duct. The current ultraslim scope is not designed for use as a cholangioscope, as it is too flexible, and it is easy to make a loop in the gastric fundus or third portion of the duodenum. There are therefore multiple published reports in the endoscopic literature with innovative suggestions on how to achieve this task. Some of the suggestions of endoscope introduction are over a guide wire, through a regular overtube, or with the help of a double-balloon overtube. However, despite use of these accessories, failure rate still remains high [3].

Another disadvantage of direct cholangioscopy is the instability of the ultraslim upper endoscope once it is inside the bile duct. All accessories supporting the scope, such as an intraductal balloon catheter, including the guide wire should be removed from the working channel of the scope to use interventional instruments. This can cause instability in the scope position. The distal tip of the scope can easily dislocate on the distal CBD or fall into the duodenum. This instability makes it difficult to perform diagnostic or therapeutic procedures such as obtaining biopsies of lesions or lithotripsy of difficult to remove biliary stones [4].

> Moreover an air embolism is a rare complication of direct POC but can be a fatal problem. Cholangitis can also occur during or after the procedure. The use of a CO_2 system instead of room air during the POC procedure and administration of antibiotics before and after the procedure are strongly recommended [5].

Finally new accessories or specialized scopes must be developed to overcome the technical disadvantages of current direct POC in order to facilitate the diagnostic and therapeutic roles of direct POC.

12.3 Dedicated Cholangioscopy (or Indirect Cholangioscopy)

Regarding POC that can be performed using a dedicated cholangioscope advanced through the accessory channel of a duodenoscope, SpyGlass (Boston Scientific, Natick, MA, USA) is the most frequently used and widely diffused probe. Similar to the SpyGlass scope is the Polyscope® (Polyscope system; Polydiagnost, Pfaffenhofen, Germany), which consists of a detachable flexible endoscope system available in 8 Fr (185 cm length) with separate optical, working/irrigation (1.2 mm), illumination, and steering channels. Although there are few differences between the two systems from technical aspects, as summarized in Table 12.1, Spyglass is preferred to polyscope, and it represents the best known tool for the management of a selected group of biliary diseases.

12.4 SpyGlass System

The first single-operator cholangioscopy (SOC) system was presented, in 2005, by Boston Scientific (Natick, MA, USA) with the name of SpyGlass Direct Visualization System (SGDVS) [6]. It was an endoscopic advanced method, based on an image acquisition system mediated by optical fibers, which significantly facilitates the diagnosis of biliary-pancreatic diseases by a single operator. It made possible the direct macroscopic visualization of lesions, allowing their microscopic characterization through targeted biopsies, and eventual treatment.

A study performed in 2007 showed that the cholangioscopy using SpyGlass (SOC-S) was superior to that of a videocholangioscope (CHF BP-30, Olympus) in terms of visualization of the four lumen quadrants and in carrying out biopsies

Table 12.1 Comparison of different systems for indirect peroral cholangioscopy

Characteristics	SpyGlass	Polyscope
Optics resolution	6000 pixels	10,000 pixels
Working channel	1.2 mm	1.2 mm
Viewing angle	70°	70°
Outer diameter	10 Fr	8 Fr
Reusable	Yes	Yes
Optical channel	No	Yes
Hermetically close		(The optical fiber doesn't need to be sterilized; this prolongs its life cycle)
Steerability	Four way	One-way (With locking of the bending and rotating of the tip)
Compatibility with existing endoscopy tower	No (You have to buy a complete endoscopy tower system)	Yes (You can use, through adapters, an existing endoscopy tower in the hospital)

(95 % CI OR, from 1.7 to 2.94; *P* <0.001). Indeed, the SpyGlass system allows to deflect the tip in the four directions [7].

In 2015 a new SOC was launched by Boston Scientific (Natick, MA, USA): SpyGlass DS (Digital Simple) Direct Visualization System. Built on the technology of the original SGDVS, the new SpyGlass DS System was designed to optimize procedural efficiency and productivity with improved ease of setup, ease of use, and image quality.

12.4.1 Equipment

The SpyGlass DS Direct Visualization System is a sterile and disposable device composed of a flexible catheter useable in a normal duodenoscope with a working channel. Compared to the previous version, an integrated digital sensor provides superior imaging, far greater resolution, and a 60 % wider field of view. The controller is an endoscopic video imaging system that combines the functionality of a camera and a LED light source. The controller receives video signals from the catheter, processes the video signals, and outputs video images to an attached monitor. It also generates and controls the illumination transmitted to the distal end of the catheter. The catheter comprises a control section, an insertion tube, and a connection cable. The control section is provided with a handle with two knobs that allow the orientation of the distal end of catheter in the four directions, with a minimum inclination of 30° in the presence of all accessories. Moreover, it owns a locking lever and a urethane band under the operator channel, which lock the system at the duodenoscope. The flexible catheter (SpyScope) consists of a Teflon device of 3.3 mm (10 Fr). It contains one working channel (1.2 mm) that allows the passage of dedicated biopsy forceps, probes for lithotripsy, or laser and guide wires, two channels (0.6 mm) for irrigation, two optical fibers to transmit illumination from the controller, and wiring to transmit video signals to the controller. The catheter is introduced through a duodenoscope that has an operating channel of at least 4.2 mm^2 (Figs. 12.1 and 12.2).

The biopsy forceps (SpyBite) are sterile and disposable accessories for sampling intraductal biopsy. They have an external diameter of 1 mm and a length of 286 cm, with an opening of 4.1 mm. The irrigation system consists of a sterile tube set connected to an irrigation pump, activated with a pedal.

12.4.2 Clinical Applications

There are different indications for SOC-S use. It can be used for diagnostic and therapeutic procedures. Among common uses, there are difficult biliary stones and macroscopic and histological typing of indeterminate biliary strictures. Less common uses are the selective guide wire placement in a bile duct, the evaluation of either stenosis after a liver transplant or filling defects of the bile ducts not characterized by other methods (MRI, ERCP, EUS), as well as resolution of multiple lithiasis. The rare uses comprise staging or endoscopic ablation of tumors, the trans-papillary gallbladder drainage, and evaluation of hemobilia.

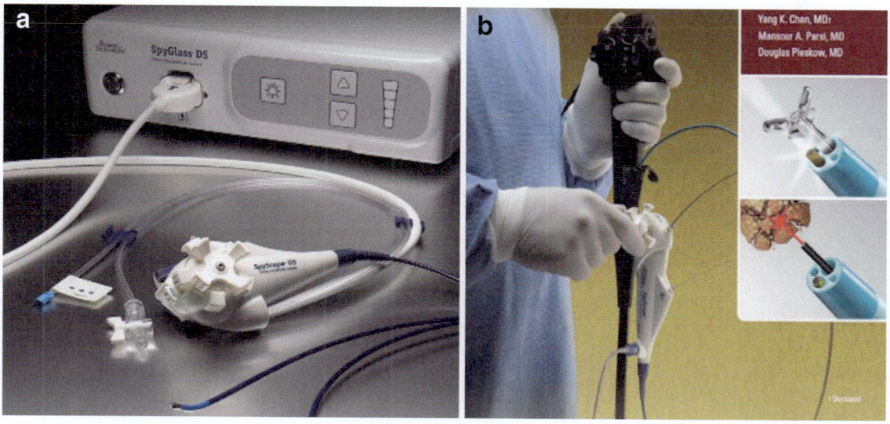

Fig. 12.1 SpyGlass DS equipments. Controller (**a**), and a flexible catheter (**b**) useable in a normal duodenoscope with a working channel

12.4.3 Treatment of Difficult Biliary Stones

Intraductal lithotripsy is the main therapeutic application of SOC-S when conventional procedures fail. The failure rate in the treatment of choledocholithiasis following standard endoscopic retrograde cholangiopancreatography (ERCP) is ranging between 8 and 16 % [8, 9]. A partial bile duct clearance depends on stones' characteristics (number, size, shape, texture, seat), the bile duct structure (shape, size, low insertion of the cystic duct), and the presence of a juxtapapillary diverticulum. Common bile duct and Wirsung lithiasis can be treated with laser (LL) or electrohydraulic lithotripsy (EHL). In such a field, the SOC-S has two important advantages. The first is to allow a direct visualization of the lumen and the stones position, avoiding duct damage. The second is to consent the correct functioning of the EHL device through the irrigation of bile ducts with the saline solution. In fact, the 1.9 Fr nitinol catheter of the EHL presents two insulated coaxial electrodes in the tip that produce sparks generating high-amplitude hydraulic pressure waves able to fragment the stones [10, 11]. The LL fragments stones using a laser beam that is delivered by means of a quartz flexible fiber introduced in the SOC-S operator channel. The pulsed application of the beam generates ion formations and free electrons at high energy with consequent spherical mechanical waves which fragment the stones [12]. A complete common bile duct drainage was achieved in 92 % of 26 patients with difficult cholelithiasis who failed three ERCP sessions with standard mechanical lithotripsy [13]. Similarly, following a mean of 1.2 sessions, a 100 % common bile duct clearance was reported by using Holmium laser lithotripsy in 60 patients with mechanical lithotripsy failure (stones average size of 23 mm), or with other conditions, such as the Mirizzi syndrome or stone impacted [14]. In a recent retrospective single-center study, a 77 % technical success in removing gallstones from the bile duct was reported [15].

The SOC-S has been used in 13 patients with cystic duct stones, including four with Mirizzi syndrome type 1, achieving complete clearance of both cystic duct and

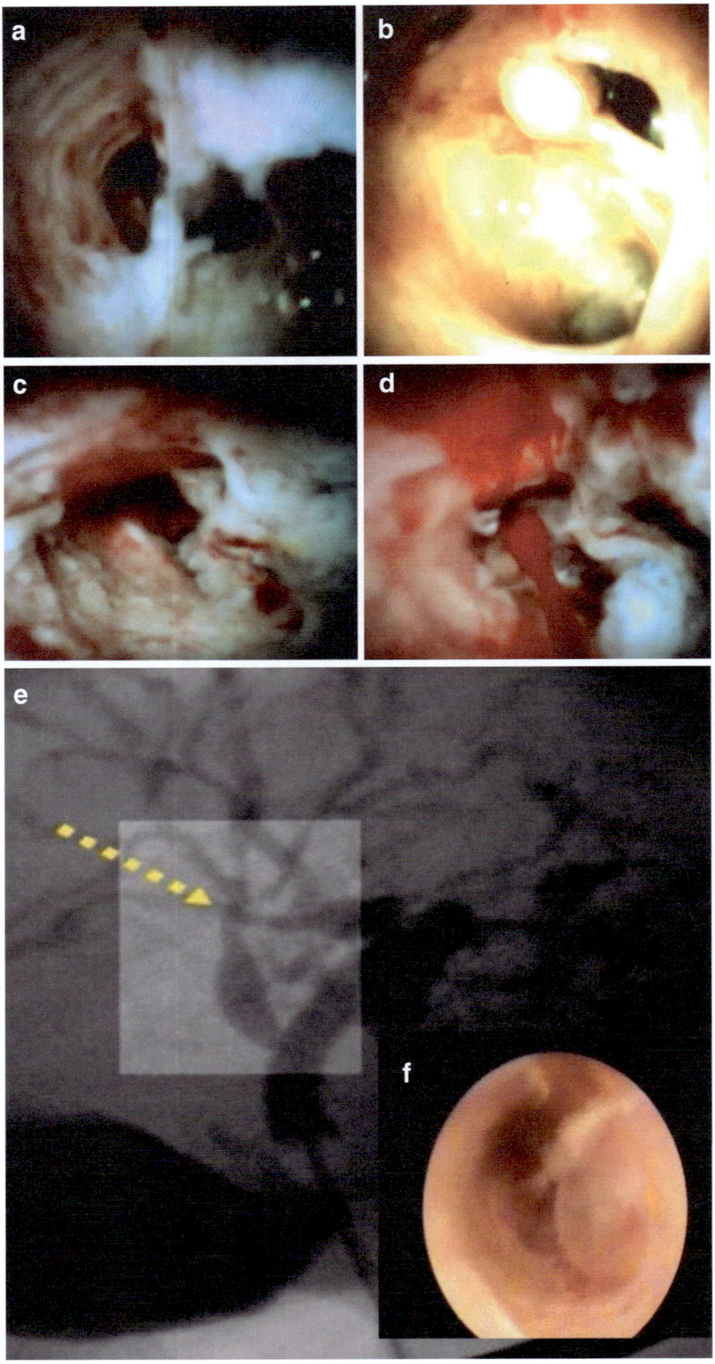

Fig. 12.2 SpyGlass DS images. (**a**) Cholangiocarcinoma of common bile duct; (**b**) a rare case of biliary cystoadenocarcinoma involving the intrahepatic left duct; (**c**, **d**) bleeding and stenotic neoplastic lesion located at hepatic hilum. A rare case of intrahepatic varices. (**e**) Stenosis of intrahepatic duct; (**f**) varices in intrahepatic duct

common bile duct in 77 % of cases [16]. In a prospective, multicenter study, 66 patients with difficult biliary stones (stones average size of 19 mm) underwent EHL (50 cases) or LL (16 cases). A complete bile ducts' clearance was achieved in all cases, with two sessions being needed in only 29 % of cases [17]. A case report showed a successful biliary lithiasis treatment with SOC-S and EHL by using an operator colonoscope in a patient with hepatic jejunostomy with Roux-en-Y reconstruction [18]. Of note, the use of SOC-S in pregnant women with gallstones allows to prevent radiological exposure [19]. Finally, a percentage of missed stones ranging between 8 and 30 % should be also taken into account, including those small stones not visible after contrast medium or masked by larger stones. These could be diagnosed and successfully treated by using the SOC-S [20, 21].

12.4.4 Treatment of Pancreatic Lithiasis

Pancreatic lithiasis is a demanding challenge for the endoscopist. Although there are only preliminary data, pancreatic lithiasis represents another promising therapeutic application of SOC-S. The efficacy of peroral pancreatoscopy with endoscope and that of SOC has been compared in series of 45 patients with main pancreatic duct (MPD) lithiasis [22]. A complete or partial clearance was obtained in 57 % and 100 % of case, respectively, without a difference between the two tools. In three patients (12 %) treated with SpyGlass, minor complications related to pancreatoscopy occurred. In a US multicenter, retrospective study on the efficacy of SOC-S in the treatment of the MPD lithiasis in 28 patients undergoing pancreatoscopy with LL was described [23]. The average size of stones was 15 mm (range: 4–32 mm). The stone removal was successful in 79 % of cases, with a partial clearance in further three (11 %) patients. Moreover, there was a good clinical outcome in 89 % of cases at 1 year follow-up, in terms of pain reduction, use of narcotics, and hospitalization. Recently, the use of SpyGlass-guided EHL was found to be a valid alternative for pancreatic lithiasis treatment in 98 patients following a failure of combined endoscopic lithotomy and extracorporeal shock wave lithotripsy (ESWL) [24].

12.4.5 Assessment of the Indeterminate Strictures of the Bile Duct

The ability to discriminate between benign and malignant biliary strictures is obviously of crucial importance in patient care management. The current radiologic methods (CT, MRI) do not provide adequate sensitive and specific diagnostic performance for all biliary-pancreatic lesions. The cytological sampling by brushing during ERCP or fine-needle aspiration (FNA) during endoscopic ultrasonography showed high specificity but modest sensitivity [25, 26]. Disappointing results were achieved even by using more performing brushes, dilation of stenosis before brushing, or gene analysis of the collected tissue [27]. Several cohort series on the use of

SOC-S in this field showed encouraging results [7]. However, the macroscopic characteristics of malignant biliary lesions are not completely standardized. Some studies on cholangioscopy with endoscope or SOC have defined highly suggestive criteria. They include the presence of dilated and tortuous vessels ("tumor vessel sign" or "capillary signs"), ulceration, nodules, exophytic or papillary excrescences, friability, and irregular surface [9, 28, 29]. On the other hand, mucosal alterations with a smooth surface or finely granular without neovascularization or intraductal masses suggest a benign condition [30]. A 61 % sensitivity and a 100 % specificity, with a 100 % interobserver agreement, for tumor vessel sign were found in a study [31]. On the contrary, another study found a good interobserver agreement with SOC only for tumoral masses, strictures, ulceration, and hyperplasia, stressing the need of validating the cholangioscopic criteria for biliary lesions [32]. When a suspected lesion is encountered, biopsies with SOC-S can be obtained by following two procedures: (1) cholangioscopy-direct biopsy obtained with the dedicated mini-forceps (SpyBite, Boston Scientific) and (2) cholangioscopy-assisted biopsy, which consists in identifying fluoroscopically the stricture area, to withdraw the cholangioscope, and to insert a standard forceps, until the stenosis under fluoroscopic guide [28]. Of note, by using the SpyBite, an adequate quantity of tissue was obtained in more than 95 % of cases [9, 13]. A prospective study involving 26 patients with indeterminate biliary strictures found that sensitivity, specificity, and accuracy of biopsies obtained with SpyBite were significantly higher as compared to either cytology or standard biopsy under fluoroscopic guidance [33]. In our experience, sampling performed with SpyBite was adequate in 97.5 % of 45 patients, with a sensitivity, specificity, and positive and negative predictive values of 93 %, 88 %, 87 %, and 94 %, respectively [34]. Another study found a 92.3 % and 74.4 % technical and clinical success, respectively, on 39 patients with indeterminate biliary strictures, and PPV and NPV as high as 100 % and 95.8 % [15].

A major challenge for the physicians is the early detection of cholangiocarcinoma in patients with primary sclerosing cholangitis (PSC). In a recent prospective observational Finnish study, the performance of the SOC-S with biopsy, brushing, and flow cytometry, in the diagnosis of indeterminate strictures in 11 patients with PSC, was evaluated. In all cases it was possible to obtain the direct biopsy sampling and cytology, with an adequate sampling in 82 % for cytology and 91 % for biopsy [35]. Similarly, the diagnostic yield of biopsies obtained by using the SpyBite was higher as compared to that of cytology in 19 patients with PSC [36].

As expected, the direct visualization with SpyGlass showed a sensitivity of 62 % for the extrinsic bile duct strictures [17], while biopsies achieved a very low (8 %) diagnostic yield [8].

In a prospective study enrolling 36 patients with indeterminate stricture of common bile duct, an adequate histological sampling was achieved in 82 % of cases, despite several hilar stenoses being present in 58 % of cases [8]. By using macroscopic evaluation, a 84 % sensitivity in diagnosing malignant lesions was observed [13].

In our study, concerning the data of our Endoscopic Unit, in Modena-Baggiovara Hospital, the direct visualization of lesions allowed to exclude seven patients with non-organic stenosis, including varices of the common bile duct or piled microcalculi [34].

In a retrospective study of 30 patients with extrahepatic cholangiocarcinoma in whom the diagnosis failed with cytology during ERCP or during EUS with FNA [37], the diagnostic accuracy of macroscopic observation with SOC-S was 77 %. Encouraging results were also reported in a recent retrospective study of 36 patients with indeterminate biliary strictures in whom the sensitivity, specificity, and diagnostic accuracy for malignant lesions using direct visualization with SOC-S and biopsy with SpyBite were 100 % and 64.2 %, 90 % and 100 %, and 96.7 % and 73.6 %, respectively [38].

A multicenter study enrolled 226 patients with indeterminate biliary strictures who underwent ERCP with SOC-S, and 140 received biopsy with SpyBite (adequacy of the sample 88 %, 20 % hilar stenosis). The sensitivity and specificity in detecting malignant stenosis was 51 % and 54 % by using only cholangiographic visualization, 78 % and 82 % for macroscopic visualization with SpyGlass, 49 % and 98 % for direct sampling of lesions with SpyBite [17].

Finally, a recent meta-analysis of eight studies on the SOC-S use for the indeterminate biliary strictures diagnosis showed that a direct visualization achieved a sensitivity of 90 % and a specificity of 87 % for malignant lesions, while the histological diagnosis following SpyBite biopsies achieved 69 % sensitivity and a 98 % specificity [39]. These data would suggest that the best use of SOC-S could be to identify macroscopically a suspicious lesion, by using macroscopic malignancy criteria, and then proceed to targeted biopsies under direct vision (cholangioscopy-direct biopsy) or indirect vision (cholangioscopy-assisted biopsy).

12.4.6 Complications

The studies on SOC-S reported an adverse event rate – especially cholangitis and pancreatitis – oscillating between 5 and 13 % (9, 10, 29, 4). It has been found that the cholangiopancreatoscopy is associated to an overall (7 % vs 2.9 %) increased procedure-related adverse event rate as compared to the simple ERCP [5]. In detail, pancreatitis, perforation, and bleeding (4.2 % vs 2.2 %) and, particularly, post-procedural cholangitis (1.0 % vs 0.2 %) were significantly higher. An overall complication rate of 7.5 %, mainly cholangitis, was also reported in another study. All adverse events resolved without sequelae. This highlights the need to offer aggressive biliary or pancreatic drainage post cholangiopancreatoscopy.

Conclusions

The cholangioscopy single operator using the digital SpyGlass system seems to be a promising and highly advantageous tool for both diagnosis and therapy of different biliary tract diseases. In detail, very interesting results have been obtained for treatment of difficult biliary stones. Moreover, the possibility of characterizing stenosis following a failure of other investigations, both macroscopically and with targeted biopsies, is of paramount importance. Further studies are required on pancreatic diseases. Research and technological development of this method, and its spread in biliopancreatic endoscopy, is expected to improve management of patients with difficult biliary and pancreatic diseases.

References

1. Moon JH, Terheggen G, Choi HJ, Neuhaus H. Peroral cholangioscopy: diagnostic and therapeutic applications. Gastroenterology. 2013;144:276–82.
2. Overhiser AJ, Sharma P. Advances in endoscopic imaging: narrow band imaging. Rev Gastroenterol Disord. 2008;8:186–93.
3. Terheggen G, Neuhaus H. New options of cholangioscopy. Gastroenterol Clin North Am. 2010;39:827–44.
4. Moon JH, Choi HJ. The role of direct peroral cholangioscopy using an ultraslim endoscope for biliary lesions: indications, limitations, and complications. Clin Endosc. 2013;46:537–9.
5. Sethi A, Chen YK, Austin GL, et al. ERCP with cholangiopancreatoscopy may be associated with higher rates of complications than ERCP alone: a single-center experience. Gastrointest Endosc. 2011;73:251–6.
6. Parsi MA. Peroral cholangioscopy in the new millennium. World J Gastroenterol. 2011;17:1–6.
7. Chen YK. Preclinical characterization of the Spyglass peroral cholangiopancreatoscopy system for direct access, visualization, and biopsy. Gastrointest Endosc. 2007;65:303–11.
8. Ramchandani M, et al. Role of single-operator peroral cholangioscopy in the diagnosis of indeterminate biliary lesions: a single-center, prospective study. Gastrointest Endosc. 2011;74:511–9.
9. Chen YK, Pleskow DK. SpyGlass single-operator peroral cholangiopancreatoscopy system for the diagnosis and therapy of bile-duct disorders: a clinical feasibility study (with video). Gastrointest Endosc. 2007;65:832–41.
10. Sievert CE, Silvis SE. Evaluation of electrohydraulic lithotripsy as a means of gallstone fragmentation in a canine model. Gastrointest Endosc. 1987;33:233–5.
11. Shah RJ, Chen YK. Techniques of peroral and percutaneous choledochoscopy for evaluation and treatment of biliary stones and strictures. Tech Gastrointest Endosc. 2007;9:161–8.
12. Hochberger J, et al. Lithotripsy of gallstones by means of a quality-switched giant-pulse neodymium:yttrium-aluminum-garnet laser. Basic in vitro studies using a highly flexible fiber system. Gastroenterology. 1991;101:1391–8.
13. Draganov PV, et al. Prospective evaluation of the clinical utility of ERCP-guided cholangiopancreatoscopy with a new direct visualization system. Gastrointest Endosc. 2011;73:971–9.
14. Maydeo A, Kwek BEA, Bhandari S, Bapat M, Dhir V. Single-operator cholangioscopy-guided laser lithotripsy in patients with difficult biliary and pancreatic ductal stones (with videos). Gastrointest Endosc. 2011;74:1308–14.
15. Tieu AH, et al. Diagnostic and therapeutic utility of SpyGlass(®) peroral cholangioscopy in intraductal biliary disease: single-center, retrospective, cohort study. Dig Endosc. 2015;27:479–85.
16. Sepe PS, et al. Single-operator cholangioscopy for the extraction of cystic duct stones (with video). Gastrointest Endosc. 2012;75:206–10.
17. Chen YK, et al. Single-operator cholangioscopy in patients requiring evaluation of bile duct disease or therapy of biliary stones (with videos). Gastrointest Endosc. 2011;74:805–14.
18. Baron TH, Saleem A. Intraductal electrohydraulic lithotripsy by using SpyGlass cholangioscopy through a colonoscope in a patient with Roux-en-Y hepaticojejunostomy. Gastrointest Endosc. 2010;71:650–1.
19. Uradomo L, Pandolfe F, Aragon G, Borum ML. SpyGlass cholangioscopy for management of choledocholithiasis during pregnancy. Hepatobiliary Pancreat Dis Int. 2011;10:107.
20. Fishman DS, Tarnasky PR, Patel SN, Raijman I. Management of pancreaticobiliary disease using a new intra-ductal endoscope: the Texas experience. World J Gastroenterol. 2009;15:1353–8.
21. Awadallah NS, Chen YK, Piraka C, Antillon MR, Shah RJ. Is there a role for cholangioscopy in patients with primary sclerosing cholangitis? Am J Gastroenterol. 2006;101:284–91.
22. Attwell AR, et al. 296 ERCP with per oral pancreatoscopy for calcific chronic pancreatitis using endoscope and catheter-based pancreatoscopes: a 10-year single center experience. Gastrointest Endosc. 2011;73:AB121–2.

23. Attwell AR, et al. ERCP with per-oral pancreatoscopy-guided laser lithotripsy for calcific chronic pancreatitis: a multicenter U.S. experience. Gastrointest Endosc. 2015;82:311–8.
24. Ito K, et al. Efficacy of combined endoscopic lithotomy and extracorporeal shock wave lithotripsy, and additional electrohydraulic lithotripsy using the SpyGlass direct visualization system or X-ray guided EHL as needed, for pancreatic lithiasis. Biomed Res Int. 2014;2014:732781.
25. Mansfield JC, Griffin SM, Wadehra V, Matthewson K. A prospective evaluation of cytology from biliary strictures. Gut. 1997;40:671–7.
26. Moreno Luna LE, et al. Advanced cytologic techniques for the detection of malignant pancreatobiliary strictures. Gastroenterology. 2006;131:1064–72.
27. Ornellas LC, Santos Gda C, Nakao FS, Ferrari AP. Comparison between endoscopic brush cytology performed before and after biliary stricture dilation for cancer detection. Arq Gastroenterol. 2006;43:20–3.
28. Shah RJ, Langer DA, Antillon MR, Chen YK. Cholangioscopy and cholangioscopic forceps biopsy in patients with indeterminate pancreaticobiliary pathology. Clin Gastroenterol Hepatol. 2006;4:219–25.
29. Fukuda Y, Tsuyuguchi T, Sakai Y, Tsuchiya S, Saisyo H. Diagnostic utility of peroral cholangioscopy for various bile-duct lesions. Gastrointest Endosc. 2005;62:374–82.
30. Shim CS, Neuhaus H, Tamada K. Direct cholangioscopy. Endoscopy. 2003;35:752–8.
31. Kim HJ, et al. Tumor vessel: a valuable cholangioscopic clue of malignant biliary stricture. Gastrointest Endosc. 2000;52:635–8.
32. Sethi A, et al. Interobserver agreement for evaluation of imaging with single operator choledochoscopy: what are we looking at? Dig Liver Dis. 2014;46:518–22.
33. Draganov PV, et al. Diagnostic accuracy of conventional and cholangioscopy-guided sampling of indeterminate biliary lesions at the time of ERCP: a prospective, long-term follow-up study. Gastrointest Endosc. 2012;75:347–53.
34. Manta R, et al. SpyGlass single-operator peroral cholangioscopy in the evaluation of indeterminate biliary lesions: a single-center, prospective, cohort study. Surg Endosc. 2013;27:1569–72.
35. Siiki A, et al. Spyglass single-operator peroral cholangioscopy seems promising in the evaluation of primary sclerosing cholangitis-related biliary strictures. Scand J Gastroenterol. 2014;49:1385–90.
36. Rey JW, et al. Efficacy of SpyGlass(TM)-directed biopsy compared to brush cytology in obtaining adequate tissue for diagnosis in patients with biliary strictures. World J Gastrointest Endosc. 2014;6:137–43.
37. Siddiqui AA, et al. Identification of cholangiocarcinoma by using the Spyglass Spyscope system for peroral cholangioscopy and biopsy collection. Clin Gastroenterol Hepatol. 2012;10:466–71; quiz e48.
38. Woo YS, et al. Role of SpyGlass peroral cholangioscopy in the evaluation of indeterminate biliary lesions. Dig Dis Sci. 2014;59:2565–70.
39. Sun X, et al. Is single-operator peroral cholangioscopy a useful tool for the diagnosis of indeterminate biliary lesion? A systematic review and meta-analysis. Gastrointest Endosc. 2015;82:79–87.

Esophageal Motility Testing: The Present and the Future

13

Nicola de Bortoli, Marzio Frazzoni, and Edoardo V. Savarino

13.1 Introduction

The primary functions of the esophagus are to transport swallowed materials from the pharynx to the stomach and to prevent the reflux of injurious gastric contents into the esophagus and airways [1]. The motor activities that allow the esophagus to accomplish these tasks are governed by complex neuromuscular interactions in three physiologically distinct neuromuscular units: the upper esophageal sphincter (UES), the body of the esophagus, and the lower esophageal sphincter (LES) [2]. Manometric techniques measure the amplitudes and timing of the pressure changes that, in general, reflect the force and timing of the circular muscle contraction or relaxation [3, 4].

Motor function can be assessed by a variety of recording techniques including radiology, scintigraphy manometry, and most recently intraluminal electrical impedance monitoring. Some of these are complementary. The gold standard, however, for the assessment of motor disorders remains manometry. Manometric measurement of esophageal pressure is the most direct method for the assessment of motor function [5]. Since its introduction in the early 1950s, esophageal manometry has contributed to a better understanding of esophageal motor function and has currently become a widely performed technique in clinical practice [6]. The first manometry systems used a catheter that contained water-perfused channels, which

N. de Bortoli
Division of Gastroenterology, Department of Translational Research and New Technology in Medicine and Surgery, University of Pisa, Pisa, Italy

M. Frazzoni
Digestive Pathophysiology Unit, Baggiovara Hospital, Modena, Italy

E.V. Savarino, MD (✉)
Division of Gastroenterology, Department of Surgery, Oncology and Gastroenterology, University of Padua, Via Giustiniani 2, 35128 Padova, Italy
e-mail: edoardo.savarino@unipd.it

R. Conigliaro, M. Frazzoni (eds.), *Diagnosis and Endoscopic Management of Digestive Diseases*, DOI 10.1007/978-3-319-42358-6_13

opened to the lumen at several points along the catheter. These water-perfused pressure channels were driven by a pneumatic pump and connected to external pressure sensors [6]. Water-perfused manometry catheters were hindered by large intervals between the pressure sensors, which could result in an inadequate assessment of sphincter pressure and peristaltic abnormalities. This shortcoming was partly overcome by adding a sleeve sensor, which measured the highest pressure exerted along a segment of several centimeters [7]. This allowed for a reliable measurement of the esophagogastric junction (EGJ), even though the EGJ moves up and down the catheter during inspiration or during swallowing. However, the esophageal pressure was still measured with a low level of detail, and the addition of more pressure channels was limited by the need of a larger diameter of the catheter and a significant amount of water being administered to a patient during the measurement. Furthermore, the response rate of water-perfused manometry is relatively low which results in difficulties when measuring rapidly changing pressures. Smaller caliber capillaries have partly overcome these shortcomings, making it now possible to create catheters with much more pressure sensors [7].

In the last 10 years, a new system to perform esophageal manometry was developed and introduced in both research and clinical setting: the high-resolution manometry. High-resolution manometry (HRM) is the current gold standard technique to assess esophageal motility. It utilizes closely spaced pressure sensors to create a dynamic representation of pressure change along the entire length of the esophagus. Data acquisition is easier than with conventional manometry, and interpretation is facilitated by esophageal pressure topography (Clouse) plots [8]. Along with the technological innovation, an international consensus process has evolved over recent years to define esophageal motility disorders using HRM, Clouse plots, and standardized metrics. This classification, titled the Chicago Classification (CC), was firstly published in 2009 [9] and updated in 2012 [10]. In recognition of many studies performed in the last years, the international HRM Working Group met in Chicago in May 2014 in conjunction with Digestive Disease Week to discuss new data in the context of working toward an update of the CC (v3.0) that was published in the first months of 2015 [11].

13.2 Where Esophageal Pressure Topography Come From?

In the 1990s, Ray Clouse and his colleagues gave birth to high-definition manometry (or high-resolution manometry) when they decreased the spacing between pressure sensing sites along the manometry catheter from 3 to 5 cm to 1 cm. Thus, they were able to increase the number of pressure sensors and to lengthen the sensing segment of the catheter so it spanned from the pharynx to the stomach. At last, it was possible to simultaneously see motor function of the upper esophageal sphincter (UES), esophagus, and lower esophageal sphincter (LES) with each swallow, giving us a complete spatial and temporal depiction of esophageal motor function for the first time [12, 13]. The true genius of his method was to convert the pressure data into a topographical plot. The convention at the time was to display manometry recordings in a two-dimensional (2-D) space with pressure waves stacked sequentially from caudal to cephalad in the y-axis. The authors added a z-axis and stacked the pressure waves sequentially in the z-axis with gastric pressures to the front and pharyngeal pressures in the back. Amplitude was therefore on the y-axis and time on the x-axis. They developed an interpolation technique that filled in pressure data between pressure waves to give a 3-D pressure contour. They then assigned colors to pressures, with high pressures represented by warmer colors (reds and yellows) and low pressures by cold colors (blues and greens). Finally, they collapsed the color contour back into a 2-D space with time on the x-axis, position relative to the nares on the y-axis, and pressure depicted as color. This is a color topographical map of esophageal pressure that has been called the Clouse plot or esophageal pressure topography (EPT). In concept, it is like topographical maps of weather radar images that assign color to atmospheric pressure. Once one is comfortable with what the EPT means, it is apparent that many motor disturbances are recognizable as distinct patterns. These tools, as will be seen later, have changed how we categorize and define esophageal motor disorders in the new millennium [12, 13].

13.3 The Present

13.3.1 Metrics and Swallow Pattern Characterization

The primary objective of the CC is to apply standardized HRM metrics to categorize esophageal motility disorders in patients with nonobstructive dysphagia and/or esophageal chest pain. The CC is based on the scoring of ten 5-ml water swallows performed in supine position. Esophagogastric junction (EGJ) relaxation, esophageal contractile activity, and esophageal pressurization are evaluated for each swallow [11].

The terms necessary to better understand the Chicago Classification are detailed in Table 13.1. Each metric has been developed to characterize a specific feature of

Table 13.1 Esophageal pressure topography metrics utilized in the Chicago Classification

Pressure topography metrics	
Metric	Description
Integrated relaxation pressure (IRP, mmHg)	Mean EGJ pressure measured with an electronic equivalent of a sleeve sensor for four contiguous or non-contiguous seconds of relaxation in the 10-s window following deglutitive UES relaxation
Distal contractile integral (DCI, mmHg-s-cm)	Amplitude × duration × length (mmHg-s-cm) of the distal esophagus contraction > 20 mmHg from proximal to distal pressure troughs
Contractile deceleration point (CDP)	Inflection point along the 30-mmHg isobaric contour where propagation velocity slows demarcating the tubular esophagus from the frenic ampulla
Distal latency (DL, s)	Interval between UES relaxation and CDP

Legend: *EGJ* esophagogastric junction, *UES* upper esophageal sphincter deglutitive esophageal function for individual test swallows. The conceptual framework for developing these metrics (and the classification in general) was that it be based on physiological principles and that identified dysfunction is prioritized in a hierarchical fashion: (i) achalasia/EGJ dysfunction, (ii) motility patterns never observed in normal subjects, and (iii) peristaltic abnormalities out of the range of normal values [11].

13.3.2 Esophagogastric Junction

During HRM analysis, EGJ pressure is dynamically monitored during normal respiration with defined axial resolution (usually 1 cm) and without artifacts attributable to swallow-induced sphincter movement [14] or to EGJ conformational changes that may spontaneously occur [15]. However, even within the domain of EPT, there are still a number of variables regarding the methodology for assessing EGJ relaxation, morphology, and competence (barrier function). Progress in the understanding of the optimal methodology for assessing the EGJ among these functional domains has been considerable with the widespread adoption of HRM into clinical practice.

With HRM and Clouse plots, the relative localization of the two constituents of the EGJ, the lower esophageal sphincter (LES) and the crural diaphragm (CD), defines EGJ morphologic subtypes [16]. The EGJ morphology was simply classified in three types: *type I EGJ morphology*, in which there is complete overlap of the CD and LES with no spatial separation evident on the Clouse plot and no double peak on the associated spatial pressure variation plot; *type II EGJ morphology*, in which the LES and CD are separated (double-peaked spatial pressure variation plot), but the nadir pressure between the two peaks does not decline to the gastric pressure; *type III EGJ morphology*, in which the LES and CD are clearly separated as evidenced by a double-peaked spatial pressure variation plot and the nadir pressure between the peaks equal to or less than the gastric pressure; with type IIIa the pressure inversion point remains at the CD level, while in type IIIb, it is located at the LES level [11]. Recently Tolone and coworkers [17] evaluated, by means of HRM and impedance with pH monitoring, 130 consecutive patients and identified 46.2 % type I EGJ, 38.5 % type II, and 15.4 % type III patients. Patients with type III EGJ had a higher number of reflux episodes (61 versus 45, $p<0.03$, versus 25, $p<0.001$), a greater mean AET (12.4 versus 4.2, $p<0.02$, *versus* 1.5, $p<0.001$), and a greater positive symptom association (75 % versus 72 %, $p=0.732$ versus 43.3 %, $p<0.02$) compared to patients with types II and I, respectively. They concluded that increasing separation between LES and CD could cause a gradual and significant increase in reflux. Thus, they demonstrated that EGJ morphology assessment may be useful to predict an abnormal impedance-pH testing in gastroesophageal reflux disease (GERD) patients [17]. Similarly, the same group [18] evaluated the vigor of EGJ and its relationship with GERD by adopting a new HRM metric, namely, the contractile integral (CI). The EGJ-CI was calculated using the distal contractile integral toolbox during three consecutive respiratory cycles. They observed that patients with a defective EGJ-CI had more frequently a positive impedance-pH monitoring or esophageal mucosal breaks at endoscopy ($p < 0.05$) than patients with a normal EGJ-CI and concluded that a defective EGJ-CI at HRM is associated with evidence of GERD at reflux monitoring or endoscopy [18]. These data reinforced the need of performing HRM to better understand the mechanisms of GERD and suggested a potential diagnostic application of HRM for GERD diagnosis, at least as complementary test, and not only for positioning the pH electrode before reflux monitoring or for excluding achalasia in case of gastroesophageal surgery, in particular anti-reflux surgery.

During swallowing, EGJ relaxation is evaluated using the integrated relaxation pressure (IRP). This has been and will continue to be defined as the mean of the 4 s (contiguous or non-contiguous) of maximal deglutitive relaxation in the 10-s window beginning at deglutitive UES relaxation. The IRP is referenced to gastric pressure. The IRP represents a realistic alternative to the "nadir LES residual pressure" obtained during a standard manometry. Lin et al. [19] evaluated in a large group of patients the difference between single-sensor-detected EGJ relaxation and IRP to diagnose achalasia. They observed that the single-sensor method of assessing EGJ relaxation had a sensitivity of only 52 % for diagnosing achalasia. The 4-s IRP using a cutoff of 15 mmHg performed optimally with 98 % sensitivity and 96 % specificity in the detection of achalasia. This is important because failing to detect impaired EGJ relaxation in these patients would result in giving them a wrong diagnosis.

13.3.3 Disorders with EGJ Outflow Obstruction

The most fundamental assessment of deglutitive contractility in the Chicago Classification is of whether or not an EGJ outflow obstruction is present as defined by an IRP > 15 mmHg. Disorders of the EGJ outflow are subdivided into achalasia subtypes and EGJ outflow obstruction based on the contractile and pressurization patterns in the body of the esophagus. Three clinically relevant subtypes of achalasia have been defined in the different versions of the Chicago Classification [9–11]: type I achalasia was characterized by 100 % failed contractions and no esophageal pressurization; type II achalasia was defined as 100 % failed contraction and panesophageal pressurization for at least 20 % of swallows; and type III achalasia was defined as the presence of preserved fragments of distal peristalsis or premature contractions for at least 20 % of the swallows [10, 11]. Some studies showed that the adoption of the Chicago Classification can improve our capability to diagnose and treat patients with achalasia. However, recent data highlighted that the use of a specific rigid cutoff (15 mmHg) to define normal from abnormal should be considered with caution. Indeed, the last iteration of the CC (v3.0) suggested assessment of EGJ relaxation by means of the median instead than by the mean value of IRP with ten swallows in order to minimize the effect of occasional outliers. Moreover, Lin et al. [19] recently showed that the critical IRP threshold may vary among achalasia subtypes and might range between 10 and 17 mmHg, specifically in type I achalasia, suggesting that IRP threshold might be reduced [19]. Similarly, Salvador and coworkers [20] observed that in a larger group of 139 patients with endoscopic, radiological, and manometric characteristics of achalasia, 10.9% of the cases had an IRP value lower than 15 mmHg. To note, the authors showed that all patients had a positive outcome after laparoscopic Heller myotomy. Therefore, they suggested that some patients might also be correctly classified as a different type of achalasia deriving on clinical, radiological, and manometric pattern even if they had a borderline IRP [20]. Finally, another important consideration is that the cutoff for the upper limit of normal is technology specific ranging from a low value of 15 mmHg for the Sierra design transducers to as high as 28 mmHg for the Unisensor design. Thus, the diagnostic accuracy for detecting EGJ outflow obstruction for each device varies and further emphasizes the need of caution when applying a rigid cutoff value.

A different condition characterized by an impaired EGJ relaxation is defined EGJ outflow obstruction (EGJ-OO). The EGJ-OO exhibits not only an IRP greater than 15 mmHg but also a preserved peristalsis and elevated intrabolus pressure above the EGJ during peristalsis [21]. The finding of an elevated intrabolus pressure proximal to the sphincter is important because it validates the physiological significance of impaired EGJ relaxation. From a physiological perspective, elevated intrabolus pressure is the consequence of the impaired relaxation. A recent work suggested that when EGJ outflow obstruction occurs as a consequence of incomplete relaxation, it is accompanied by a relative increase in the ratio of peristaltic amplitude in the distal part of the esophagus, whereas this is not the case with mechanical obstruction [22]. With the term EGJ-OO, the CC includes a heterogeneous group of patients with some individuals having an incomplete phenotype of achalasia or an undetected mechanical cause of EGJ-OO such as hiatus hernia, esophageal stenosis, or eosinophilic esophagitis. Consequently, it is a patient group that merits further evaluation with mucosal biopsies and imaging studies to exclude inflammatory or malignant etiologies, be that with computerized tomography or endoscopic ultrasound. Only after these possibilities have been fully explored should it be accepted as atypical achalasia [23]. On this topic, van Hoeij et al. [24] evaluated 34 patients with primary EGJ-OO. They concluded that EGJ-OO is an unclear motility disorder with poor clinical significance. Indeed, the authors observed that 10% of patients had unrelated symptoms and 15% had spontaneous symptom relief. Moreover, one hundred percent of patients showed no stasis during esophageal radiogram, whereas treated patients showed a beneficial response to botox injections. Finally, less than 10% of patients developed achalasia during follow-up [24].

13.3.4 EPT Metrics to Score Individual Swallows

The main HRM deglutitive peristaltic metrics used to evaluate esophageal contractile function are the distal contractile integral (DCI) and the distal latency (DL) (Fig. 13.1, Table 13.1) [10, 11]. They are used to characterize each of the ten 5-ml test swallows in order to obtain the final diagnosis. In particular, the DL physiologically represents an indirect measurement of deglutitive inhibition and thus of normal peristalsis. The DL is measured as the interval from UES relaxation to the

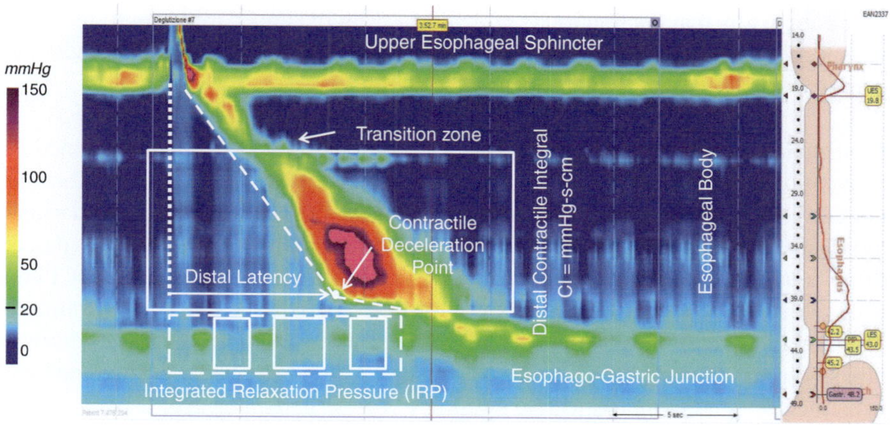

Fig. 13.1 High-resolution manometry tracing showing an example of a peristaltic wave. In the picture are well-represented both upper and lower esophageal sphincters and the swallowing-induced lower esophageal sphincter relaxation

Table 13.2 Characterization of esophageal contractility

Contraction vigor (20-mmHg isobaric contour)	
Failed	DCI <100 mmHg-s-cm
Weak	DCI >100 mmHg-s-cm but <450 mmHg-s-cm
Ineffective	Failed or weak
Normal	DCI >450 mmHg-s-cm but <8000 mmHg-s-cm
Hypercontractile	DCI >8000 mmHg-s-cm
Contraction pattern	
Premature	DL <4.5 s
Fragmented	Large break (>5 cm length) in the 20-mmHg isobaric contour with DCI >450 mmHg-s-cm
Intact	Not achieving the above diagnostic criteria
Intrabolus pressure pattern (30-mmHg isobaric contour)	
Panesophageal pressurization	Uniform pressurization of >30 mmHg extending from UES to EGJ
Compartmentalized esophageal pressurization	Pressurization of >30 mmHg extending from the contractile front to EGJ
EGJ pressurization	Pressurization restricted to the zone between the LES and CD in conjunction with the LES-CD separation
Normal	No bolus pressurization >30 mmHg

Legend: *DCI* distal contractile integral (mmHg-s-cm), *DL* distal latency (s), *EGJ* esophagogastric junction, *LES* lower esophageal sphincter, *CD* crural diaphragm

contractile deceleration point (CDP) [10, 11]; a value less than 4.5 s defines a premature contraction. The contractile vigor is measured by using the DCI. This metric applies an algorithm to quantify the contractile pressure exceeding 20 mmHg for the region spanning from the transition zone to the EGJ [10, 11]. As described in Table 13.2, the integrity of the contraction associated with each swallow describes how completely that contraction is propagated from the upper sphincter to the EGJ, irrespective of the vigor of the contraction or latency. These qualifiers fall under the contraction pattern that is subsequently characterized.

Contraction Vigor Although an ineffective contraction was originally defined in conventional manometry on the basis of low-amplitude peristalsis, this criterion was not used to define weak peristalsis in the v2.0 of the CC [10]. The CC v3.0 clarified the distinction between contractile vigor and pattern and opted to clearly separate these concepts, basing the evaluation of contractile vigor entirely on the DCI and using a cutoff value of 100 mmHg-s-cm for failed peristalsis and a cutoff value of 450 mmHg-s-cm for weak peristalsis. The value for the weak peristalsis was derived directly from the study of Xiao and coworkers [25] that showed a positive percent agreement in predicting ineffective swallows of 83 % and a negative percent agreement of 90 % in a validation sample of 100 patients. Both failed and weak peristaltic contractions are ineffective. At the other extreme of contractile vigor, it was accepted to keep the cutoff for hypercontractility at 8000 mmHg-s-cm, but to eliminate the "hypertensive" designation for contractions with DCI between 5000 [10] and 8000 mmHg-s-cm, because it has no apparent clinical significance [11].

Contraction Pattern Hence, the CDP (the inflection point in the contractile front propagation velocity in the distal esophagus) is a key landmark in the assessment of the contraction pattern. However, in some instances like atypical peristaltic architecture or compartmentalized pressurization, the CDP can be difficult to localize, and so far the HRM Working Group decided to add two caveats for localizing the CDP in the last version of CC: (i) the CDP must be localized to within 3 cm of the LES, and (ii) in instances of compartmentalized pressurization, the CDP needs to be localized along an isobaric contour line of greater magnitude than the compartmentalized intrabolus pressure. Moreover, the HRM Working Group defined that breaks in the 20-mmHg isobaric contour should be considered into the chapter of "contraction pattern." Kumar et al. [26] observed that small breaks (<3 cm) in the 20-mmHg isobaric contour are frequently encountered in normal subjects, and therefore the HRM Working Group suggested that these should be considered normal [11]. On the other hand, Roman et al. [27] showed that large breaks (>5 cm) in the 20-mmHg isobaric contour were significantly more common in patients with dysphagia than in controls (14 % versus 4 %, $p=0.02$), and this concept was considered in the CC v3.0. Finally, in a recent study, Porter et al. [28] adopted the term "fragmented" to characterize those contractions with a large break in the 20-mmHg isobaric contour, but normal or elevated DCI (>450 mmHg-s-cm).

13.3.5 Major Motility Disorders

Major motility disorders are defined as patterns of motor function that are not encountered in controls in the context of normal EGJ relaxation. The hierarchical Chicago Classification v3.0 is reported in Table 13.3 [11].

Table 13.3 The Chicago Classification v3.0

Achalasia and EGJ outflow obstruction	Criteria
Type I achalasia (classic achalasia)	Elevated median IRP (>15 mmHg[a]), 100 % failed peristalsis (DCI < 100 mmHg-s-cm) *Premature contractions with DCI values less than 450 mmHg-s-cm satisfy criteria for failed peristalsis*
Type II achalasia (with esophageal compression)	Elevated median IRP (>15 mmHg[a]), 100 % failed peristalsis, panesophageal pressurization with ≥20 % of swallows *Contractions may be masked by esophageal pressurization, and DCI should not be calculated*
Type III achalasia (spastic achalasia)	Elevated median IRP (>15 mmHg[a]), no normal peristalsis, premature (spastic) contractions with DCI >450 mmHg-s-cm with ≥20 % of swallows *May be mixed with panesophageal pressurization*
EGJ outflow obstruction	Elevated median IRP (>15 mmHg[a]), sufficient evidence of peristalsis such that criteria for types I–III achalasia are not met[b]
Major disorders of peristalsis (not encountered in normal subjects)	
Aperistalsis (absent contractility)	Normal median IRP, 100 % failed peristalsis *Achalasia should be considered when IRP values are borderline and when there is evidence of esophageal pressurization* *Premature contractions with DCI values less than 450 mmHg-s-cm meet criteria for failed peristalsis*
Distal esophageal spasm (DES)	Normal median IRP, ≥20 % premature contractions with DCI >450 mmHg-s-cm[a]. Some normal peristalsis may be present
Hypercontractile esophagus (jackhammer)	At least two swallows with DCI >8000 mmHg-s-cm[a, c] *Hypercontractility may involve, or even be localized to, the LES*
Minor disorders of peristalsis (characterized by contractile vigor and contraction pattern)	
Ineffective esophageal motility (IEM)	≥50 % ineffective swallows *Ineffective swallows can be failed or weak (DCI < 450 mmHg-s-cm)* *Multiple repetitive swallow assessment may be helpful in determining peristaltic reserve*
Fragmented peristalsis	≥50 % fragmented contractions with DCI > 450 mmHg-s-cm
Normal esophageal motility	Not fulfilling any of the above classifications

Modified from Kahrilas et al. [11]

[a]Cutoff value dependent on the manometric hardware; this is the cutoff for the Sierra device

[b]Potential etiologies: early achalasia, mechanical obstruction, esophageal wall stiffness, or manifestation of hiatal hernia

[c]Hypercontractile esophagus can be a manifestation of outflow obstruction as evident by instances in which it occurs in association with an IRP greater than the upper limit of normal

Aperistalsis It (absent peristalsis) is defined by the combination of a normal IRP and 100 % failed contractions [11]. As mentioned previously, the contractions with DCI <100 mmHg-s-cm meet the criteria for failed peristalsis, but type I achalasia should be considered in cases of borderline IRP [19].

Distal Esophageal Spasm (DES) It should be considered when 20 % or more esophageal contractions resulted premature with a DL value lower than 4.5 s [29] in a context of normal EGJ relaxation [11].

Hypercontractile Disorders The definition of hypercontractile esophagus (jackhammer esophagus, Fig. 13.2) is, in the last version of CC, identified as the only one hypercontractile disorder of the esophageal contraction [11]. The jackhammer esophagus (the nickname is quietly explicative) was previously defined as the occurrence of at least one swallow with DCI >8000 mmHg-s-cm in the CC v2.0 [30]. However, more recently, the HRM Working Group observed that an 8000-mmHg-s-cm DCI might occur in control subjects, and the previously indicated threshold of one swallow was insufficient and of uncertain relevance. Thus, the Working Group proposed to define jackhammer esophagus as the occurrence of >20 % of swallows with a DCI >8000 mmHg-s-cm and normal latency. Further, the authors of CC v3.0 clarified that the hypercontractility can involve the LES or even might be restricted to the LES. In keeping, the authors suggested that it is necessary to expand the DCI measurement including the EGJ in such instances [11].

13.3.6 Minor Motility Disorders

The clinical significance of minor motility disorders continues to be debated. The prior classification for "peristaltic abnormalities" encountered significant dissatisfaction in the clinical community because of its complexity and unclear relevance. In the place of "peristaltic abnormalities" [10], the new version of CC v3.0 adopted the terminologies "ineffective esophageal motility," popularized in conventional manometric diagnoses, and "fragmented peristalsis" [11].

Ineffective Esophageal Motility (IEM) In 2008, Blonski et al. [31], by means of conventional manometry, defined ineffective esophageal motility (IEM) on the

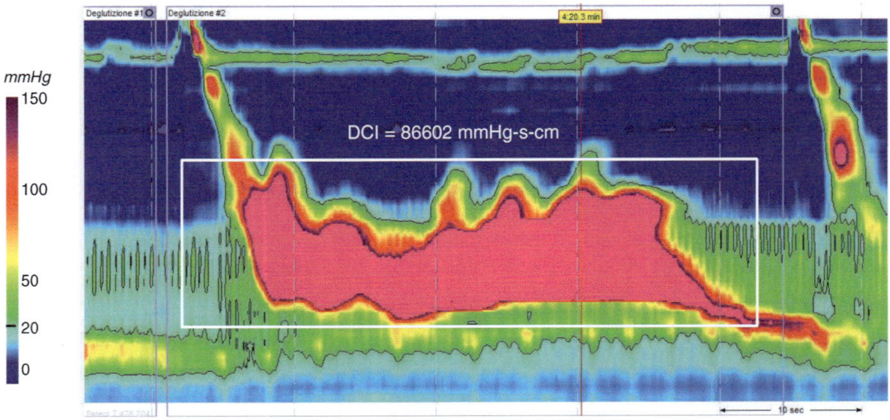

Fig. 13.2 High-resolution manometry tracing showing an example of jackhammer esophagus

basis of 50 % or more ineffective esophageal swallows which were in turn defined as esophageal contractions exhibiting amplitudes <30 mmHg at pressure sensors positioned 3 or 8 cm above the LES. The unifying feature of swallows contributing to the diagnosis of IEM is poor bolus transit in the distal esophagus. Thus, the Working Group proposed to define IEM as ≥50 % ineffective swallows based on a DCI <450 mmHg-s-cm, in accordance with Xiao and coworkers' results [25]. No distinction need to be made between failed swallows and weak swallows, thereby eliminating the former designation of "frequent failed peristalsis."

Fragmented Persistalsis The Working Group proposed to define "fragmented peristalsis" as ≥50 % fragmented contractions (large breaks >5 cm in the 20-mmHg isobaric contour) with the added stipulation of not meeting IEM criteria. Large breaks are significantly more common in patients with dysphagia than in controls (14 versus 4 %, $p=0.02$) [27]. It has been shown that the proportion of failed or fragmented contractions was greater in patients with GERD than in controls [28, 31]. The new definitions of the minor disorders of peristalsis are detailed in Table 13.3 [11].

13.4 The Future

13.4.1 The Near Future: Multiple Rapid Swallows

The recent introduction in clinical and research practice of HRM and impedance-manometry has represented a major advance in defining and characterizing esophageal motor abnormalities in GERD patients [32–34]. Several studies have shown that esophageal dysmotility prevalence parallels the increasing severity of GERD presentation [35–37], and, of particular relevance, those patients had failed and hypotensive peristaltic contractions, which resulted in incomplete esophageal emptying [36, 38]. Moreover, intermittent and nonspecific alterations of esophageal motility are frequently encountered in patients with GERD. However, the true impact and frequency of these abnormalities are not clear, even because standard manometric protocols based on single wet swallows are affected by intrinsic limitations, considering that active esophageal contractions may not be necessary to allow liquid transport, especially if it happens in the upright-seated position [39]. On that ground, recent studies highlighted the importance of including provocative tests, aimed at increasing esophageal workload, during HRM studies, in order to enhance the description and interpretation of esophageal motility [40, 41].

Multiple rapid swallows (MRS) that consist in the administration of five swallows (1–2 ml per swallow) in rapid sequence (less than 10 s) represent the simplest provocative maneuver. Indeed, when multiple swallows are rapidly administered, esophageal peristalsis is deeply inhibited, and pronounced LES relaxation ensues. After the last swallow of the series, a robust esophageal contraction is expected [42]. Abnormal responses consist of incomplete inhibition (when contraction fragments are seen during the period of expected inhibition) or suboptimal contraction (when the post-MRS sequence fails to demonstrate augmentation of smooth muscle contraction) [42, 43]. In particular, Shaker et al. [44] showed that the strength of smooth muscle contraction augments almost twofold with MRS in normal controls and that lack of strong contraction is significantly more prevalent in GERD patients who develop postoperative dysphagia [43, 44]. Therefore, this alteration is considered to represent an inadequate peristaltic reserve of the esophageal smooth muscle [43]. To date, Martinucci and coworkers showed an inverse correlation between MRS response and acid exposure time in patients with negative endoscopy heartburn [45]. Considering these data, MRS has been proposed to be included in routine HRM studies. Indeed, it is simple, cheap, and easy to perform, and, above all, assessing the response to such a provocative test may increase the ability of HRM studies to detect clinically relevant esophageal dysfunction in patients with minor defects of peristalsis or with dysphagia without any finding of achalasia or EGJ-OO. This "low-volume challenge test" should be also suggested in patients with GERD-related symptoms to better define which patients will develop impairment of esophageal clearance. Finally, swallow challenges during the HRM study such as free drinking or a test meal, to trigger motility abnormalities, may improve the diagnostic yield of the study.

13.4.2 Future Role of the HRM Working Group

The real goal of the HRM Working Group is to update the classification every 3 years according to the main literature research projects. This is required to maintain a classification that takes into account relevant new developments in the esophageal motility pathophysiology. The future aim of the HRM Working Group will be to consider pharyngeal and UES functions that are still not included in the CC v3.0. Recent studies suggest the utility of combined impedance-HRM, but not HRM by itself, in detecting the main mechanism involved in GERD pathogenesis, which is the transient lower esophageal sphincter relaxation (Fig. 13.3), and in predicting the risk of aspiration in patients with oropharyngeal swallowing disorders [46–48]. Impedance measurement might also complement the analysis of esophageal function in patients without significant pressure abnormalities to evaluate the impact of esophageal body motility on bolus flow [49, 50] and might also be incorporated into future versions of the CC. Prospective trials taking into account provocative tests such as MRS, applesauce, and solid meal are needed to better recognize borderline diagnostic conditions. Finally, outcome studies about medical and surgical treatment of esophagogastric junction (both in GERD and in achalasia) are necessary.

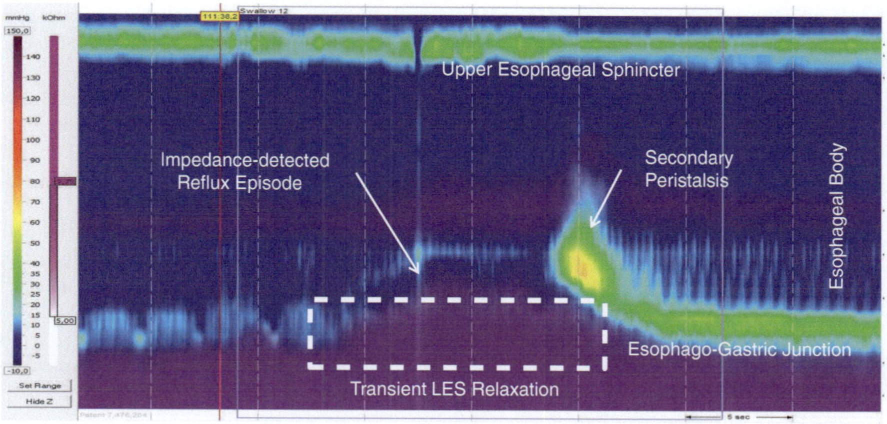

Fig. 13.3 High-resolution impedance-manometry tracing showing an example of a transient lower esophageal sphincter relaxation accompanied by an impedance-detected reflux episode

References

1. Crane RK, editor. Gastrointestinal physiology II. Baltimore: University Park Press; 1977.
2. Miller AJ. The neuroscientific principles of swallowing and dysphagia. San Diego: Singular Pub. Group; 1999.
3. Code CF. An Atlas of esophageal motility in health and disease. Springfield: Thomas; 1958.
4. Fransen G, Valembois P. Basic data anatomy and embryology. In: Vantrappen G, Hellemans J, editors. Diseases of the Esophagus. New York: Springer; 1978. p. 1–15.
5. Murray JA, Clouse RE, Conklin JL. Component of the standard oesophageal manometry. Neurogastroenterol Motil. 2003;15:591–606.
6. Butin JW, Olsen AM, Moersch HJ, Code CF. A study of esophageal pressures in normal persons and patients with cardiospasm. Gastroenterology. 1953;23:278–93.
7. Dent J. A new technique for continuous sphincter pressure measurement. Gastroenterology. 1976;71:263–7.
8. Soudagar AS, Sayuk GS, Gyawali CP. Learners favor high resolution oesophageal manometry with better diagnostic accuracy over conventional line tracings. Gut. 2012;61(6):798–803.
9. Pandolfino JE, Fox MR, Bredenoord AJ, et al. High-resolution manometry in clinical practice: utilizing pressure topography to classify oesophageal motility abnormalities. Neurogastroenterol Motil. 2009;21(8):796–806.
10. Bredenoord AJ, Fox M, Kahrilas PJ, et al. Chicago classification criteria of esophageal motility disorders defined in high resolution esophageal esophageal pressure topography (EPT). Neurogastroenterol Motil. 2012;24 Suppl 1:57–65.
11. Kahrilas PJ, Bredenoord AJ, Fox M, Gyawali CP, Roman S, Smout AMJP, Pandolfino JE, International High Resolution Manometry Working Group. The Chicago Classification of esophageal motility disorders, v3.0. Neurogastroenterol Motil. 2015;27(2):160–74.
12. Clouse RE, Staiano A. Topography of the esophageal peristaltic pressure wave. Am J Physiol. 1991;261(4 Pt 1):G677–84.
13. Clouse RE, Staiano A, Alrakawi A, Harolan A. Application of topographical methods to clinical esophageal manometry. Am J Gastroenterol. 2000;95:2720–30.

14. Pandolfino JE, Ghosh SK, Zhang Q, Jarosz A, Shah N, Kahrilas PJ. Quantifying EGJ morphology and relaxation with high-resolution manometry: a study of 75 asymptomatic volunteers. Am J Physiol Gastrointest Liver Physiol. 2006;290:G1033–40.
15. Bredenoord AJ, Weusten BL, Timmer R, Smout AJ. Intermittent spatial separation of diaphragm and lower esophageal sphincter favors acidic and weakly acidic reflux. Gastroenterology. 2006;130:334–40.
16. Pandolfino JE, Kim H, Ghosh SK, et al. High-resolution manometry of the EGJ: an analysis of crural diaphragm function in GERD. Am J Gastroenterol. 2007;102(5):1056–63.
17. Tolone S, de Cassan C, de Bortoli N, Roman S, Galeazzi F, Salvador R, Marabotto E, Furnari M, Zentilin P, Marchi S, Bardini R, Sturniolo GC, Savarino V, Savarino E. Esophagogastric junction morphology is associated with a positive impedance-pH monitoring in patients with GERD. Neurogastroenterol Motil. 2015;27(8):1175–82.
18. Tolone S, de Bortoli N, Marabotto E, de Cassan C, Bodini G, Roman S, Furnari M, Savarino V, Cocimo L, Savarino E. Esophagogastric junction contractility for clinical assessment in patients with GERD: a real added value? Neurogastroenterol Motil. 2015;27(10):1423–31.
19. Lin Z, Kahrilas PJ, Roman S, et al. Refining the criterion for an abnormal integrated relaxation pressure in esophageal pressure topography based on the pattern of esophageal contractility using a classification and regression tree model. Neurogastroenterol Motil. 2012;24(8):e356–63.
20. Salvador R, Savarino E, Pesenti E, Spadotto L, Capovilla G, Cavallin F, Galeazzi F, Nicoletti L, Merigliano S, Costantini M. The impact of Heller myotomy on integrated relaxation pressure in esophageal achalasia. J Gastrointest Surg. 2016;20(1):125–31.
21. Scherer JR, Kwiatek MA, Soper NJ, Pandolfino JE, Kahrilas PJ. Functional esophagogastric junction obstruction with intact peristalsis: a heterogeneous syndrome sometimes akin to achalasia. J Gastrointest Surg. 2009;13:2219–25.
22. Gyawali CP, Kushnir VM. High-resolution manometric characteristics help differentiate types of distal esophageal obstruction in patients with peristalsis. Neurogastroenterol Motil. 2011;23:502–e197.
23. Kahrilas PJ, Peters JH. Evaluation of esophagogastric junction using high resolution manometry and esophageal pressure topography. Neurogastroenterol Motil. 2012;24(1):11–9.
24. van Hoeij FB, Smout AJ, Bredenoord AJ. Characterization of idiopathic esophagogastric junction outflow obstruction. Neurogastroenterol Motil. 2015;27(9):1310–6.
25. Xiao Y, Kahrilas PJ, Kwasny MJ, Roman S, Lin Z, Nicodeme F, Lu C, Pandolfino JE. High-resolution manometry correlates of ineffective esophageal motility. Am J Gastroenterol. 2012;107:1647–54.
26. Kumar N, Porter RF, Chanin JM, Gyawali CP. Analysis of intersegmental trough and proximal latency of smooth muscle contraction using high-resolution esophageal manometry. J Clin Gastroenterol. 2012;46:375–81.
27. Roman S, Lin Z, Kwiatek MA, Pandolfino JE, Kahrilas PJ. Weak peristalsis in esophageal pressure topography: classification and association with dysphagia. Am J Gastroenterol. 2011;106:349–56.
28. Porter R, Kumar N, Drapekin J, Gyawali CP. Fragmented smooth muscle contraction segments on high resolution manometry: a marker of esophageal hypomotility. Neurogastroenterol Motil. 2012;24:763–8.
29. Pandolfino JE, Roman S, Carlson D, et al. Distal esophageal spasm in high-resolution esophageal pressure topography: defining clinical phenotypes. Gastroenterology. 2011;141(2):469–75.
30. Roman S, Pandolfino JE, Chen J, Boris L, Luger D, Kahrilas PJ. Phenotypes and clinical context of hypercontractility in high resolution pressure topography (EPT). Am J Gastroenterol. 2012;107:37–45.
31. Martinucci I, de Bortoli N, Giacchino M, Bodini G, Marabotto E, Marchi S, Savarino V, Savarino E. Esophageal motility abnormalities in gastroesophageal reflux disease. World J Gastrointest Pharmacol Ther. 2014;5(2):86–96.

32. Pandolfino JE, Roman S. High-resolution manometry: an atlas of esophageal motility disorders and findings of GERD using esophageal pressure topography. Thorac Surg Clin. 2011;21:465–75.
33. Savarino E, Tutuian R. Combined multichannel intraluminal impedance and manometry testing. Dig Liver Dis Off J Ital Soc Gastroenterol Ital Assoc Stud Liver. 2008;40:167–73.
34. Savarino E, Giacchino M, Savarino V. Dysmotility and reflux disease. Curr Opin Otolaryngol Head Neck Surg. 2013;21:548–56.
35. Savarino E, Gemignani L, Pohl D, Zentilin P, Dulbecco P, Assandri L, Marabotto E, et al. Oesophageal motility and bolus transit abnormalities increase in parallel with the severity of gastro-oesophageal reflux disease. Aliment Pharmacol Ther. 2011;34:476–86.
36. Diener U, Patti MG, Molena D, Fisichella PM, Way LW. Esophageal dysmotility and gastroesophageal reflux disease. J Gastrointest Surg Off J Soc Surg Aliment Tract. 2001;5:260–5.
37. Kahrilas PJ, Dodds WJ, Hogan WJ, Kern M, Arndorfer RC, Reece A. Esophageal peristaltic dysfunction in peptic esophagitis. Gastroenterology. 1986;91:897–904.
38. Lee J, Anggiansah A, Anggiansah R, Young A, Wong T, Fox M. Effects of age on the gastroesophageal junction, esophageal motility, and reflux disease. Clin Gastroenterol Hepatol Off Clin Pract J Am Gastroenterol Assoc. 2007;5:1392–8.
39. Simren M, Silny J, Holloway R, Tack J, Janssens J, Sifrim D. Relevance of ineffective oesophageal motility during oesophageal acid clearance. Gut. 2003;52:784–90.
40. Gyawali CP, Bredenoord AJ, Conklin JL, Fox M, Pandolfino JE, Peters JH, Roman S, et al. Evaluation of esophageal motor function in clinical practice. Neurogastroenterol Motil. 2013;25:99–133.
41. Basseri B, Pimentel M, Shaye OA, Low K, Soffer EE, Conklin JL. Apple sauce improves detection of esophageal motor dysfunction during high-resolution manometry evaluation of dysphagia. Dig Dis Sci. 2011;56:1723–8.
42. Fornari F, Bravi I, Penagini R, Tack J, Sifrim D. Multiple rapid swallowing: a complementary test during standard oesophageal manometry. Neurogastroenterol Motil Off J Eur Gastrointest Motil Soc. 2009;21:718–e741.
43. Stoikes N, Drapekin J, Kushnir V, Shaker A, Brunt LM, Gyawali CP. The value of multiple rapid swallows during preoperative esophageal manometry before laparoscopic antireflux surgery. Surg Endosc. 2012;26:3401–7.
44. Shaker A, Stoikes N, Drapekin J, Kushnir V, Brunt LM, Gyawali CP. Multiple rapid swallow responses during esophageal high-resolution manometry reflect esophageal body peristaltic reserve. Am J Gastroenterol. 2013;108:1706–12.
45. Martinucci I, Savarino EV, Pandolfino JE, Russo S, Bellini M, Tolone S, Tutuian R, Roman S, Furnari M, Frazzoni M, Macchia L, Savarino V, Marchi S, de Bortoli N. Vigor of peristalsis during multiple rapid swallows is inversely correlated with acid exposure time in patients with NERD. Neurogastroenterol Motil. 2016;28(2):243–50.
46. Omari TI, Dejaeger E, van Beckevoort D, Goeleven A, Davidson GP, Dent J, Tack J, Rommel N. A method to objectively assess swallow function in adults with suspected aspiration. Gastroenterology. 2011;140:1454–63.
47. Omari TI, Kritas S, Cock C, Besanko L, Burgstad C, Thompson A, Rommel N, Heddle R, et al. Swallowing dysfunction in healthy older people using pharyngeal pressure-flow analysis. Neurogastroenterol Motil. 2014;26:59–68.
48. Omari TI, Papathanasopoulos A, Dejaeger E, Wauters L, Scarpellini E, Vos R, Slootmaekers S, Seghers V, et al. Reproducibility and agreement of pharyngeal automated impedance manometry with videofluoroscopy. Clin Gastroenterol Hepatol. 2011;9:862–7.
49. Lin Z, Imam H, Nicodeme F, Carlson DA, Lin CY, Yim B, Kahrilas PJ, Pandolfino JE. Flow time through esophagogastric junction derived during high-resolution impedance-manometry studies: a novel parameter for assessing esophageal bolus transit. Am J Physiol. 2014;307:G158–63. pii:ajpgi.00119.2014.
50. Rommel N, Van Oudenhove L, Tack J, Omari TI. Automated impedance manometry analysis as a method to assess esophageal function. Neurogastroenterol Motil. 2014;26:636–45.

14 The Diagnostic Yield of Novel Parameters in Reflux Monitoring

Nicola de Bortoli, Marzio Frazzoni, and Edoardo Savarino

The principles of impedance were first applied to the gastrointestinal tract in 1991. MII testing was approved by the US Food and Drug Administration for esophageal functional testing in 2002. Impedance measures change in resistance (Ohms) of alternating electrical current passing through pairs of metal rings on a catheter. In the empty esophagus, baseline current is conducted between the rings by ions on the mucosa. Because impedance catheters have multiple sets of impedance-measuring rings, bolus movement and direction (antegrade or retrograde) can be assessed [1].

MII-pH monitoring is performed using a polyvinyl catheter (diameter 2.3 mm) equipped with an antimony pH electrode and several cylindrical electrodes, with a length of 4 mm, placed at intervals of about 2 cm to measure the electrical impedance of the esophageal contents at multiple levels along the longitudinal axis of the esophagus [2]. Each pair of adjacent electrodes represents an impedance-measuring segment corresponding to one recording channel. The catheter is positioned with the pH electrode 5 cm above the LES and the six impedance recording channels at 3, 5, 7, 9, 15, and 17 cm above the manometrically defined lower esophageal sphincter (LES). The overall recording time lasts 24 h.

MII-pH provides a detailed characterization of each reflux event including chemical (acid and non-acid reflux) and physical properties (liquid, mixed, gas) [3]

N. de Bortoli, MD (✉)
Division of Gastroenterology, Department of Translational Research and New Technology in Medicine and Surgery, University of Pisa, Cisanello Hospital, Via Paradisa 2, 56124 Pisa, Italy
e-mail: nick.debortoli@gmail.com

M. Frazzoni
Digestive Pathophysiology Unit, Baggiovara Hospital, Modena, Italy

E. Savarino
Division of Gastroenterology, Department of Surgery, Oncology and Gastroenterology, University of Padua, Padua, Italy

R. Conigliaro, M. Frazzoni (eds.), *Diagnosis and Endoscopic Management of Digestive Diseases*, DOI 10.1007/978-3-319-42358-6_14

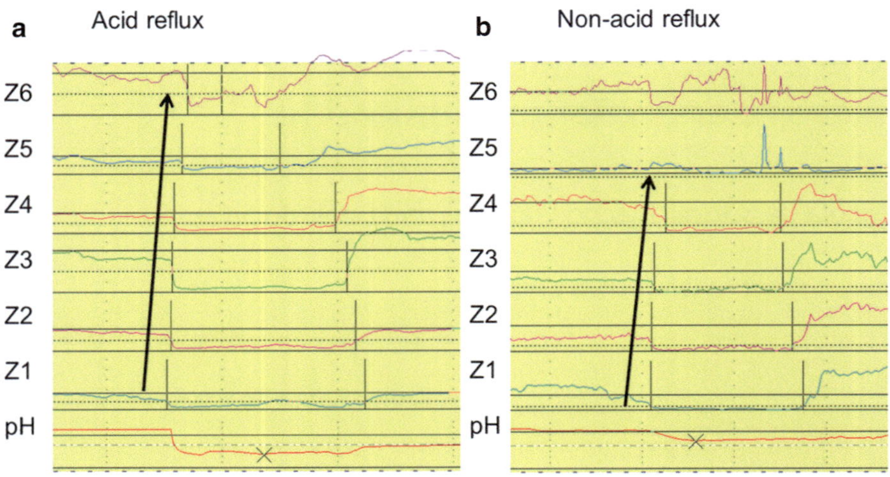

Fig. 14.1 Example of two different reflux events: (**a**) acid reflux event that involves both distal and proximal channels with a contemporary drop of esophageal pH below 4; (**b**) non-acid reflux event that involves distal channels only, the pH does not drop below 4. *Z1-Z6* impedance detection channels

(Fig. 14.1). To date, nonacid reflux represents the majority of reflux episodes in patients with gastroesophageal reflux disease (GERD) on proton pump inhibitor (PPI) therapy [4, 5]. Indeed, the total number of reflux episodes is not affected by the acid-suppressive therapy, and weakly acidic refluxes account for approximately 90 % of all reflux episodes on PPI thus representing a potential mechanism underlying failure of PPI treatment in patients with reflux-related symptoms [6, 7]. Moreover, MII-pH monitoring, as well as pH-metry alone, provides the opportunity to assess the temporal relationship between the occurrence of refluxes and the onset of symptoms [8, 9]. The relationship between symptoms and reflux events can be evaluated with symptom index (SI) and symptom association probability (SAP) that are the most commonly employed symptom indices being used [9].

Based on esophageal pH monitoring, NERD patients with a physiological esophageal acid exposure time (AET) and a close temporal relationship between symptoms and reflux events have been defined as hypersensitive to acid stimuli. On the other hand, in line with Rome III criteria, patients with heartburn, normal upper endoscopy, physiological AET, negative correspondence between symptoms and refluxes, and who fail to respond to PPIs are defined as functional heartburn (FH) [10–12]. In this regard, the advent of MII-pH monitoring improved the diagnostic yield of GERD patients mainly by identifying a positive SAP or SI with weakly acidic or weakly-alkaline refluxes [13–19] both in PPI-responsive and in PPI-refractory patients [20, 21]. Indeed, pH-only monitoring and response to PPI therapy underestimate GERD when with MII-pH criteria [20, 22, 23].

On the other hand, all available diagnostic tests for GERD have some limitations. MII-pH drawbacks are mainly due to the day-to-day variability of the test [24–26]. Additionally, the reflux-symptom correlation in patients with GERD who do not respond to PPI therapy is actually calculated with SI or SAP also if their validity is still uncertain [27, 28]. Recently Zerbib et al. [29] described that MII-pH findings are not always able to predict response to PPIs in patients with reflux-related typical symptoms when the test is performed off-PPI therapy.

Regarding the clinical utility of pathophysiological investigations in patients with heartburn, we described a group of patients (more than 19 % of the whole population enrolled) with heartburn totally suppressed by PPI therapy, in which GERD was not diagnosed with conventional MII-pH criteria [30]. These data suggest that PPI response alone should not always be considered sufficient for GERD diagnosis [30]. Notably, patients with non-erosive reflux disease (NERD) are pathophysiologically heterogeneous and should be accurately studied by means of MII-pH to define the best therapeutic approach [31]. Indeed, a meta-analysis showed that reportedly low response rate in NERD is likely the result of inclusion within this umbrella term of patients with reflux-unrelated heartburn [32].

Recently, the ability of MII-pH testing to better understand GERD's pathophysiology has been improved through the introduction of up-and-coming parameters such as the post-reflux swallow-induced peristaltic wave (PSPW) index, which stand for the efficacy of esophageal chemical clearance [33], and the nocturnal baseline impedance values (MNBI), which indicates impairment of esophageal mucosa integrity [34].

Frazzoni [33], firstly, defined PSPW as an antegrade 50 % drop in impedance relative to the pre-swallow baseline originating in the most proximal impedance sites, reaching all the distal impedance sites, and followed by at least 50 % return to the baseline in all the distal impedance sites (bolus exit) (Fig. 14.1) [35]. Post-reflux swallows not reaching the distal impedance sites and/or not followed by return to the baseline were excluded. To limit overlap with spontaneous swallowing (64 swallows h^{-1}, approximately 1 min^{-1}) [36] and considering the latency period of salivary gland response to esophageal acidification (10–15 s) [37], only PSPWs occurring within 30 s from the end of reflux episodes were taken into account (Fig. 14.2).

Impairment of esophageal chemical clearance could represent specific mechanism involved in GERD pathophysiology. PSPW index has been showed to be significantly lower in patients with reflux esophagitis and NERD than in healthy controls or in patients functional heartburn (FH), i.e., with reflux-unrelated heartburn. Moreover, this parameter is not altered after medical or surgical therapy [33]. Moreover, Frazzoni et al. [38] showed that patients with PPI-refractory heartburn/regurgitation and refractory reflux esophagitis were associated with a more severe impairment of chemical clearance but similar levels of acid exposure when compared with those patients with healed reflux esophagitis. Adequate acid suppression was found in the majority of patients with refractory reflux esophagitis who did not record any benefit from further PPI escalation [38]. These data confirmed that both contact time of esophageal mucosa with acidic/weakly acidic refluxate and impairment of chemical clearance (PSPW index) play a relevant role in the pathogenesis of refractory reflux esophagitis.

Frazzoni et al. [39] also evaluated the PSPW index in patients with short-segment Barrett's esophagus with or without mucosal dysplasia. They observed that the

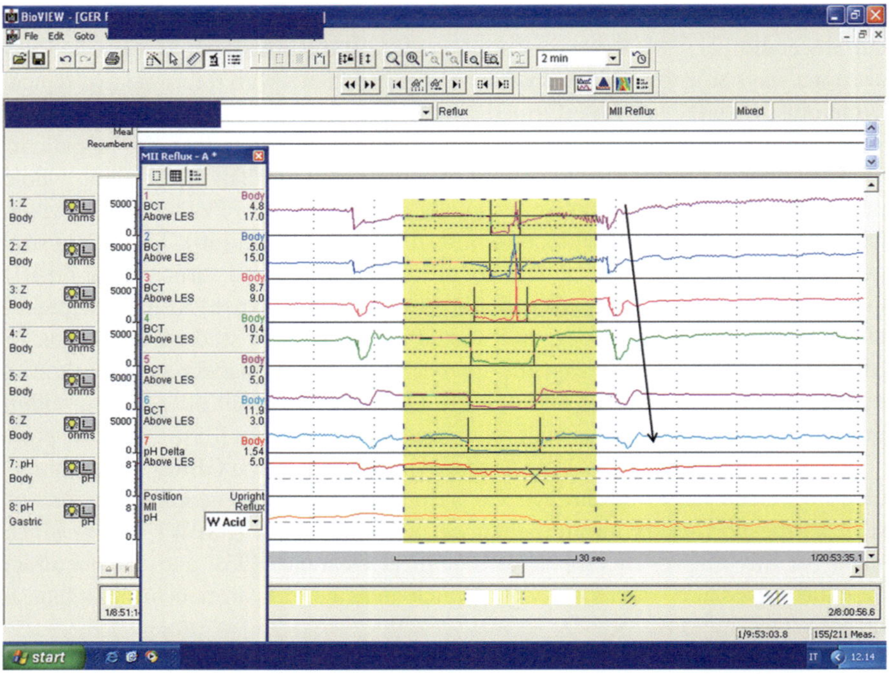

Fig. 14.2 Impedance-pH tracing showing a weakly acidic reflux followed by a swallow-induced peristaltic wave (*arrow*)

PSPW index was significantly lower in patients with than in patients without dysplasia at the time of surveillance (15 %, vs. 32 %; $p=0.001$) and at the time of diagnosis too. Statistical analysis showed that a PSPW index <26 % was predictive of incident dysplasia with a 75 % accuracy.

First of all, Farrè and coworkers [34] tested for the first time the hypothesis that multichannel intraluminal impedance (MII) might be a suitable tool for the assessment of esophageal mucosal integrity, by performing in vivo experiments of acid perfusion in rabbits and humans. They also analyzed impedance-pH tracings from patients with GERD. These authors showed that impedance baseline values reflect the status of the esophageal mucosa both in an animal model and in healthy volunteers, indicating that MII is a useful tool to evaluate the esophageal mucosa integrity. They confirmed that patients with erosive and non-erosive esophagitis had a lower impedance baseline compared to healthy volunteers [34].

Further, Kessing et al. [40] described lower values of baseline impedance levels in distal esophagus in patients with abnormal esophageal AET rather than in healthy volunteers (HVs). The authors described a negative correlation between baseline impedance levels and esophageal AET [40]. Woodland et al. [41] observed that, within both NERD and FH, patients who showed a positive acid sensitivity test had lower baseline impedance than those who did not. Of note, the authors found that a subgroup of patients with FH, despite having a normal MII-pH study and a negative response to proton pump inhibitors (PPIs), had baseline impedance values very similar to those of patients with NERD.

These studies evaluated baseline impedance values during the upright period of 24-h MII-pH analysis. Frequently these authors described some difficulties to obtain data on baseline impedance values excluding frequent swallows and reflux events. We recently dedicated our interest in baseline impedance values, and we decided to calculate the baseline value during overnight rest. It seemed easier and less affected from sampling errors. During sleeping esophageal mucosa collapses on the MII-pH probe, allowing a more accurate assessment of the real impedance in the esophageal mucosa. Nocturnal baseline impedance was assessed from the most distal impedance channel. Three 10-min time periods (around 1.00 am, 2.00 am, and 3.00 am) were selected, and the mean baseline for each period was computed with the aid of the software. Time periods including swallows, refluxes, and pH drops were avoided. The mean of the three measurements was manually calculated to obtain a parameter that we defined mean nocturnal baseline impedance (MNBI). In a large group of patients with GERD typical symptoms, negative endoscopy, and normal pathophysiological characteristics (normal AET and number of refluxes, negative SI and SAP), we observed that patients with a good symptom relief after PPI therapy had lower baseline impedance values than PPI-refractory patients with normal pathophysiological characteristics (FH) [42]. FH patients showed similar baseline value than HVs. Moreover, we observed similar results analyzing PSPW index: it was lower in responders than in nonresponders and in HVs. A direct linear correlation between PSPW and baseline impedance values was found [42].

After that preliminary study, de Bortoli et al. [43] decided to extend these analyses to patients with a 24-h MII-pH diagnosis of hypersensitive esophagus (HE) (normal AET and number of reflux events but positive correlation between symptoms and refluxes as established by both positive SI and SAP analyses) [43]. The authors confirmed previous results observed with MNBI and PSPW index: both parameters were lower in patients with HE and those with positive response to PPI therapy but normal pathophysiological findings (FH-PPI responder) compared to healthy controls and FH-PPI non-responders. These results suggest that both MNBI and PSPW index can be helpful to diagnose GERD in patients with heartburn even when SI and SAP are negative or inconclusive [43].

More recently Frazzoni and coworkers [44] aimed to assess the diagnostic accuracy of MNBI and PSPW index in a large multicenter case series of patients with PPI-responsive heartburn. All patients were evaluated after discontinuing PPI-therapy for 1 month. The authors retrospectively studied 68 patients with erosive esophagitis and 221 patients with NERD and compared their result with those observed in 50 healthy controls. In receiver operating characteristic analysis, the area under curve of the PSPW index (0.977; 95 % confidence interval, 0.961–0.993) was significantly greater than that of the other impedance-pH parameters in identifying patients with reflux disease ($P<.001$). The PSPW index and the MNBI resulted able to identify patients with erosive reflux disease with the highest level of sensitivity (100 % and 91 %, respectively), as well as the 118 pH-positive (99 % and 86 %) and 103 pH-negative (77 % and 56 %) cases of NERD. The PSPW index and the MNBI identified pH-negative NERD with the highest level of sensitivity; values were 82 % and 52 % for the 65 SAP-positive and/or SI-positive cases and 68 % and 63 % for the 38 SAP-negative and SI-negative cases. Diagnoses of NERD were confirmed by pH-only criteria, including those that were positive on the basis of the SAP or SI, for 165 of 221 cases (75 %) and by impedance-pH criteria for 216 of 221 cases (98 %) (P=.001). The authors concluded that the PSPW index and the MNBI increase the diagnostic yield of impedance pH monitoring of patients with reflux disease [44].

Similar results were described by Kandulsky et al. [45]; they observed that baseline impedance values might differentiate patients with ERD or NERD from patients with FH (78 % sensitivity and 71 % specificity) in a population of patients with proton pump inhibitor-refractory reflux related symptoms. Low levels of baseline impedance were associated with greater esophageal acid exposure and dilation of intercellular spaces, confirming that baseline impedance should be considered as a marker of mucosal integrity [45].

Currently, PPI resistance is the real challenge in GERD [46]. However, it has been claimed that between 10 and 40 % of patients with typical reflux symptoms (heartburn/regurgitation) remain symptomatic on a standard dose of PPIs, and many of them will continue to experience symptoms on even high doses of PPIs [47].

What constitutes refractory GERD remains an area of controversy. Most investigators believe that only patients with GERD who exhibit partial or lack of response to PPIs twice daily should be considered as PPI failures [47]. Furthermore, regurgitation persists in many patients despite PPI therapy [48], often awakening patients at night.

Management of PPI-refractory GERD patients is a challenging task. Baclofen could be helpful as add-on therapy with PPIs, but its use is limited by poor tolerability [49] and it is not approved for GERD management. In patients with documented GERD who do not respond sufficiently to PPI therapy, laparoscopic Nissen fundoplication represents the currently suggested treatment modality to overcome PPI failures [50].

Frazzoni et al. [51] aimed to assess reflux parameters in refractory GERD patients before and after EsophyX or laparoscopic fundoplication and their relationship with symptoms. The authors evaluated patients on PPI therapy before intervention and off PPI therapy 3 months after intervention by means of MII-pH monitoring. Distal and proximal refluxes were significantly reduced postoperatively in the surgical but not in the endoscopic (EsophyX) group. The esophageal acid exposure time was normal in 50 % of cases after EsophyX and in 100 % of cases after surgery (P=0.033). They concluded that EsophyX fundoplication was significantly less effective than laparoscopic fundoplication in improving reflux parameters and in inducing symptom remission in patients with refractory GERD [51].

The same working group [52] aimed to evaluate reflux parameters and their relationship with symptoms before and after laparoscopic fundoplication, on and off PPI therapy, respectively, in patients with PPI-unresponsive heartburn/regurgitation and with a positive symptom-reflux association and/or abnormal reflux parameters detected on PPI therapy. The authors described that esophageal AET (100 %) as well as the number of total (77 %) and proximal reflux (95 %) events and of acid (92 %) and weakly acidic (65 %) refluxes decreased significantly after surgery in patients with refractory GERD. The authors concluded that laparoscopic fundoplication improves acid and weakly acidic reflux parameters when compared with PPI therapy and strongly support that surgical option should be considered in PPI failures patients with GERD confirmed with pathophysiological test [52].

In a recent study, normal reflux parameters and sustained symptom remission at a 3-year follow-up, i.e., GERD cure, were achieved with laparoscopic fundoplication in 90 % of patients with PPI-refractory GERD as diagnosed by on-PPI impedance-pH monitoring [53]. Interestingly, this study shows that weakly acidic refluxes are the main determinants of PPI refractoriness: preoperatively, positive symptom/reflux indexes and abnormal reflux parameters were mainly associated with weakly acidic refluxes; postoperatively, persistent remission of heartburn/regurgitation was associated with total/subtotal abolition of weakly acidic refluxes [53].

On-PPI impedance-pH monitoring is warranted in all PPI-refractory patients before laparoscopic fundoplication in order to establish a cause-and-effect relationship between reflux and heartburn/regurgitation persisting despite PPI therapy; indeed, no reflux pattern can be demonstrated associated with PPI failure at off-PPI testing [29]. Impedance-pH monitoring should always be preceded by esophageal manometry to rule out severe esophageal motility disorders. Surgery is indicated in patients with abnormal impedance-pH parameters and/or positive symptom-reflux associations. When symptom reflux correlation (SI/SAP) fails, PSPW index and MNBI appear ready for prime time. Their applicability and reproducibility are very high, [44] and few additional minutes only are required for their calculation during visual analysis of tracings. Currently, visual analysis of impedance-pH tracings is necessary because automated software analysis is not accurate enough [54]. PSPW index and MNBI appear particularly useful when GERD diagnosis is in doubt, i.e., when esophageal AET and the number of total refluxes are normal and SAP and SI are negative or discordant, or the patient denies symptoms during the impedance-pH study or admits poor accuracy in symptom recording: in these instances, when PSPW index and/or MNBI values are abnormal, GERD diagnosis cannot be dismissed (Fig. 14.3). SAP and SI should not be abandoned, however, as there is some evidence that they can predict positive outcome following laparoscopic fundoplication [53, 55, 56]. Whether PSPW index and MNBI can predict response to antireflux interventions remain an open issue to be addressed in future studies.

To conclude, MNBI and PSPW index might be considered up-and-coming parameters that can be helpful to better investigate patients with GERD-related symptoms, particularly when symptom-reflux association indexes fail to do it. These parameters make pathophysiological sense and certainly deserve a chance in redeeming the clinical value of ambulatory pH-impedance testing. For sure, further researches are needed to determine if normal MNBI and PSPW index in the setting of normal pH and normal conventional impedance parameters would be the benchmark for diagnosis of functional esophageal symptoms. Other confounders in the assessment of these parameters need to be evaluated, for instance, the contribution of abnormal motor function or esophageal dilation. Recently Gyawali [57] suggested that software tools need to be

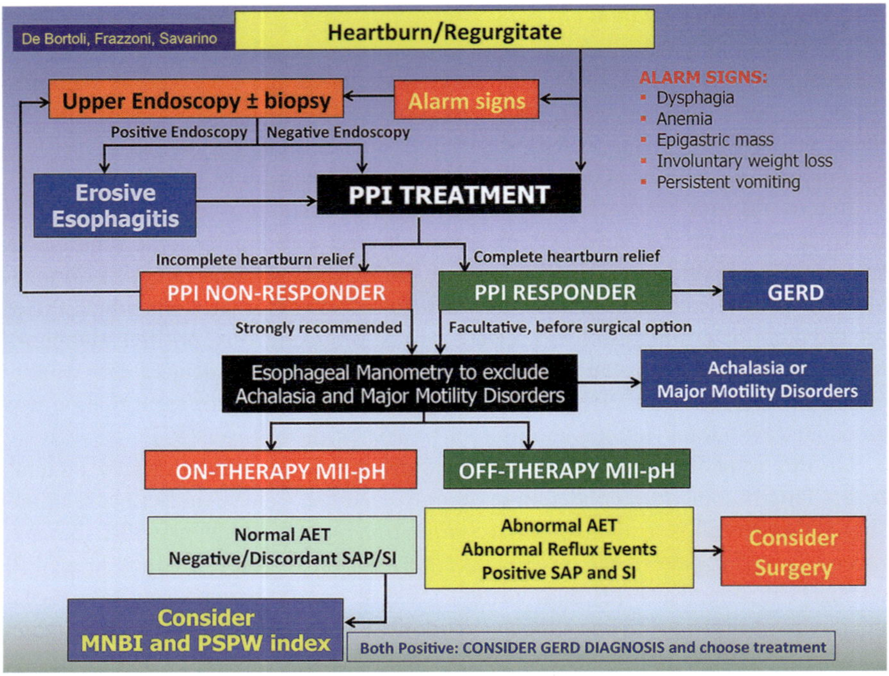

Fig. 14.3 Diagnostic algorithm for patients with typical reflux symptoms

developed by companies marketing pH-impedance to simplify calculation of these parameters, as both MNBI and PSPW index need to be rigorously studied and potentially adapted for clinical use in the short term.

References

1. Dolder M, Tutuian R. Laboratory based investigations for diagnosing gastroesophageal reflux disease. Best Pract Res Clin Gastroenterol. 2010;24(6):787–98. Epub 2010/12/04. eng.
2. Bredenoord AJ, Pandolfino JE, Smout AJ. Gastro-oesophageal reflux disease. Lancet. 2013;381(9881):1933–42. Epub 2013/03/13. eng.
3. Zentilin P, Iiritano E, Dulbecco P, Bilardi C, Savarino E, De Conca S, et al. Normal values of 24-h ambulatory intraluminal impedance combined with pH-metry in subjects eating a Mediterranean diet. Dig Liver Dis. 2006;38(4):226–32. Epub 2006/02/17. eng.
4. Frazzoni M, Savarino E, Manno M, Melotti G, Mirante VG, Mussetto A, et al. Reflux patterns in patients with short-segment Barrett's oesophagus: a study using impedance-pH monitoring off and on proton pump inhibitor therapy. Aliment Pharmacol Ther. 2009;30(5):508–15. Epub 2009/06/13. eng.
5. Boeckxstaens GE, Smout A. Systematic review: role of acid, weakly acidic and weakly alkaline reflux in gastro-oesophageal reflux disease. Aliment Pharmacol Ther. 2010;32(3):334–43. Epub 2010/05/25. eng.
6. Mainie I, Tutuian R, Shay S, Vela M, Zhang X, Sifrim D, et al. Acid and non-acid reflux in patients with persistent symptoms despite acid suppressive therapy: a multicentre study

using combined ambulatory impedance-pH monitoring. Gut. 2006;55(10):1398–402. Pubmed Central PMCID: 1856433, Epub 2006/03/25. eng.

7. Zerbib F, Roman S, Ropert A, des Varannes SB, Pouderoux P, Chaput U, et al. Esophageal pH-impedance monitoring and symptom analysis in GERD: a study in patients off and on therapy. Am J Gastroenterol. 2006;101(9):1956–63. Epub 2006/07/20. eng.
8. Savarino E, Zentilin P, Tutuian R, Pohl D, Gemignani L, Malesci A, et al. Impedance-pH reflux patterns can differentiate non-erosive reflux disease from functional heartburn patients. J Gastroenterol. 2012;47(2):159–68. Epub 2011/11/01. eng.
9. Bredenoord AJ, Weusten BL, Smout AJ. Symptom association analysis in ambulatory gastro-oesophageal reflux monitoring. Gut. 2005;54(12):1810–7. Pubmed Central PMCID: 1774780, Epub 2005/11/15. eng.
10. Fass R, Fennerty MB, Vakil N. Nonerosive reflux disease–current concepts and dilemmas. Am J Gastroenterol. 2001;96(2):303–14. Epub 2001/03/10. eng.
11. Martinez SD, Malagon IB, Garewal HS, Cui H, Fass R. Non-erosive reflux disease (NERD)–acid reflux and symptom patterns. Aliment Pharmacol Ther. 2003;17(4):537–45. Epub 2003/03/08. eng.
12. de Bortoli N, Martinucci I, Bellini M, Savarino E, Savarino V, Blandizzi C, et al. Overlap of functional heartburn and gastroesophageal reflux disease with irritable bowel syndrome. World J Gastroenterol WJG. 2013;19(35):5787–97. Pubmed Central PMCID: 3793133, Epub 2013/10/15. eng.
13. Savarino E, Zentilin P, Tutuian R, Pohl D, Casa DD, Frazzoni M, et al. The role of nonacid reflux in NERD: lessons learned from impedance-pH monitoring in 150 patients off therapy. Am J Gastroenterol. 2008;103(11):2685–93. Epub 2008/09/09. eng.
14. Shay S, Tutuian R, Sifrim D, Vela M, Wise J, Balaji N, et al. Twenty-four hour ambulatory simultaneous impedance and pH monitoring: a multicenter report of normal values from 60 healthy volunteers. Am J Gastroenterol. 2004;99(6):1037–43. Epub 2004/06/08. eng.
15. Sifrim D, Castell D, Dent J, Kahrilas PJ. Gastro-oesophageal reflux monitoring: review and consensus report on detection and definitions of acid, non-acid, and gas reflux. Gut. 2004;53(7):1024–31. Pubmed Central PMCID: 1774114, Epub 2004/06/15. eng.
16. Blondeau K, Tack J. Pro: impedance testing is useful in the management of GERD. Am J Gastroenterol. 2009;104(11):2664–6. Epub 2009/11/06. eng.
17. Bredenoord AJ, Weusten BL, Timmer R, Conchillo JM, Smout AJ. Addition of esophageal impedance monitoring to pH monitoring increases the yield of symptom association analysis in patients off PPI therapy. Am J Gastroenterol. 2006;101(3):453–9. Epub 2006/02/09. eng.
18. Savarino E, Pohl D, Zentilin P, Dulbecco P, Sammito G, Sconfienza L, et al. Functional heartburn has more in common with functional dyspepsia than with non-erosive reflux disease. Gut. 2009;58(9):1185–91. Pubmed Central PMCID: 2719081, Epub 2009/05/23. eng.
19. de Bortoli N, Martinucci I, Savarino E, Franchi R, Bertani L, Russo S et al. Lower pH values of weakly acidic refluxes as determinants of heartburn perception in gastroesophageal reflux disease patients with normal esophageal acid exposure. Dis Esophagus. 2016;29(1):3–9. Epub 2014/09/13. Eng.
20. Frazzoni M, Conigliaro R, Mirante VG, Melotti G. The added value of quantitative analysis of on-therapy impedance-pH parameters in distinguishing refractory non-erosive reflux disease from functional heartburn. Neurogastroenterol Motil. 2012;24(2):141–6, e87.
21. Frazzoni M, Conigliaro R, Melotti G. Weakly acidic refluxes have a major role in the pathogenesis of proton pump inhibitor-resistant reflux oesophagitis. Aliment Pharmacol Ther. 2011;33(5):601–6. Epub 2011/01/05. eng.
22. Savarino E, Tutuian R, Zentilin P, Dulbecco P, Pohl D, Marabotto E, et al. Characteristics of reflux episodes and symptom association in patients with erosive esophagitis and nonerosive reflux disease: study using combined impedance-pH off therapy. Am J Gastroenterol. 2010;105(5):1053–61. Epub 2009/12/10. eng.
23. Savarino E, Marabotto E, Zentilin P, Frazzoni M, Sammito G, Bonfanti D, et al. The added value of impedance-pH monitoring to Rome III criteria in distinguishing func-

tional heartburn from non-erosive reflux disease. Dig Liver Dis. 2011;43(7):542–7. Epub 2011/03/08. eng.
24. Savarino E, Zentilin P, Frazzoni M, Cuoco DL, Pohl D, Dulbecco P, et al. Characteristics of gastro-esophageal reflux episodes in Barrett's esophagus, erosive esophagitis and healthy volunteers. Neurogastroenterol Motil. 2010;22(10):1061–e280. Epub 2010/06/19. eng.
25. Zentilin P, Dulbecco P, Savarino E, Giannini E, Savarino V. Combined multichannel intraluminal impedance and pH-metry: a novel technique to improve detection of gastro-oesophageal reflux literature review. Dig Liver Dis. 2004;36(9):565–9. Epub 2004/10/06. eng.
26. Pandolfino JE, Vela MF. Esophageal-reflux monitoring. Gastrointest Endosc. 2009;69(4):917–30, 30 e1. Epub 2009/03/03. eng.
27. Hershcovici T, Wendel CS, Fass R. Symptom indexes in refractory gastroesophageal reflux disease: overrated or misunderstood? Clin Gastroenterol Hepatol. 2011;9(10):816–7. Epub 2011/07/28. eng.
28. Slaughter JC, Goutte M, Rymer JA, Oranu AC, Schneider JA, Garrett CG, et al. Caution about overinterpretation of symptom indexes in reflux monitoring for refractory gastroesophageal reflux disease. Clin Gastroenterol Hepatol. 2011;9(10):868–74. Epub 2011/07/26. eng.
29. Zerbib F, Belhocine K, Simon M, Capdepont M, Mion F, Bruley des Varannes S, et al. Clinical, but not oesophageal pH-impedance, profiles predict response to proton pump inhibitors in gastro-oesophageal reflux disease. Gut. 2012;61(4):501–6. Epub 2011/10/15. eng.
30. de Bortoli N, Martinucci I, Savarino E, Bellini M, Bredenoord AJ, Franchi R, et al. Proton pump inhibitor responders who are not confirmed as GERD patients with impedance and pH monitoring: who are they? Neurogastroenterol Motil. 2014;26(1):28–35. Epub 2013/09/03. eng.
31. Savarino E, Zentilin P, Savarino V. NERD: an umbrella term including heterogeneous subpopulations. Nat Rev Gastroenterol Hepatol. 2013;10(6):371–80. Epub 2013/03/27. eng.
32. Weijenborg PW, Cremonini F, Smout AJ, Bredenoord AJ. PPI therapy is equally effective in well-defined non-erosive reflux disease and in reflux esophagitis: a meta-analysis. Neurogastroenterol Motil. 2012;24(8):747–57, e350. Epub 2012/02/09. eng.
33. Frazzoni M, Manta R, Mirante VG, Conigliaro R, Frazzoni L, Melotti G. Esophageal chemical clearance is impaired in gastro-esophageal reflux disease–a 24-h impedance-pH monitoring assessment. Neurogastroenterol Motil. 2013;25(5):399–406, e295. Epub 2013/01/31. eng.
34. Farre R, Blondeau K, Clement D, Vicario M, Cardozo L, Vieth M, et al. Evaluation of oesophageal mucosa integrity by the intraluminal impedance technique. Gut. 2011;60(7):885–92. Epub 2011/02/10. eng.
35. Tutuian R, Vela MF, Balaji NS, Wise JL, Murray JA, Peters JH, et al. Esophageal function testing with combined multichannel intraluminal impedance and manometry: multicenter study in healthy volunteers. Clin Gastroenterol Hepatol. 2003;1(3):174–82.
36. Bredenoord AJ, Weusten BL, Timmer R, Smout AJ. Reproducibility of multichannel intraluminal electrical impedance monitoring of gastroesophageal reflux. Am J Gastroenterol. 2005;100(2):265–9.
37. Shafik A, El-Sibai O, Shafik AA, Mostafa R. Effect of topical esophageal acidification on salivary secretion: identification of the mechanism of action. J Gastroenterol Hepatol. 2005;20(12):1935–9. Epub 2005/12/13. eng.
38. Frazzoni M, Bertani H, Manta R, Mirante VG, Frazzoni L, Conigliaro R, et al. Impairment of chemical clearance is relevant to the pathogenesis of refractory reflux oesophagitis. Dig Liver Dis. 2014;46(7):596–602.
39. Frazzoni M, Bertani H, Conigliaro R, Frazzoni L, Losi L, Melotti G. Neoplastic progression in short-segment Barrett's oesophagus is associated with impairment of chemical clearance, but not inadequate acid suppression by proton pump inhibitor therapy. Aliment Pharmacol Ther. 2014;40(7):835–42. Epub 2014/08/05. eng.
40. Kessing BF, Bredenoord AJ, Weijenborg PW, Hemmink GJ, Loots CM, Smout AJ. Esophageal acid exposure decreases intraluminal baseline impedance levels. Am J Gastroenterol. 2011;106(12):2093–7. Epub 2011/08/17. eng.

41. Woodland P, Al-Zinaty M, Yazaki E, Sifrim D. In vivo evaluation of acid-induced changes in oesophageal mucosa integrity and sensitivity in non-erosive reflux disease. Gut. 2013;62(9):1256–61. Epub 2012/06/23. Eng.
42. Martinucci I, de Bortoli N, Savarino E, Piaggi P, Bellini M, Antonelli A, et al. Esophageal baseline impedance levels in patients with pathophysiological characteristics of functional heartburn. Neurogastroenterol Motil. 2014;26(4):546–55. Epub 2014/01/18. eng.
43. de Bortoli N, Martinucci I, Savarino E, Tutuian R, Frazzoni M, Piaggi P et al. Association between baseline impedance values and response proton pump inhibitors in patients with heartburn. Clin Gastroenterol Hepatol. 2015;13(6):1082–8. Epub 2014/12/17. Eng.
44. Frazzoni M, Savarino E, de Bortoli N, Martinucci I, Furnari M, Frazzoni L, et al. Analyses of the post-reflux swallow-induced peristaltic wave index and nocturnal baseline impedance parameters increase the diagnostic yield of patients with reflux disease. Clin Gastroenterol Hepatol. 2016;14(1):40–6. Epub 2015/07/01. Eng.
45. Kandulski A, Weigt J, Caro C, Jechorek D, Wex T, Malfertheiner P. Esophageal intraluminal baseline impedance differentiates gastroesophageal reflux disease from functional heartburn. Clin Gastroenterol Hepatol. 2015;13(6):1075–81.
46. Cicala M, Emerenziani S, Guarino MP, Ribolsi M. Proton pump inhibitor resistance, the real challenge in gastro-esophageal reflux disease. World J Gastroenterol. 2013;19(39):6529–35. Pubmed Central PMCID: 3801364.
47. Fass R, Sifrim D. Management of heartburn not responding to proton pump inhibitors. Gut. 2009;58(2):295–309. Epub 2009/01/13. eng.
48. Broeders JA, Rijnhart-de Jong HG, Draaisma WA, Bredenoord AJ, Smout AJ, Gooszen HG. Ten-year outcome of laparoscopic and conventional nissen fundoplication: randomized clinical trial. Ann Surg. 2009;250(5):698–706. Epub 2009/10/06. eng.
49. Sifrim D, Zerbib F. Diagnosis and management of patients with reflux symptoms refractory to proton pump inhibitors. Gut. 2012;61(9):1340–54. Epub 2012/06/12. eng.
50. Kahrilas PJ, Shaheen NJ, Vaezi MF, American Gastroenterological Association I, Clinical P, Quality Management C. American Gastroenterological Association Institute technical review on the management of gastroesophageal reflux disease. Gastroenterology. 2008;135(4):1392–413, 413 e1–5.
51. Frazzoni M, Conigliaro R, Manta R, Melotti G. Reflux parameters as modified by EsophyX or laparoscopic fundoplication in refractory GERD. Aliment Pharmacol Ther. 2011;34(1):67–75.
52. Frazzoni M, Conigliaro R, Melotti G. Reflux parameters as modified by laparoscopic fundoplication in 40 patients with heartburn/regurgitation persisting despite PPI therapy: a study using impedance-pH monitoring. Dig Dis Sci. 2011;56(4):1099–106. Epub 2010/08/26. eng.
53. Frazzoni M, Piccoli M, Conigliaro R, Manta R, Frazzoni L, Melotti G. Refractory gastroesophageal reflux disease as diagnosed by impedance-pH monitoring can be cured by laparoscopic fundoplication. Surg Endosc. 2013;27(8):2940–6. Epub 2013/02/26. Eng.
54. Roman S, Bruley des Varannes S, Pouderoux P, Chaput U, Mion F, Galmiche JP, et al. Ambulatory 24-h oesophageal impedance-pH recordings: reliability of automatic analysis for gastro-oesophageal reflux assessment. Neurogastroenterol Motil. 2006;18(11):978–86.
55. Patel A, Sayuk GS, Gyawali CP. Parameters on esophageal pH-impedance monitoring that predict outcomes of patients with gastroesophageal reflux disease. Clin Gastroenter Hepatol. 2015;13(5):884–91. Epub 2014/08/28. Eng.
56. Desjardin M, Luc G, Collet D, Zerbib F. 24-hour pH-impedance monitoring on therapy to select patients with refractory reflux symptoms for antireflux surgery. A single center retrospective study. Neurogastroenterol Motil. 2016;28(1):146–52.
57. Gyawali CP. Redeeming clinical value of esophageal pH impedance monitoring. Clin Gastroenterol Hepatol. 2016;14(1):47–9.

MIX
Papier aus verantwortungsvollen Quellen
Paper from responsible sources
FSC® C105338

If you have any concerns about our products,
you can contact us on
ProductSafety@springernature.com

In case Publisher is established outside the EU,
the EU authorized representative is:
Springer Nature Customer Service Center GmbH
Europaplatz 3, 69115 Heidelberg, Germany

Printed by Libri Plureos GmbH
in Hamburg, Germany